Pelvic Floor Disorders for the Colorectal Surgeon

Edited by

Ian Lindsey

Karen Nugent

Tony Dixon

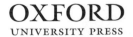

OXFORD
UNIVERSITY PRESS

OXFORD

UNIVERSITY PRESS

Great Clarendon Street, Oxford OX2 6DP

Oxford University Press is a department of the University of Oxford.
It furthers the University's objective of excellence in research, scholarship,
and education by publishing worldwide in

Oxford New York

Auckland Cape Town Dar es Salaam Hong Kong Karachi
Kuala Lumpur Madrid Melbourne Mexico City Nairobi
New Delhi Shanghai Taipei Toronto

With offices in

Argentina Austria Brazil Chile Czech Republic France Greece
Guatemala Hungary Italy Japan Poland Portugal Singapore
South Korea Switzerland Thailand Turkey Ukraine Vietnam

Oxford is a registered trade mark of Oxford University Press
in the UK and in certain other countries

Published in the United States
by Oxford University Press Inc., New York

© Oxford University Press, 2011

The moral rights of the author have been asserted
Database right Oxford University Press (maker)

First published 2011

British Library Cataloguing in Publication Data
Data available

Library of Congress Cataloging in Publication Data
Data available

Typeset in Minion by Glyph International Bangalore, India
Printed in Great Britain
on acid-free paper by
CPI Antony Rowe, Chippenham, Wiltshire

ISBN 978–0–19–957962–4

10 9 8 7 6 5 4 3 2 1

Foreword

It is a pleasure to be invited to write a foreword for *Pelvic Floor Disorders for the Colorectal Surgeon*. Functional disorders comprise at least one quarter of all colorectal referrals. They are therefore an extremely important part of the practice of the colorectal surgeon. Some, such as rectal prolapse, have been managed fairly successfully for a long time, but others, for example, various forms of defaecation disorder have not been so amenable to treatment. This is partly due to ignorance of the pathophysiology of functional disorders and the added psychological state of the patient in some cases.

The whole field has changed remarkably in the last ten years. The nihilistic attitude prevalent in the past has given way to a more rational approach based on the analysis of pathophysiology by investigation. Physiological testing has been available since the 1960s, but recent advances in imaging have improved our understanding of some of the disorders of defaecation and continence. These have helped to throw light on the interface between anatomical deformity and dysfunction. It was held by some that anatomical correction did not correspond to symptomatic relief. This is no longer tenable since identification of particular clinical subgroups by investigation, such as some patients with internal rectal prolapse for example, has resulted in a more selective and therefore more successful approach to management.

There have also been important technical developments, which have shown clear benefit. Perineal and endoanal surgical techniques for external and internal prolapse have been used for many years but these have been supplemented by stapling techniques to treat haemorrhoids and rectocele. There is now a great deal of information on the effectiveness of stapling, some of which has been obtained from randomized prospective controlled trials. Sacral nerve stimulation has had a dramatic effect on the outlook of patients with incontinence whereby half the patients not responding to medical treatment can be maintained in a satisfactory manner for many years. We now have an algorithm for the treatment of incontinence, which has transformed the outcome of many patients. Similarly there is movement in constipation. Progress has been made in the identification of subgroups with improved classification. The role of surgery has been redefined while sacral nerve stimulation offers hope to up to half the patients with slow transit constipation who do not respond to medical treatment.

The subject is therefore not only clinically important but also intellectually interesting since it is a growth area, which offers many opportunities for research for the benefit of patients. The appearance of *Pelvic Floor Disorders for the Colorectal Surgeon* is timely owing to the need for a comprehensive text in the field given the progress made in the last few years. It updates knowledge in all fields of functional disorders of the pelvic floor with emphasis on the integration of modern imaging and physiological testing with the clinical features.

The book is a multi-author work consisting of 24 chapters from 23 contributors, including colorectal surgeons, radiologists and pain specialists, drawn from the young consultant cadre in the United Kingdom and continental Europe. The three editors are experts who have themselves contributed to knowledge in the field. Chapters are illustrated by clear black and white photographs and line drawings and contain a comprehensive bibliography, which will be a great resource to the reader. The book is divided into three parts including organization and diagnosis, the conditions themselves, and the various techniques available to treat them. The reader is given a modern approach, which aims to break through some of the traditional attitudes with a freshness that is rarely seen when describing functional disease. There is a sense of optimism, which is inspiring.

The book will be essential reading for anyone interested in functional colorectal disorders of the pelvic floor. It will therefore be invaluable to colorectal surgeons, but also to other practitioners including gastroenterologists, radiologists and general practitioners with an interest, specialist nurses, trainees and medical students.

R John Nicholls

RJ Nicholls MA (Cantab), M.Chir, FRCS(Eng), EBSQ(Coloproctology), hon FRCP(Lond), hon FACS , hon FRCSE, hon FRCS(Glasg), hon fellow ASCRS, Emeritus Consultant Surgeon, St Mark's Hospital, London Visiting Professor, Imperial College, London

Preface

This small textbook of colorectal pelvic floor disorders originated to fill the need for a current and practical resource. Pelvic floor practice is changing rapidly, but textbooks covering chronic constipation or faecal incontinence have not kept up; they still cover topics such as subtotal colectomy for slow transit constipation, and division of the puborectalis muscle for anismus, yet they fail to adequately cover (or sometimes even recognise) internal rectal prolapse. We recognise this because many of these editions sit on our shelves. In one sense this is the nature of textbooks compared to scientific journals, but it also highlights a generational change in pelvic floor practice. We make no apologies for being current.

The layout of the book is in three sections. The first provides an organizational and diagnostic approach to pelvic floor problems that is conceptual in scope. The second details the patho-anatomical and physiological entities that this diagnostic approach will throw up and describes their management. The third is more technical, covering key new diagnostic and therapeutic procedures and their results.

We hope that the reader finds this work stimulating and thought-provoking, and that it gently forces him or her to critically analyse some of their own cherished views, and those more widely established, on colorectal pelvic floor practice.

Ian Lindsey, Karen Nugent, Tony Dixon

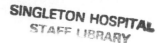
Table of contents

Contributors list

Oleh Babyak
European Coloproctology Center,
Vienna, Austria

Andrew Paul Baranowski
Consultant in Pain Medicine
NHNN, University College
London Hospitals
Foundation Trust,
London, UK

Brigitta Boller
European Coloproctology Center,
Vienna, Austria

Steven Brown
Consultant in General Surgery
Sheffield Teaching Hospitals,
Sheffield, UK

Will Chambers
Frenchay Hospital,
Bristol, UK

Rowan Collinson
Consultant Colorectal Surgeon
Auckland City Hospital,
Auckland, New Zealand

Christopher Cunningham
Consultant Colorectal Surgeon,
Oxford Pelvic Floor Centre,
Department of Colorectal Surgery,
Churchill and John Radcliffe Hospitals,
Oxford, UK

Volodymyr Denysenko
European Coloproctology Center,
Vienna, Austria

Tony Dixon
Frenchay Hospital,
Bristol, UK

Martijn P. Gosselink
Senior Surgical Resident,
Department of Surgery,
Erasmus MC,
Rotterdam, The Netherlands

Chris Harmston
Consultant Colorectal Surgeon
University Hospital Coventry
Coventry, UK

Roel Hompes
U.Z. Gasthuisberg,
Leuven, Belgium

Mike Jarrett
Consultant Colorectal Surgeon,
Kingston upon Thames, UK

David Jayne
Consultant in General Surgery,
Leeds General Infirmary,
Leeds, UK

Oliver M. Jones
Consultant Colorectal Surgeon,
Oxford Pelvic Floor Centre,
Department of Colorectal Surgery,
Churchill and John Radcliffe Hospitals,
Oxford, UK

Henry Kwok
Clinical Colorectal Fellow
Auckland City Hospital,
Auckland, New Zealand

Ian Lindsey
Consultant Colorectal Surgeon,
Oxford Pelvic Floor Centre,
Department of Colorectal Surgery,
Churchill and John Radcliffe Hospitals,
Oxford, UK

Mark Mercer-Jones
Consultant in Colorectal Surgery,
Queen Elizabeth Hospital,
Gateshead, Newcastle, UK

Karen Nugent
Senior Lecturer,
Honorary Consultant Surgeon
Southampton General Hospital,
Southampton, UK

Sophie Pilkington
Specialist Registrar in
Colorectal Surgery,
Southampton University Hospitals
NHS Trust,
Southampton, UK

Marianne Starck
Department of Surgery,
Malmö University Hospital,
Queen Elizabeth Hospital,
Malmö, Sweden

Niels Wijffels
Consultant in General Surgery,
Zuwe Hofpoort Ziekenhuis,
Woerden, The Netherlands

Part A

Approaches

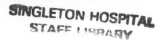

Chapter 1

Establishing and developing a pelvic floor service: the multidisciplinary team and the approach to patient assessment

Chris Cunningham

Introduction

Interest in pelvic floor and functional bowel disease has varied over the years. The 1980s saw considerable enthusiasm for surgical intervention in the form of subtotal colectomy for slow transit constipation, and postanal repair for incontinence. These subsequently lost appeal as long term results and morbidity were disappointing. There followed a quiet period where the combination of constipating agents and enemas formed the cornerstone of faecal incontinence management, and stoma formation was reserved for those with intractable problems. Interventions such as dynamic graciloplasty failed to capture the support of surgeons generally, who were perhaps disconcerted by technical difficulties, inconclusive benefits, and not inconsiderable morbidity. The main benefit appeared to be in highly motivated and well supported patients and it lacked applicability to the general population with end-stage faecal incontinence. Obstructed defaecation was occasionally improved with rectocele repair; but there was uncertainty as to the role of rectal intussusception, which was erroneously suggested to be a normal variant, or at least only an epiphenomenon of constipation. Through much of this period functional bowel disease and pelvic floor disorders were regarded as Cinderella topics failing to capture the interest of surgeons and trainees and becoming the reserve of a few zealots in specialist centres.

However, the spectrum of therapeutic options in pelvic floor conditions has increased enormously in the last decade. Sacral nerve stimulation has transformed the treatment of faecal incontinence for many patients, providing a tremendous option to those previously committed to stoma formation or a life of meticulous conservative management. Efforts to manage constipation and obstructed defaecation have dramatically improved with newer procedures to correct internal rectal prolapse (or intussusception) such as laparoscopic ventral rectopexy or perhaps more controversially stapled transanal rectal resection (STARR) or Transtar. There is also exciting evidence that correction of significant rectal intussusception may have a role in improving faecal incontinence, hinting at an alternative and hitherto unrecognized pathogenesis of incontinence. Technologies such as implanted artificial sphincters are appealing and likely to gain wider application as technical issues relating to infection and device erosion are conquered. All of this means that the delivery of a modern pelvic floor service is more demanding and complex than ever, but also appealing. There are benefits in developing subspecialty interest and expertise, and a multidisciplinary platform to implement an effective service. A comprehensive prospective audit of practice, particularly related to patient selection, outcome, and quality of life, is vital to avoid repeating past mistakes from overzealous and often morbid interventions for functional disorders.

Many surgical approaches in modern pelvic floor practice involve minimally invasive techniques which appeal to clinicians and patients alike. However, these approaches are still associated with significant expense and potential morbidity. Their use must be tempered by the fact that benign conditions are being treated with the aim of improving quality of life. The balance of risk versus benefit must be fully understood by patients and clinicians, and realistic expectations set out before treatment gets underway.

Establishing and developing a pelvic floor service

An effective pelvic floor service requires a few basic components. The first and most obvious is an interest and training in managing this group of patients who can be challenging and demanding. The second relates to basic diagnostic infrastructure either within one's own institution or readily available close by in a referral centre. Finally, one needs to create a multidisciplinary environment where individuals can be counselled and advised of diagnosis, treatment options and realistic outcomes.

The multidisciplinary team

The pelvic floor multidisciplinary team (MDT) needs to be inclusive. Core membership should include a pelvic floor physiologist and a specialist nurse who undertake diagnostic evaluation of pelvic floor abnormalities, and introduce and optimize conservative management at an early stage. Surgical input from the colorectal and urogynaecological teams is essential, and it is very useful to have close links with the obstetric department. In Oxford midwives and physiotherapists dealing with postpartum pelvic floor rehabilitation regularly attend the Pelvic Floor Centre. A dedicated dietician is valuable to reinforce the advice given through biofeedback; to ensure that the unit presents consistent and accurate advice; and to manage more challenging cases. Specialist radiologist involvement is required for expert interpretation and training in the use of studies such as defaecating proctography and dynamic pelvic magnetic resonance imaging (MRI), although routine reporting of these studies should be within the skill set of pelvic floor surgeons.

It is valuable to have regular contributions from a medical gastroenterologist with a dysmotility interest, although they need not be core members. There is a large shared population between pelvic floor clinics and medical gastroenterology clinics; many males and nulliparous females present through medical gastroenterology clinics, often with symptoms attributed to severe irritable bowel syndrome (IBS). Engagement of a medical gastroenterologist enables a ready flow of these patients to the pelvic floor MDT and is also valuable in optimizing management of patients with combined pathologies.

Finally, the pelvic floor MDT needs access to expertise in chronic pain management, pain rehabilitation, and psychological and psychiatric assessment and treatment. Whilst this is only required in an minority of patients, it is clear that those with complex issues, particularly those related to chronic pain and previous interventions, often need a novel approach to managing the physical and psychological aspects of their condition; this is only possible with appropriate experts. The importance of the MDT cannot be overstated and it is the basis for rigorous case presentation and discussion, consensus decision making, and mutual education.

Initially, it may be reasonable for the MDT to meet on a monthly basis to discuss interesting or challenging cases and to provide follow up on previously discussed clinical problems and decisions. This is an excellent environment for the team to develop expertise collectively. An alternative strategy, particularly if the practice increases, is to combine the MDT with the pelvic floor clinic. This makes for effective delivery of MDT decisions and allows efficient assessment of patients by different specialties in one clinic.

Clinic environment

Although a pelvic floor service can be absorbed into a regular colorectal surgical clinic, the creation of a dedicated specialist pelvic floor clinic offers several advantages. At a practical level it allows key members of the MDT to be present in the clinic simultaneously; this may become the environment for an efficient MDT meeting. In general, patients with pelvic floor abnormalities require more time for the establishment of trust for suitable clinical assessment, and a review with discussion of results and the proposed treatment plan. Commitment to a dedicated clinic facilitates this with the allocation of generous time slots creating an environment where teaching and training can be encouraged. Furthermore, in the present climate, many trainees are searching for comprehensive experience in pelvic floor disorders and the provision of a focus for this is rewarded by the presence of interested juniors and visitors.

Finally, in a developing service the provision of a dedicated pelvic floor clinic gives the service an identity to which other clinicians will more readily refer in the knowledge that patients are going to experience a level of assessment that is unsustainable in a general colorectal service. It is inevitable that developing and promoting a specialist interest and expertise in pelvic floor conditions will lead to many referring clinicians unburdening themselves of difficult patients with complex histories and often unsuccessful or even deleterious previous surgical interventions. Any trained colorectal surgeon can offer a 'fair weather' pelvic floor service but, in the author's opinion, it is the ability to absorb and manage these complex and difficult patients effectively that is the defining feature of a specialist clinic. As noted above, this extends beyond the skill and remit of most pelvic floor specialists and often requires input from psychologists, pain specialists and rehabilitation experts.

Asking the right questions

In many areas of surgical practice the traditional approach of obtaining a history, with careful examination leading to appropriate investigations, has been overturned in the rush to exclude cancer and meet targets with 'direct to test' protocols. However, in pelvic floor practice these principles remain the bedrock of clinical assessment for which there is no short cut. Many patients are referred with the primary aim of excluding important conditions such as colorectal cancer and inflammatory bowel disease. The ability and indeed the desire to unearth underlying pelvic floor pathology or dysfunction is dependent on a careful history and, putting it simply, asking the right questions. For example, one must look deeper into why a 70-year-old woman presents with constipation and haemorrhoidal symptoms. Concern over cancer may be an issue precipitating the presentation but most of these patients when questioned will have longstanding issues relating to bowel function that can be attributed to pelvic floor dysfunction.

Clues to this are found in a bowel habit that has become intrusive with repeated visits to the toilet through incomplete emptying, the requirement to assist defaecation by supporting the perineum or posterior vaginal wall, or the presence of post defaecatory soiling in the absence of significant urge incontinence. These are some key factors that suggest pre-existing pelvic floor problems, frequently resulting from rectal intussusception. The reason behind this presentation may be deterioration due to progressive pathology or just concern that these symptoms may represent sinister disease. This is the first point of decision making. Is this patient coping with these symptoms and is there any need to pursue investigations of pelvic floor function once risk of sinister pathology is excluded? It would be inappropriate to perform proctography in every elderly lady who presents with constipation, but equally inappropriate to deny a population thorough assessment and the option of best conservative management, or even surgery, when they are reassured they have no sinister disease. The balance depends on healthcare resources as well as patient expectations and demands.

One of the values of a dedicated pelvic floor clinic is that the general colorectal clinic environment can act as a filter for patients in whom further assessment is deemed appropriate and desired. In practical terms this is helpful as it allows the clinician to sow the seeds that there may be a remediable pelvic floor problem and offer preliminary advice regarding possible investigations and conservative management. Most of this can be done through patient information leaflets with recourse to reliable and trusted websites. This gives the patient some time to consider their problems and whether they wish to pursue investigations. The management of most pelvic floor conditions benefits from a period of contemplation and consideration.

An essential aim is to obtain a clear and honest pelvic floor history. The skilled interviewer may have to offer some leading questions to encourage patients to describe the details of their troubles and identify if there are any underlying psychological issues such as previous abuse. Many of these patients have been seen by numerous doctors in the past and part of the role of a coordinated pelvic floor clinic is to make them feel that they are being taken seriously and their difficulties are understood. It can be useful for the consultation to be shared between a surgeon and a pelvic floor clinical nurse specialist, setting the scene to then allow the nurse and patient further time if necessary. Structured questionnaires can be valuable in making sure that all areas are covered, particularly when trainees or less experienced nursing staff are involved.

A systematic approach to history taking, particularly with routine incorporation of a quality of life instrument, also lays the foundation to a system of structured prospective data collection and audit. Examples of a simple structured questionnaire (Wexner constipation and FISI) are shown in tables 1.1 and 1.2. Standard history questionnaires logically extend to standardized means of follow-up assessment with quality of life instruments. There are more of these available than symptoms and it is unusual that one finds the ideal questionnaire, however, regular use of mainstream, validated quality of life questionnaires reap rewards when describing and publishing patient outcomes.

How do pelvic floor patients present?

Patient groups

Patients presenting to pelvic floor clinic fall into two broad groups. The largest group comprises parous women whose symptoms are, broadly speaking, secondary to the consequences of pregnancy and childbirth. The other includes men and nulliparous women, where the underlying aetiology is usually more obscure; arising from previous surgical misadventure, connective tissue or neuromuscular abnormalities, or from predominantly behavioural or psychological origins. Many of these patients have been labelled as suffering from IBS or having behavioural peculiarities that often date from teenage years. Inevitably there is some overlap between these groups, not least for the simple reason that previously nulliparous women with connective tissue disorders also have babies. The background to pelvic floor and gastrointestinal disorders can have roots in significant life events, such as an eating disorder and psychological distress as well as physical and emotional abuse. This should be borne in mind particularly, but not exclusively, in those affected at an early age. Patients present with a wide spectrum of conditions, the most prevalent being constipation and obstructed defaecation, faecal incontinence, prolapse, and pelvic pain.

Chronic constipation

Constipation means different things to different people, but the common thread is that defaecation is difficult or reduced in frequency. Broadly speaking functional constipation can arise from slow transit colonic constipation (uncommon), evacuation problems (common) or a combination where colonic transit may be delayed as a secondary consequence. Patients are often referred for exclusion of sinister pathology and this of course should be the priority. This may be all that the patient wishes and it is simple and important to establish this at an early stage to avoid unnecessary investigation. Most patients with constipation arising from pelvic floor dysfunction will describe difficult evacuation with a feeling of incomplete emptying necessitating repeat visits to the toilet. This is frequently associated with a need to support the perineum and posterior vaginal wall or resort to 'digitation'. These symptoms can become

Table 1.1 Constipation Questionnaire (Wexner)

In the last 4 weeks, or typically for you,

1. How frequently have your bowels opened?

0	1–2 times per 1–2 days	2	once per week	4	more than once per month
1	twice per week	3	less than once per week		

2. How often have you had anal/rectal/coccyx pain before, during or after opening your bowels?

0	never	2	sometimes	4	always
1	rarely	3	usually		

3. How often have you felt that your bowels are incompletely emptied, like you didn't finish?

0	never	2	sometimes	4	always
1	rarely	3	usually		

4. How often have you had abdominal pain because of difficulty with your bowels?

0	never	2	sometimes	4	always
1	rarely	3	usually		

5. How long would you typically spend in the lavatory trying to go?

0	less than 5 minutes	2	10–20 minutes	4	more than 30 minutes
1	5–10 minutes	3	20–30 minutes		

6. Do you need to do the following to help you move your bowels, and how often? (circle which, and the frequency)

0	no assistance needed	1	laxatives	2	enemas, suppositories or digital assistance (placing a finger in the vagina, anus or between to help empty bowels)

7. On average, how often would you revisit the lavatory because you hadn't completely emptied your bowels?

0	never	2	3–6 times a day	4	9+ times a day
1	1–3 times a day	3	6–9 times a day		

8. For how many years have you had difficulty evacuating your bowel?

0	less than 1 year	2	5–10 years	4	more than 20 years
1	1–5 years	3	10–20 years		

Table 1.2 Incontinence Questionnaire (FISI)

In the last 4 weeks, or typically for you,					
1. How often have you had an accidental or involuntary loss or leakage of bowel gas?					
0	never	6	once a week	11	once a day
4	1–3 times a month	8	twice or more a week	12	twice or more a day
2. How often have you had an accidental or involuntary loss or leakage of mucous?					
0	never	5	once a week	10	once a day
3	1–3 times a month	7	twice or more a week	12	twice or more once a day
3. How often have you had an accidental or involuntary loss or leakage of liquid stool?					
0	never	10	once a week	17	once a day
8	1–3 times a month	13	twice or more a week	19	twice or more once a day
4. How often have you had an accidental or involuntary loss or leakage of solid stools?					
0	never	10	once a week	16	once a day
8	1-3 times a month	13	twice or more a week	18	twice or more once a day

intrusive, and not infrequently patients adopt a protracted routine of toileting before embarking on the day's activities. Management with osmotic laxatives can be very effective in this group and it is important to introduce these simple measures at an early stage and perhaps avoid unnecessary investigation and treatment. However, if patients are prescribed laxatives alone for a longstanding, embarrassing illness they are struggling to come to terms with, they can get the false impression that they are being 'fobbed off'. Therefore, it is important that follow up is organized to test the efficacy of any trial of conservative treatment; this can act as a point of commencement of investigations should the trial fail.

Patients with slow transit constipation generally do not experience an urge or call to stool. In contrast to the pelvic discomfort of obstructed defaecation there is often an absence of symptoms but ultimately bloating, heaviness, and abdominal discomfort tend to be prominent features. Some of these patients will experience alternating bowel function associated with abdominal cramps and distension. This picture is more in keeping with constipation predominant IBS, but further investigation of pelvic floor function can identify underlying dysfunction. In Oxford, about 30% of patients with a high-grade internal rectal prolapse coming to surgery have a diagnosis of IBS mentioned in the GP's original referral letter; the true rate is almost certainly higher (1). In such patients with IBS, we found that eliciting at least one of the following four symptoms predicted 95% of high-grade internal rectal prolapse coming to surgery: faecal incontinence, 'digitation', incomplete evacuation and toilet revisiting.

Faecal incontinence

Isolated faecal incontinence accounts for about 25% of referrals to the Oxford Pelvic Floor Centre. It may be associated with urgency, occur as a passive event, or be mixed. Urge incontinence is also a feature of rectal pathology such as proctitis or carcinoma in which case 'wet wind' is a common feature. Patients with urge incontinence will tend to describe occasional disastrous events of major incontinence and they are typically unable to control flatus and loose stool. The threat of urge incontinence understandably leads to anxiety, which in many patients aggravates faecal urgency leading to a dreadful cycle which can be socially crippling. Passive incontinence is more typical of deficient internal sphincter function or anatomical deformity such as a fistula or scarring from previous surgery. The pattern varies enormously. For some it is little more than unpredictable staining of underwear or the unwitting release of small pellet stools, for others the problem is post defaecatory leakage and difficult anal hygiene. Those with anorectal prolapse or rectal intussusception have a variable pattern, with urge, passive leakage, or post defaecatory leakage, or some combination of these. Many patients will have mixed patterns of faecal incontinence because of a combination of underlying pelvic floor pathophysiologies.

Mixed symptoms

Presentation with mixed obstructed defaecation and faecal incontinence is not unusual although this may seem initially counter-intuitive. This has been attributed to passive loss of stool that remains in the rectum, perhaps trapped in a rectocele, after ineffective rectal evacuation. Many of these patients have only marginally reduced anal sphincter pressures which are out of keeping with the degree of faecal incontinence. It is also common to see a relatively thickened internal sphincter, again, perhaps at odds with the clinical presentation of faecal incontinence. Traditionally these patients have been offered techniques to improve rectal evacuation, biofeedback, or enemas and constipating agents to reduce faecal loss. However, difficult evacuation, passive incontinence, and post defaecatory soiling are features of internal rectal prolapse. The mechanism may be simply mechanical with leakage of stool from an incompletely emptied rectum with a weak sphincter, but a more complex process of high-grade internal rectal prolapse leading to passive incontinence through the recto-anal inhibitory reflex may also function. Investigations often show a thickened internal sphincter and near normal sphincter pressures which may define those who are less likely to develop external rectal prolapse. In any event, correction of internal rectal prolapse with laparoscopic ventral rectopexy is effective at improving continence, with several published series to support this (2–5).

Chronic pelvic pain

Chronic pelvic or perineal pain is a misery for patients and their families and a real challenge for the pelvic floor specialists. Most of these patients have been through a selection of clinics, particularly urology, gynaecology, orthopaedic and colorectal. Many will have seen pain specialists and be using treatments or mechanisms to help cope with symptoms. Referral to a pelvic floor clinic will usually be the result of some tenuous connection with bowel function and sadly many patients will not be improved significantly. However, it is important to have a strategy to approach this problem in a systematic fashion and, in common with most tertiary assessments, this is gained from returning to careful assessment of the fundamentals; establishing the onset, nature, duration, and the natural history of the pain is essential. In many circumstances the description of pain becomes a confused amalgamation of the original pathology (eg endometriosis, childbirth, pelvic prolapse) and the results of previous surgical interventions; and a clear history is often not available. It is important to exclude unusual serious causes and thorough assessment under anaesthesia and MRI scanning is most useful in this regard. The approach must have a multidisciplinary base and time with a clinician or specialist nurse can be invaluable in disentangling the origin of symptoms. Clues to an anorectal source may be found in a history suggesting a link to difficult evacuation. Detailed appraisal of pelvic floor pain is discussed in chapter 6.

Clinical assessment

General physical and abdominal examination is important. Assessment of fitness may be a major determinant of how far to pursue investigations and treatment, particularly surgical interventions. Patients with obesity and diabetes are more prone to pelvic floor problems but also the complications of intervention. Optimization of underlying medical problems should be encouraged. In extreme obesity, correction of this may be more important than any efforts directed to the pelvic floor, even if considering surgery for obesity.

In the UK it is traditional to examine patients in the left lateral position to assess the perineum and anorectum. This has limitations in pelvic floor assessment as inspection of the vaginal introitus is limited and the consequences of gravity are less obvious, even allowing for straining and bearing down. For this reason, examination with the aid of a gynaecological couch has much to advocate it and is routine in many parts of Europe. The traditional 'knees to elbows' or all fours approach in the USA gives good access for anal procedures in the consulting room or office but is less helpful at assessing for prolapse. For the moment the standard of care in the UK is examination in the left lateral position which appears to be culturally acceptable to the population of colorectal surgeons.

Careful inspection of the perineum will identify obvious scarring and deformity as a result of previous interventions or childbirth. Morphology of the perineum has been described by Nivatvongs and it may be useful to record this (6). The anus may be gaping from obstetric injury or pelvic neuropathy, or tight with evidence of spasm or a bulky internal sphincter. The presence of soiling, excoriation, tags and haemorrhoids is relevant. It is essential to include a dynamic component to the examination, asking the patient to bear down or push. Here we observe the nature of the movement and if it appears coordinated and appropriate. Understandably many patients are reluctant to unleash the full effort in doing this for fear of incontinence and it can be worth repeating at the end of the examination as the individual becomes more relaxed. The amount of perineal descent or ballooning should be noted as well as the presence of vaginal prolapse.

Palpation around the anus will give an impression of sphincter bulk, spasm and signs of obstetric or surgical trauma. Digital rectal examination is undertaken gently and it is valuable to ask the patient to bear down again, squeeze, and relax. It is worth repeating cycles of this in an effort to allow the patient to relax a little and become accustomed to what is a rather unusual request. One obtains a good idea of pelvic floor coordination and recruitment of other muscles such as the gluteals to compensate for a deficient pelvic floor. An impression of paradoxical contraction of the puborectalis muscle may also be detected. Digital examination allows assessment of: the sphincter bulk; any evidence of previous damage to, and the quality of, the perineal body and posterior vaginal wall; and any rectocele. With the finger above the sphincter mechanism it is again useful to ask the patient to bear down and in this position one may be aware of a poorly supported anterior rectal wall and the presence of internal rectal prolapse as the descending intussusceptiens strikes the examining finger. A bulky, retroverted or fibroid uterus may also be felt to intrude significantly into the rectum at this level. A vaginal tampon or ring pessary can interfere with pelvic floor assessment and if convenient should be removed.

Inspection and digital rectal examination are followed by inspection using rigid sigmoidoscopy, excluding mucosal disease and occasionally allowing assessment of a high take off rectal intussusception; however, the return in pelvic floor assessment is limited. A short proctoscope/anoscope is valuable in assessment of haemorrhoid and mucosal prolapse particularly with the patient pushing down in an effort to expel the proctoscope. A good impression of full thickness internal prolapse can also be obtained as the proctoscope is delivered through the anus. In patients with a history suggestive of external prolapse its absence at routine examination is not unusual and the best approach is to re-examine on a commode after a reasonable period of straining.

Are investigations required?

Many patients referred to a tertiary practice will have already had colonic investigations to exclude sinister pathology. The tenacity with which this is undertaken varies enormously but in the author's practice complete colonic assessment by colonoscopy is preferred; and in the elderly, flexible sigmoidoscopy and minimum prep. computerised tomography (CT) of the colon is a reasonable compromise. Patients in the over 70s group, who form a major component of a pelvic floor practice, have significant incidental findings of colorectal pathology and it is a tenet of functional practice to exclude organic pathology first.

Assessment of the pelvic floor varies between surgeons and institutions but in the author's opinion a standardized approach is important, not least as it helps to objectively define groups of patients and their responses to treatment in what is still an evolving practice with areas of considerable controversy. Basic assessment should include anorectal physiology and anal ultrasound. Objective physiology measurements cannot always be estimated accurately from digital assessment in clinic and recording of baseline function before undertaking interventions is sensible; if postoperative outcome is disappointing then reference to preoperative measurements is valuable. The presence of normal resting and squeeze pressures in patients with incontinence perhaps points to rectal intussusception as a cause rather than primary sphincter function. Relative subtleties such as rectal compliance, rectoanal inhibitory reflex, and balloon expulsion tests are perhaps less reliable, but abnormalities in these areas no doubt contribute to the overall assessment of the patient's function.

Key points

- Dedicated specialty pelvic floor clinics are the ideal environment for pelvic floor practice
- Symptom complexes are often subtle and partly hidden
- Multidisciplinary teamwork facilitates good clinical practice

Editor's summary

This handbook covers all aspects of pelvic floor practice compiled by clinicians with large volume practices in the subspeciality. It provides a solid foundation for the development of a pelvic floor service at an exciting time, with the development of new techniques and a more thorough understanding of underlying pathologies. One of the most important elements in creating a mature pelvic floor service is acceptance that not all patients will benefit from surgical intervention; and a central role of the pelvic floor clinic and MDT is to identify this group and concentrate efforts on non-operative approaches to improving symptoms or coping with conditions. In all aspects of medical practice, patients and doctors accept that most treatments and all operations carry risks and there is a particularly fine balance in managing quality of life issues with pelvic floor conditions.

It is important for professional and medico-legal reasons that all conservative measures have been explored thoroughly before proceeding with surgical treatment. We have all witnessed patients whose symptoms are no better after a sphincter repair, and then find a manageable solution in careful dietary manipulation, exercise, and use of constipating agents. It is clear that the best approach is optimization before surgery. This can be difficult, because it is easier for a surgeon with a limited infrastructure to perform an operation than to undertake six sessions of biofeedback. An assessment of the risk of making the patient worse must be considered. The patient who is seeking to improve quality of life must be aware of the chances of a poor outcome that will result in an impaired status. Chronic pain after staple anopexy; pelvic sepsis or urgency after STARR; and bowel injury or mesh erosion after rectopexy are just a few outcomes that, although rare, may destroy quality of life. In the author's opinion, the road towards surgical intervention must demonstrate due consideration to these risks which must be grasped by the patient. The answer to the patient's question, 'Could it make me worse?' often helps to determine if a patient proceeds with surgery. This is an exciting time in pelvic floor surgery and the delivery of optimum assessment and treatment to patients will be provided within the context of robust multidisciplinary teams, strengthened by comprehensive training and education, and guided by honest audit and reporting.

References

1. Wijffels N, Collinson R, Cunningham C, Lindsey I. Internal rectal prolapse: occult by name, occult by nature. *Colorect Dis* 2008; **10**(suppl.2):16 [abstract].

2. Lazorthes F, Gamagami R, Cabarrot P, Muhammad S. Is rectal intussusception a cause of idiopathic incontinence? *Dis Colon Rectum* 1998; **41**(5):602–5.

3. Schultz I, Mellgren A, Dolk A, Johansson C, Holmstrom B. Continence is improved after the Ripstein rectopexy. Different mechanisms in rectal prolapse and rectal intussusception? *Dis Colon Rectum* 1996; **39**(3):300–6.

4. Slawik S, Soulsby R, Carter H, Payne H, Dixon AR. Laparoscopic ventral rectopexy, posterior colporrhaphy and vaginal sacrocolpopexy for the treatment of recto-genital prolapse and mechanical outlet obstruction. *Colorectal Dis* 2008; **10**(2):138–43.

5. Collinson R, Wijffels N, Cunningham C, Lindsey I. Laparoscopic ventral rectopexy for internal rectal prolapse: short-term functional results. *Colorectal Dis* 2010; **12**:97–104.

6. Nivatvongs S, Fang DT, Kennedy HL. The shape of the buttocks. A useful guide to selection of anesthesia and patient position in anorectal surgery. *Dis Colon Rectum* 1983; **26**:85–6.

Chapter 2

Radiological workup

Brigitta Boller, Oleh Babyak, and
Volodymyr Denysenko

Introduction

This work will review the use of imaging studies in the assessment of the pelvic floor
disorders in patients with obstructed defecation syndrome (ODS) symptoms. It is a
summary of the diagnostic experience in the field of pelvic floor disorders that we have
accumulated over the last 10 years with more than 4000 patients. We believe that in
most cases a pelvic floor pathology is not caused by a solitary disorder. Only the anatomical definitions per se are solitary, eg rectocele, cystocele, enterocele, mucosal and
rectal prolapse. The situations we deal with in daily practice are of a higher complexity
with at least two concurrent disorders. The evaluation of their interaction matched
to the patient's symptoms is the key to this work and is essential for successful
diagnosis.

Diagnostic approach

The following diagnostic procedure was developed for patients with ODS symptoms:

1. Sonography of the abdomen
2. Endosonography of the anterior rectal wall/dorsal vaginal wall
3. Endosonography of the anal canal
4. Double-contrast irrigoscopy
5. Colonic transit time
6. Dynamic examination of the pelvic floor

   In this chapter we briefly look at colonic transit time and then concentrate on the
dynamic examination of the pelvic floor (dynamic pelvicography).

Colonic transit time

The colonic transit time examination is performed in patients who suffer from chronic
constipation. It is used to distinguish functional slow transit constipation (a disorder
of transport through the bowel) from mechanical defaecation obstruction. There is
no special preparation necessary. However, in the days before the examination no
laxatives should be taken.

Procedure

The patient takes a daily capsule containing 10 radiopaque markers over a period of six days. On the seventh day a plain abdominal X-ray is taken, the intestinal markers are counted, and the intestinal transit time calculated. If the latter is more than 72 hours, the transit time is considered to be slow. The segmental distribution of markers in the colon can be interpreted to give an idea of segmental transit.

Significance

The measurement of colonic transit time alone cannot give a definitive diagnosis. Like other studies in the area of the pelvic floor, it is interpreted in the light of other findings. It is important to emphasize the interdisciplinary character of pelvic floor disorders and the need for cooperation between doctors looking after each of the three compartments.

The validity of colonic transit study is further limited by the fact that some studies have shown that colonic transit time varies in the same patient, and a long transit time is not necessarily associated with symptoms of constipation.

Dynamic pelvicography

Definition

The definition of 'defaecography' was first given in 1952. At that time the first work on defaecography was published by Dr Wallden (1). Then Broden and Snellman described this method in 1968 (2). The still image of the filled rectum produced by this diagnostic procedure saw little development until the end of the 1990s. Work since 1999 has improved the whole diagnostic approach in this field in general, and defaecography in particular. This has helped to develop a new way of looking at the pelvic floor and its pathology. There are said to be three pelvic floor compartments, but here we consider them as one integrated whole. This is the very basis of the diagnostic approach. All three compartments are examined in one dynamic procedure to best simulate and visualize the act of emptying as close to reality as possible. It is called dynamic pelvic floor examination because all the pelvic floor organs are being examined and evaluated. The sense of dynamic pelvicography is as a representation of the anatomical and functional components in disorders of the pelvic floor.

It is performed to provide:

- Objective correlation of subjective patient complaints and of the clinical examination
- Visualization of the anatomical and functional disorders
- Information for guidance on the choice of the therapy

Another important point about dynamic pelvicography is its role as a documentary record of the patient's problem: the recorded sequence is a baseline document which can be later referred to as the basis for therapy in case of postoperative problems.

Preparation and method

Prior to the examination female patients are asked about possible pregnancy. Due to the relatively high radiation dose, examination of young patients is avoided if possible. The radiation dose is relatively high in pelvicography because defaecation takes several minutes, during which the examiner relies heavily on fluoroscopy. Moreover, in the lateral projection, the pelvis is the broadest part of the body, resulting in the need for high entrance exposure. Therefore pelvicography is among those radiological procedures associated with a considerable, but not extreme radiation dose.

For at least three days before the examination, no laxatives, enemas, suppositories, laxative teas, or homeopathic remedies for constipation may be used. It is very important that the contrast medium is not a liquid as it would have an enema effect. Liquid in the rectum is not the physiological norm and may stress the continence mechanism, which may result in abnormal contractions of anal and pelvic floor muscles at rest. The ideal contrast medium needs to simulate stool in weight and consistency. To contrast small bowel and colon a barium sulphate suspension for oral and rectal contrast is used. 24 hours before the examination one half of the powder is dissolved in 0.25–1.5 litre of water and taken orally. The second half is taken about three hours before the examination. Meals and drugs, other than above-mentioned, can be taken regularly. Immediately before the examination the bladder is filled with a non-ionic water soluble contrast medium for the urinary bladder, the vagina is contrasted with barium (3). Then barium paste is injected into the rectum until the patient experiences discomfort due to rectal distension, which causes a physiological urge to empty. The examination can now be started (4). The patient is sat on a commode as comfortably as possible. The commode must be radiolucent and properly attached to the fluoroscopic table and able to permit both lateral and frontal projections (5). Disposable plastic bags are used to collect excreted barium paste. Radiographic lead filters are used to cut out flare. The latter can especially be a problem in the lower part of the image, particularly in the obese patient. An anteroposterior (AP) view is also taken because it often gives more information on the position and form of rectoceles and enteroceles than the lateral view. It can be also useful to attach a radiographic ruler beneath the bag in the midline of the commode for exact and direct measurements on the X-ray films.

The special value of the physiological (upright) position (6) during the examination is the natural pressure of the abdomen, the weight of the intestine, and the influence of gravity. These criteria play a crucial role when comparing this X-ray method to dynamic magnetic resonance imaging (MRI) undertaken mostly in the supine position. MRI machines with a sitting position are quite rare and expensive.

A total of four images are made as well as an X-ray video of the emptying process. For the first image the patient is asked to completely relax the pelvic floor musculature and anal sphincter (including puborectalis and external sphincter). The next image is made with a deliberate contraction of these muscles. The third image is carried out during attempts at straining (7). The patient is also asked to press digitally to empty. The defaecation process and the emptying of the bladder are recorded radiologically. One more image is made after emptying (the patient must strain). Thereafter these four images are evaluated.

Common findings

Below are the most common findings which can be efficiently differentiated:

- Mucosal prolapse (intrarectal and intra-anal)
- Intussusception

- ◆ Rectocele
- ◆ Hypermobile and descended perineum
- ◆ Wall prolapse or external prolapse
- ◆ Enterocele (physiological (functional) and pathological (anatomically persistent))
- ◆ Sigmoidocele
- ◆ Colpocele
- ◆ Pelvic floor dissynergy (paradoxical puborectalis contraction)

Mucosal prolapse (intrarectal and intra-anal)

Mucosal prolapse represents sliding down of folds of the rectal mucosa, which have partly lost their functionality. Intrarectal mucosa folds remain in the rectum while intra-anal mucosal prolapse protrudes into the anal canal. A certain degree of mucosal prolapse during defaecation straining is a physiological event whereby the mucosa prolapses into the anal canal during passage of the rectal contents. In normal individuals this is corrected by contraction of the pelvic floor muscles. Sometimes, however, it is difficult to differentiate rectal mucosal prolapse from a rectal intussusception. In many circumstances the differentiation is based on subjective quantification of the anterior rectal wall folds.

Rectal Intussusception

Intussusception is an invagination of the rectal wall of more than 2 cm (8,9). There are circular, assymetrical, single or double intussusceptions (Fig. 2.1). There are two kinds of morphologically distinguished intussusceptions:

1. Intrarectal intussusception is an invagination of the rectal wall into the rectum. It usually causes almost no discomfort.
2. Intra-anal intussusception is an invagination of the rectal wall into the anal canal. It sometimes remains asymptomatic, but mostly causes an obstruction of the anal canal (10), causing the so-called obstructed defaecation syndrome (ODS).

Rectocele

A rectocele is an extension and corresponding bulging of the rectal wall (11). It can be traced back to overstraining, mostly as a result of stretching and overloading in ODS. The rectum bends towards the slightest resistance. Hence, most often, ventral rectoceles can be found (Fig. 2.1). With a rectocele we measure:

1. Position: ventral, lateral, dorsal
2. Position in relation to the surrounding organs; impression and/or displacement of those
3. Deformation during the emptying process.

Lateral rectoceles are quite common and sometimes one can find dorsal rectoceles. Ventral rectoceles or ventral combined with dorsal ones are most commonly found. An anteroposterior view during the examination is a great help in such cases. The top of the rectocele is a vector direction of the pressing force which normally should

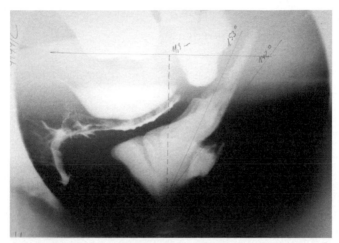

Fig. 2.1 Rectocele and intussusception.

be directed into the anal canal. In the case of a rectocele there is a protrusion of the anterior rectal wall into the posterior vaginal wall, which occurs when straining to defaecate. After defaecation the residual rectal contents are left in the protrusion (12). In the course of time, the contractility of the anterior rectal wall pushes the residue back into the rectal ampoule, resulting in a repeated sensation of rectal fullness and hence the urge to empty the rectum (13). This explains why patients with a rectocele complain of repeated defaecation.

Hypermobile and descended perineum

A hypermobile perineum is a perineum which moves more than normal during evacuation (9). We consider this a compensatory mechanism. With increasing age a descending of the abdominal and pelvic organs can lead to a change in the normal balance. A very common risk factor for the development of pelvic descent is chronic constipation with laxative abuse. It can also occur in women after several pregnancies and complicated deliveries, or after hysterectomy. The pelvic hypermobility results in the nerves and muscles being overstretched and gradually losing their function.

In contrast to the hypermobile perineum we distinguish the descended perineum. In this case the pelvic floor is very latent with almost no mobility. This is already a decompensated disorder as a result of the progressive loss of muscle elasticity and denervation of the rectum. This situation was observed in patients who had been suffering from constipation for many years.

Wall prolapse or external prolapse

This type of prolapse is considered to be the most advanced form of a prolapse, when the rectal wall protrudes through the anal canal with all its layers. It can also build a pouch with the small bowel loops of an enterocele (Fig. 2.2).

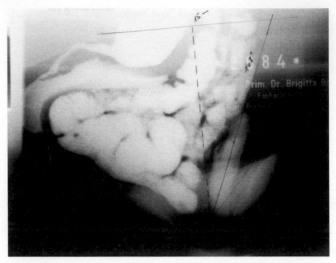

Fig. 2.2 Enterocele.

Enterocele (physiological (functional) and pathological (anatomically persistent))

If the small bowel loops protrude into the Douglas pouch, it is called an enterocele (14). It is often difficult to clearly distinguish pathological and physiological enteroceles. The quality of these disorders are measured by a functional mechanism. Once again a compensatory character becomes important. A physiological enterocele we regard as a functional one, which works like a stamp and helps to expel the faeces. It does not protrude between the vagina and the rectum. A pathological enterocele does not play any compensatory role (Fig. 2.2). We believe that due to heavy straining it dissects the wall between vagina and rectum and loses its auxiliary function. Patients with a pathological enterocele have a sense of incomplete evacuation, with symptoms similar to the patients who have ODS. Often there is no associated rectal disorder at all. Frequently a pathological enterocele can be found in women after hysterectomy. In this case dynamic pelvicography is mandatory in the preoperative workup if a patient is to be surgically treated (15).

Sigmoidocele

A sigmoidocele is a prolapse of redundant sigmoid colon into the Douglas pouch. It is not as common as an enterocele.

Colpocele

If the vagina is not descended and stays in the anatomically correct position, it can become indented by a rectocele. However, with a descended pelvic floor and a redundant rectum a change in the position of the vagina can be observed. The vagina moves to an almost horizontal position, and a protrusion of the rectum under the vagina is seen. At the same time all the pelvic floor organs seem to change their anatomical axes and position. In this case the dorsal wall of the vagina is not indented by the rectocele, and, therefore no colpocele is observed. One gets an impression that the organs move in the direction of least resistance.

Pelvic floor dyssynergy (paradoxical puborectalis contraction)

The pelvic floor comprises, among other things, a muscle plate. Of this muscle plate, the most powerful and important muscle is the puborectalis. Together with the anal sphincter it is responsible for continence. During defaecation both the external anal sphincter and puborectalis muscle relax to enable evacuation. If this coordination is abnormal the muscles do not relax and may even contract more than usual; this results in the anal canal staying closed or not opening not wide enough to enable evacuation. When the abnormality is caused by the anal sphincter we call it anismus. When the puborectalis muscle contracts abnormally, we call it a paradoxical puborectalis contraction. As a consequence, the impression of the puborectalis muscle persists and the anorectal angle decreases insufficiently (9). The anorectal junction remains closed, and the patient is unable to expel the rectal contents despite repeated and subjectively adequate straining (Fig. 2.3).

Pelvic floor dissynergy is common amongst shop-assistants or teachers who may not be able to go to the toilet when they need to. Therefore they have to 'hold back'. Physiologically they overstrain their puborectalis muscle in this manner. It is believed that patients with paradoxical puborectalis contraction have forgotten how to empty physiologically. They must learn to do so again with the help of biofeedback therapy.

Evaluation

Normal findings

To understand any possible pathology we must look at normal defaecation first. When the patient is asked to squeeze, the levator ani muscles, especially the puborectalis,

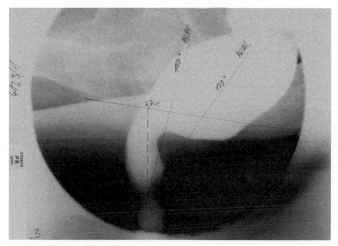

Fig. 2.3 Pelvic floor dissynergy.

contract maximally. This event causes an impression at the posterior border of the anorectal junction and an acute anorectal angulation. Then the patient is asked to relax the levator ani muscles. At this stage the puborectalis muscle is still contracted, but less than during squeezing, as can be seen by a partial decrease of the impression, as well as a slight decrease of the anorectal angle and a slight descent of the anorectal junction. When the patient is requested to defaecate, further obliteration of the impression, decrease of the anorectal angle, descent of the anorectal junction and widening of the anal canal can be seen. At the end of defaecation the rectal ampulla should be empty and there should be no further urge to defaecate.

Abnormal findings

In the relaxed position before the examination

In the relaxed state, postoperative changes/deformation of the rectal wall can be seen. Even before the examination a paradoxical compression of the puborectalis muscle can be seen (ARAP ≥ ARAC). We can also observe deformation of the anterior rectal wall in the form of a rectocele.

During squeeze

At squeeze no significant changes can normally be seen, except for the rectocele, although a pathologically low excursion of the pelvic floor muscles may indicate a decompensated descending of the pelvic floor.

At straining

At straining, rectal wall prolapse and rectocele reach their maximum size/length. The type of an enterocele (pathological/physiological) can be reliably evaluated; other disorders such as pelvic floor dyssynergy, anismus, excessive widening of the rectum, changing of the axes of the organs, pathology of the uterus/vagina (corresponding cystocele and colpocele), and uterine descent can be well visualized.

At the end of the examination

At the end of the examination, after emptying, the residual rectocele and the reduction of the wall prolapse are documented. Depending on the measurements we can judge whether the disorder is compensated or decompensated. We conclude that a disorder is compensated when, for instance, an intra-anal intussusception has reduced to an intrarectal intussception (from 4–5 to 2–3 cm). Regarding an enterocele we can see whether it is physiological (functional) or pathological, the latter being anatomically persistent. This means that if an enterocele dissects the rectovaginal wall and stays in between the rectum and vagina, even after the examination, we call it a pathological enterocele. Otherwise we call it a functional or physiological enterocele, when the small bowel loops move upwards after the straining.

Our standard pelvicography procedure also includes several types of measurements. These measurements cannot be regarded as reliable or significant in all cases. The anatomical position of the pelvic organs is very individual and there are hardly any reference data which allow comparison, even within a consistent group of patients. The reasons are obvious: we have patients of different ages, physique, profession, lifestyle etc. In order to bring at least some comparable data into the diagnostic procedure

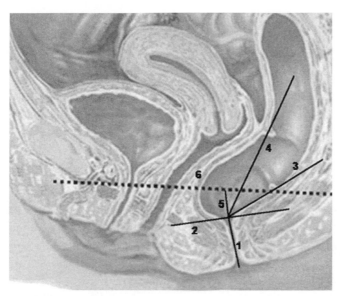

Fig. 2.4 Anorectal angles.

an evidence line is used; the pubococcygeal line. In terms of anatomy this line links the lowest part of the pubic bone with the lower edge of the coccyx, thus giving a constant to compare the results with normal findings.

In Figure 2.4 the following parameters are found (16,17):

1. Length of the anal canal (line 1); in a situation with decompensated disorder the pelvic floor musculature is shortened and widened through mechanical compression. This would indicate weakened muscle elasticity and tone.

2. Border anus/rectum (line 2); an important line for measurements of perineal descent (line from the middle of the rectum/anus border to the pubococcygeal line).

3. Angle ARAP: the angle between the anal canal (line 1) and a line tangential to the lower 1/3 of the rear rectal wall (line 3).

4. Angle ARAC: the angle between the anal canal (line 1) and a line tangential to the middle of the rectum at the level of the transverse fold (line 4). With paradoxical contraction of the puborectalis muscle, the ARAP angle is always larger than the ARAC angle (relevant only in the relaxed state or during straining).

5. Distance from the anorectal border to the pubococcygeal line (line 5): this is an important parameter for evaluation of the pelvic floor musculature and its mobility.

6. The evidence line (dotted line 6)–the pubococcygeal line–is a static, unchangeable anatomical unit. Using this line, one can measure pelvic floor descent and judge the mobility of the pelvic floor. In a normal patient approximately 1/3 of the rectum is expected to be under this line, with the remaining 2/3 above it. In contrast, in patients with a descended perineum 2/3 or even the whole rectal ampulla can lie under the evidence line.

7. Width of the anal canal (during emptying); the anal canal gets wider during emptying because of mechanical pressure. An abnormally wide anal canal can be related to low internal anal sphincter tone: incontinence could be an issue (18,19).

8. A line parallel to the ischial tuberosity can be regarded as an additional auxiliary line in questionable findings (not shown here).

Relevant states for the measurement of pelvic floor descent:

1. Relaxed position

2. Squeeze

3. Maximum straining during emptying.

The following parameters are evaluated:

1. Maximum excursion: position during emptying minus position during squeeze.

2. Excursion during straining: straining position minus relaxed position.

3. Deformation during the emptying process.

Discussion

Dynamic pelvicography, ie the dynamic examination of the pelvic floor organs, including urinary bladder, vagina, small bowel, colon and rectum, is probably the best imaging diagnostic method for the study of pathological changes in the pelvic floor. It allows judgements to be made on the mobility of the pelvic floor, pathological functions of the musculature, and changes to the form and axis of the organs. It provides important parameters for the deformation and morphology of pelvic floor organs; and can also show compensated and decompensated disorders as well as development of internal hernias–enteroceles probably being the most important and often overlooked.

With this method the organs of the pelvic floor are examined under physiological conditions (20). We have to stress here the subjectivity of the word 'physiological'. On the one hand, one might be critical about how physiological retrograde filling of the rectum and other pelvic floor organs is when they are being filled from bottom to top. One the other hand this method simulates the filling of the pelvic floor organs for the purpose of imaging diagnostics, especially taking the time limitation of the whole procedure into consideration. As an alternative examination method there is dynamic MRI which is substantially more time-consuming and expensive.

There is a large variation in the patterns of anorectal function among healthy individuals. There is also a large variation in the measurements of the parameters of anorectal function. Therefore, caution should be taken when these measurements are interpreted, and the measurements should not be used as the only criteria for treatment. (21,22)

Anatomical abnormalities of the rectal wall, such as intussusception, rectocele, and mucosal prolapse can occur in asymptomatic patients; the demonstration of rectal wall changes in the absence of defaecatory disorders is of no greater importance than the accidental demonstration of an oesophageal hernia. However, changes in the shape of the anorectal region during defaecation should be considered abnormal. These changes do not necessarily cause symptoms; whether or not they will progress to a clinical disorder needs further investigation.

Key points

+ In most cases, a pelvic floor disorder is not caused by a solitary disorder or pathology
+ Dynamic pelvicographic examination of the pelvic floor organs (bladder, vagina, small bowel, colon and rectum) is the most appropriate diagnostic method for studying these multiple pathological changes
+ The organs of the pelvic floor are examined under conditions as close as possible to physiological conditions giving an anatomical and functional representation of the disordered pelvic floor
+ Dynamic pelvicography allows good documentation of dysfunction justifying indications for therapy
+ An alternative examination, dynamic MRI, is substantially more time-consuming and costly.

Editor's summary

High quality dynamic proctography remains the 'gold standard' in the assessment of pelvic floor disorders and, where possible, three or four phase evaluation is preferred to provide a fuller assessment. We believe dynamic MRI does not offer normal physiological conditions because it assesses evacuation in the supine position, without the influence of gravity in an embarrassed patient. Surgeons with a pelvic floor interest cannot fully grasp the pathology of disordered defaecation without directly visualising the studies themselves. Without this, the report becomes largely meaningless. Proctography does have its drawbacks, particularly in the over-diagnosis of anismus and under-diagnosis of prolapse disease. If the study is at odds with the clinical story and physical examination an examination under anaesthetic (EUA) will usually clarify. An interested radiographer can provide a quality personalized service.

References

1. Wallden L. Defecation block in cases of deep rectogenital pouch. *Acta Chir Scand* 1952; **165**: 1–121.
2. Broden B, Snelman B Procidentia of the rectum studied with cineradiography: a contribution to the discussion of causative mechanism. *Dis Col Rectum* 1968; **11**: 330–47.
3. Archer B. Contrast Medium Gel for Marking Vaginal Position during Defecography. *Radiology* 1992; **182**: 278–79.
4. Poon F, Lauder J, Finlay I. Technical report: Evacuating proctography - A simplified technique. *Clin Radiol* 1991; **44**(2): 113–6.
5. Hyland GJ. Defaecating video proctography. *J Audiov Media Med* 1988; **11**: 91–93.

6. Eckberg O, Nylander G, Fork FT. Defecography. *Radiology* 1985; **155**: 45–48.

7. Goei R, van Engelshoven J, Schouten H, Baeten CG, Stassen C. Anorectal function: defecographic measurement in asymptomatic subjects. *Radiology* 1989; **173**: 137–41.

8. Bartolo DC, Bartram Cl, Ekberg O, Fork FT, Kodner I, Kuijpers JH, et al.. Proctography. Symposium. *Int J Colorectal Dis* 1988; **3**: 67–89.

9. Shorvon PJ, Mchugh S, Diamant NE, Somers S. Defecography in normal volunteers: results and implications. *Gut* 1989; **30**: 1737–49.

10. Karlbom U, Nilsson S, Pahlman L, Graf W. Defecographic study of rectal evacuation in constipated patients and control subjects. *Radiology* 1999; **210**: 103–8.

11. Agachan F, Pfeifer J, Wexner S. Defecography and proctography. *Dis Col Rectum* 1996; **39**: 899–905.

12. Freimanis MG, Wald A, Caruana B. Evacuation proctography in normal volunteers. *Invest Radiol* 1991; **26**(6): 581–5.

13. Mahieu P, Pringot J, Bodart P. Defecography: II. Contribution to the diagnosis of defecation disorders. *Abdom Imaging* 1984; **9**: 253–61.

14. Halligan S, Bartram C, Hall C, Wingate J. Enterocele revealed by simultaneous evacuation. Proctography and peritoneography: does 'defecation bloc' exist? *Am J Roentgenol* 1996; **167**: 461–6.

15. Kelvin F, Maglinte D, Hornback J, Benson T. Pelvic prolapse: assessment with evacuation proctography (defecography). *Radiology* 1992; **184**: 547–51.

16. Felt-Bersma RJ, Luth WJ, Janssen JJ, Meuwissen SG. Defecography in patients with anorectal disorders. *Dis Col Rectum* 1990; **33**(4): 277–84.

17. Selvaggi F, Pesce G, Scotto Di Carlo E. Evaluation of normal subjects by defecographic technique. *Dis Col Rectum* 1990; **33**(8): 698–702.

18. Nelsen M, Buron B, Christiansen J, Hegedüs V. Defecographic. Findings in patients with anal incontinence and constipation and their relation to rectal emptying. *Dis Col Rectum* 1993; **36**(9): 806–9.

19. Klauser AG, Ting KH, Mangel E. Interobserver agreement in defecography. *Dis Col Rectum* 1994; **37**(12):1310–6.

20. Jones H, Swift R, Blake H. A prospective audit of the usefulness of evacuating proctography. *J Am Coll Surgeons* 1998; **80**(1): 40–45.

21. Bartram CI, Turnbull GK, Lennard-Jones JE. Evacuation proctography: An investigation of rectal expulsion in 20 subjects without defecatory disturbance. *Abdom Imaging* 1988; **13**(1): 72–80.

22. Skomorowska E, Hegedüs V, Christiansen J. Evaluation of perineal descent by defaecography. *Int J Colorectal Dis* 1988; **3**(4): 191–4.

Chapter 3

Anorectal physiology

Henry Kwok and Rowan Collinson

Background

The anorectum is responsible for the control of defaecation and maintenance of continence. Proper function requires integration of the pelvic floor, rectal compliance, and pelvic sensorimotor function. Disorders of the anorectum often have complex pathophysiology and manifest in a number of ways, in particular rectal outlet obstruction, faecal incontinence (FI) and pain. These conditions are gaining increasing attention, in part due to their increasing prevalence in the aging Western population. Recent systematic reviews have estimated the prevalence of constipation to be up to 25% (1) and that of FI in the order of 11–15% (2).

Anorectal physiology testing supplements a thorough pelvic examination. Digital rectal examination performed by an experienced clinician can reveal useful information such as resting tone and squeeze pressure, with correlations to manometry reportedly as high as 72% (3). However, the reliability of clinical examination has been brought to question, with overall sensitivities and specificities as low as 63% and 57% respectively reported (4). As a result, a wide range of tests exist to objectively assess anorectal function to supplement clinical examination. From their basic beginnings, technological developments have improved the ease of use of these procedures in clinical practice and their ability to mimic real-life situations. These tests have contributed much to our understanding of anorectal disorders, and now form an integral part of the research and management of these conditions in the following ways:

- Quantifying the severity of anorectal disorders
- Identifying contributing factors to anorectal disorders
- Predicting natural history of disorders
- Selecting patients for treatment
- Tailoring treatment options to the underlying disorders
- Predicting and assessing treatment outcome.

Routine outpatient anorectal tests are listed in Table 3.1. There is significant overlap between these modalities and they complement each other in the work up of anorectal disorders. With a few obvious exceptions (e.g. MRI, DPG), most of these tests can be performed in the anorectal physiology laboratory at the same time as the primary consultation.

Table 3.1 Routine tests in outpatient anorectal physiology evaluation

Functional tests	Structural tests
Anal manometry	Endoanal ultrasound (EAUS)
Rectal and anal sensation	Defecating proctogram (DPG)
Rectal balloon expulsion	Dynamic magnetic resonance imaging (MRI)
Rectal compliance	
Anorectal neurophysiology	

Setup of anorectal physiology laboratory

Testing is performed in the outpatient setting. It is important that efforts be made to ensure patient privacy and comfort due to the invasive and potentially socially-embarrassing nature of the procedures. Screens, curtains and well-placed changing areas all help to put the patients at ease.

A trained gastrointestinal physiologist or nurse specialist is central to the running of the laboratory, and performance of testing. They may also administer non-surgical treatments, such as pelvic floor physiotherapy and biofeedback. Clinical oversight should be provided by a colorectal surgeon with an interest. A multidisciplinary meeting for discussion of complex cases is strongly recommended. To minimize inter- and intra-observer variability the laboratory must have well-maintained equipment, stable staffing and well-established protocols, preferably based on internationally-agreed guidelines.

Proformas should be used to standardize the collection of patient history and physical findings. They allow the construction and maintenance of accurate computerized databases, which facilitate research and performance audit. Proformas should include validated symptom scoring systems. Examples for FI include the St Marks Incontinence Score (Table 3.2) and the Wexner Continence Grading Scale (5). For obstructed defaecation (OD) and constipation, the Obstructed Defecation Score (ODS) (6) and the Cleveland Clinic Constipation Score (7) serve a similar function.

Table 3.2 St Mark's Incontinence Score (from Vaizey et al. 1999) (5)

Clinical condition	Never	Rarely	Sometimes	Weekly	Daily
Incontinence to solid stool	0	1	2	3	4
Incontinence to liquid stool	0	1	2	3	4
Incontinence to gas	0	1	2	3	4
Alteration in lifestyle	0	1	2	3	4
Symptoms				No	Yes
Need to wear a pad or plug				0	2
Taking constipating medicines				0	2
Lack of ability to defer defaecation for 15 minutes				0	4

Symptom-specific quality of life indices also exist (eg Faecal Incontinence Quality of Life (FIQL) scale (8)), and should ideally also be collected.

Anal manometry

Technique

Anal manometry assesses anal sphincter function by measuring anal canal pressure by way of an intra-anally situated pressure transducer. Different types of manometric transducer include the balloon catheter, the water-perfused tube catheter and the solid-state microtransducer (9). The transducer is attached to a computer processor and display, which can be anything from very basic (hand-held, giving a simple numerical value for the pressure) to a conventional personal computer with dedicated software allowing advanced data analysis and storage (Fig. 3.1a–c). Depending on the catheter used, anal canal pressures are measured using either a stationary or a pull-through technique (9). A recent clinical comparison of different transducer types found little variation in their performance (10), meaning that cost-effective choices are possible, depending on the needs of the physiology laboratory. During a pull-through technique, the catheter tip is placed 6 cm into the anal verge and the pressures

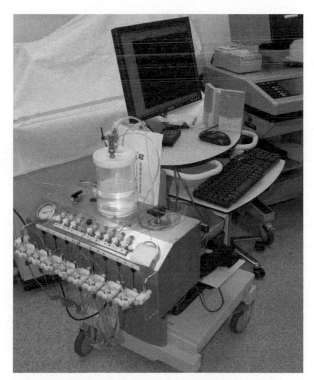

Fig. 3.1.a Anorectal manometry equipment: eight channel transducer system (PIP-4-8SS; Mui Scientific, Ontario, Canada) connected to PC.

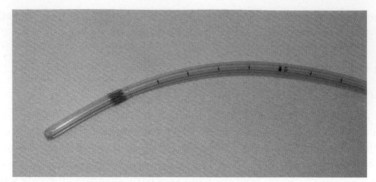

Fig. 3.1.b Anorectal manometry equipment: tip of a water-perfused nine-lumen vector manometry catheter with 3.9-mm external diameter (used with 3.1a above) (MED 2280; Mediplus, High Wycombe, UK).

are recorded for every 1 cm the catheter is withdrawn. One has to be mindful that a rapid pull-through can induce reflexive sphincter contractions and false measurements (9). Basic measurements usually include:

- anal sphincter function—resting sphincter pressure, squeeze sphincter pressure, and duration of squeeze
- estimation of the functional length of the anal sphincter
- anorectal pressure responses during abrupt increases in intra-abdominal pressure eg cough
- changes in anal pressure during attempted defaecation ('bearing down')
- recto-anal inhibitory reflex (RAIR)—discussed later

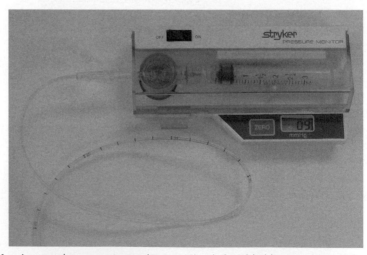

Fig. 3.1.c Anorectal manometry equipment: Simple hand-held manometry device. The Stryker Intra-compartmental Pressure monitor (Stryker Instruments, Kalamazoo, MI, USA) connected to a water-filled balloon-tipped catheter (tip not shown).

Table 3.3 Example of anal length and pressures in normal subjects (from Rao et al. 1999) (11)

	All (n = 45)	Male (n = 19)	Female (n = 26)
Length of anal sphincter (cm)	3.7 (3.6–3.8)	4.0 (3.8–4.2)*	3.6 (3.4–3.8)
Max. anal rest pressure (mm Hg)	68 (62–74)	72 (64–80)	65 (56–74)
Max. squeeze pressure (mm Hg)	164 (150–178)	193 (175–211)*	143 (124–162)

Data given as mean (95% CI). *p < 0.05 male vs female

As an example, Table 3.3 lists the normal pressures and sphincter lengths in 45 healthy subjects, between 22 and 62 years old (11).

Utility

In the maintenance of normal continence, the internal anal sphincter (IAS) contributes the majority of the constant resting tone (12). The external anal sphincter (EAS) is also tonically active, but is most active and necessary at times of raised intra-abdominal pressure (12). With active squeeze, much of the pressure is generated by the EAS with contribution from the puborectalis muscle (13). Resting pressure reflects IAS function and the squeeze pressure reflects EAS function.

Anal pressures can be recorded during dynamic manoeuvres such as coughing or Valsalva. During these manoeuvres which raise intra-abdominal pressure, a reflex response results in an increase in EAS activity. The absence of this response may be indicative of diseases of sacral neural plexuses (11,14). Conversely, it is normal for the anal pressure to decrease as the anal sphincter relaxes with straining. This is particularly relevant in the evaluation of OD, as an absent or reversed response may indicate anal non-relaxation or anismus (15).

In EAS fatigability testing, the patient is asked to squeeze the anal sphincter for 40 seconds; the ability to maintain the squeeze pressure is recorded as the 'fatigability index'. It has been proposed that poor EAS endurance may be linked to FI (16), although there is not universal agreement on this (17).

Anal manometry also has an important role in preoperative assessment in patients considered for surgical procedures which may affect continence, such as ileal pouch-anal anastomosis, ultralow anterior resection, or fistulotomy. The findings may guide selection of the appropriate operation, and allow interpretation of post-operative functional outcomes.

Other anal manometry tests

High-resolution manometry

This emerging technique uses closely-spaced solid-state sensors to simultaneously measure circumferential pressures in the rectum and throughout the anal canal, avoiding the need for a pull-through manoeuvre. It has up to sixteen circumferential channels positioned at any given level, providing measurements that are not affected by circumferential asymmetry (18). Further data are required to determine if it is superior to conventional manometry, given the significant cost implications.

Ambulatory anal manometry

Developed in the late 1980s, this technique allows prolonged manometric recording in ambulant subjects. It has contributed significantly to our understanding of the daily variations in anorectal activity, in particular anal sampling activity (19,20). It is used to correlate anorectal pressure patterns with episodes of anorectal events, such as anal seepage or major FI. Two methods are commonly used–pressure microtransducers or a multiport perfused sleeve sensor (9). Electromyography of the EAS can also be simultaneously recorded. Despite its promise, this technique primarily remains a research tool, due in part to its cost and logistic considerations.

Rectal and anal sensation

Rectal balloon distension test

The simple apparatus for this test is a latex balloon mounted on the end of a catheter. The balloon is incrementally inflated in the rectum, typically at a rate of 1 ml/sec, and the rectal sensory threshold to distension can be quantitated. Commonly three measurements are made (21):

- The 'first constant sensation' (FCS): the minimal balloon volume perceived by the patient.
- The 'desire to defecate volume' (DDV): with increasing insufflation, the volume at which the urge to defaecate is induced.
- The 'maximum tolerated volume' (MTV): reached when patient experiences discomfort and intense desire to defaecate.

As an example of normative values, those used by a single anorectal laboratory (21,22) are listed in Table 3.4. It is important to note that sensation of rectal distension is not only mediated by the rectal wall itself, but is also by the concurrent stretch of the pelvic floor muscles, as demonstrated by the ability of patients who have undergone proctectomy and colo-anal anastomosis to perceive balloon distension (23).

Table 3.4 Example of normative values for rectal balloon sensation test (from Gladman et al. 2003 and Chan et al. 2005) (21,22)

		First constant sensation (ml)	Desire to defaecate volume (ml)	Maximum tolerated volume (ml)
Normal	Male	40–110	70–190	140–270
	Female	20–70	60–160	90–270
Hyposensitivity	Male	> 160	> 230	> 315
	Female	> 120	> 210	> 325
Hypersensitivity	Male		< 70	< 140
	Female		< 60	< 90

Rectal sensation of distension is under the influence of several factors. It is a function of the compliance/relaxation of the rectal wall, extrinsic neural pathways such as afferent nerve function and/or central afferent mechanisms, and even abnormalities in perceptual and behavioural processes (22). Rectal balloon distension cannot distinguish between these factors. Therefore it is a screening test that can only label a patient as having rectal hypersensitivity, rectal hyposensitivity, or normal rectal distension sensation.

Abnormal rectal distension thresholds have been implicated in a variety of organic and functional anorectal disorders. Rectal hypersensitivity (heightened perception of rectal distension) is seen in conditions that reduce rectal compliance (eg colitis) but true rectal hypersensitivity can also occur as a primary phenomenon, for example in the irritable bowel syndrome (24).

On the other hand, rectal hyposensitivity (diminished perception of rectal distension) is most often observed in patients with constipation or OD (25,26). This may be relevant in several situations, such as poor outcome in patients undergoing colectomy for slow-transit constipation and patients undergoing sphincter reconstruction for FI (21). In the context of FI however, the rectal sensory threshold can either be elevated, reduced or even normal (12).

In practice, balloon sensation testing can provide an estimate of whether the patient has normal or altered rectal sensation. To really elucidate further the possible aetiology of altered rectal sensitivity, the rectal barostat is necessary. However, simple rectal balloon sensation has also been used to monitor treatment progress in patients undergoing biofeedback therapy for both rectal hyper- and hypo-sensitivity; the normalization of the rectal sensory threshold has been shown to correlate with success of these treatments (27,28).

Recto-anal inhibitory reflex (RAIR)

Normally, rectal distention causes a reflex relaxation of the IAS to allow rectal content to reach the anal mucosa, where it is thought to be 'sampled' to discriminate its consistency and necessity to be evacuated. This is referred to as the recto-anal inhibitory reflex. This reflex can be reproduced experimentally by a rapid inflation of a rectal balloon with simultaneous measurement of anal pressure. A normal response is a transient decrease in resting anal pressure by > 25% (Fig. 3.2) (29). The key role of RAIR testing is in the detection of congenital Hirschsprung's disease (28) and some acquired conditions such as systemic sclerosis, (30) where the reflex is absent.

Anal mucosal sensation

In the anal mucosal electro-sensitivity test, an electrode-tipped catheter is used to stimulate the anal mucosa at 1cm intervals by a constant current. The threshold at which the current becomes perceptible by the patient is recorded, as the intensity of the current (in mAmps) is increased (31). However, on its own it cannot distinguish between a sensory deficit of the nerve endings in the anal canal versus a peripheral nerve (ie pudendal nerve) deficit. Currently its routine use is not widely supported, as independently it does not add any more information that the less complex investigations discussed above (32).

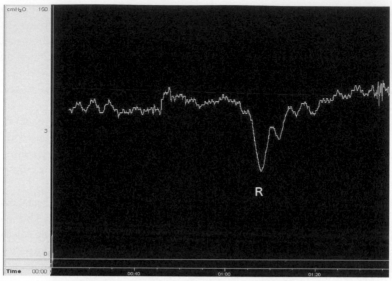

Fig. 3.2 Example of the RAIR (R. denotes the point where IAS relaxation is recorded as a drop in pressure, followed by a steady return to baseline IAS pressure).

Balloon expulsion test

In the balloon expulsion test, a 60 ml saline-filled balloon is inserted into the patient's rectum and the patient is instructed to expel the balloon on a seated commode in privacy in one minute. Patients with OD are unable to expel the balloon (33). In this case, the volume of the balloon can be increased until the patient feels that they can expel the balloon. Failure to expel a balloon that has been filled to cause constant sensation is indicative of anismus (34). This test has been used to predict outcome of colectomy in severe idiopathic constipation, by selecting out patients with significant OD (35).

Rectal compliance

If rectal sensory thresholds are derived using simple rectal balloon distension, they do not always reflect true rectal afferent sensory function, because they do not take account of the other important variables of rectal compliance and relaxation. This can be overcome by controlling the balloon insufflation with a barostat, an electromechanical device that delivers isobaric rectal distention using a highly compliant polyethylene balloon (Fig. 3.3). Using this device and proper technique, the sensory thresholds are measured independent of rectal compliance. Likewise it can calculate rectal compliance by calculating the change in rectal pressure in relation to the change in volume ($\Delta V/\Delta P$), usually by way of step-wise isobaric rectal distensions at 2 mmHg increments.

Regarding rectal hyposensitivity, recent work has demonstrated two distinct groups–one with normal compliance and impaired sensation (reflecting impaired afferent nerve function) and the other with abnormally increased compliance

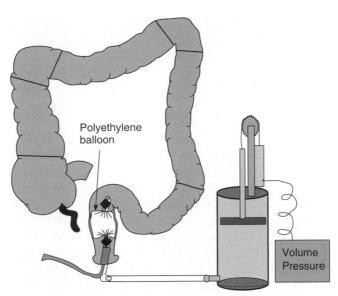

Polyethylene balloon

**Volume
Pressure**

Fig. 3.3 A rectal barostat assembly. A highly compliant polyethylene balloon is inflated by a barostat, which monitors intraballoon pressure and volume. Reproduced with permission from Bharucha AE. Update of tests of colon and rectal structure and function. *J Clin Gastroenterol*. 2006 Feb;**40**(2):96–103.

(excessive rectal laxity) (36). In some of the latter group, there may be a demonstrable anatomical abnormality such as megarectum (37). While treatment with bowel retraining, biofeedback and sacral nerve stimulation have all been reported (36), the above subgrouping may further enable tailoring of treatment modalities. This is an area of ongoing research.

Rectal hypersensitivity is seen in patients where compliance is obviously altered such as ulcerative colitis or following rectal irradiation, but is also seen in a more idiopathic manner in diarrhoea-predominant irritable bowel syndrome and urge faecal incontinence (12). In the case of the latter, this has implications for the rational management of these patients various available pharmacological, neuromodulatory, and surgical options.

Neurophysiology and testing

The neuromuscular activity of the anorectal structures and pelvic floor is governed by both somatic and autonomic activity. According to basic neurophysiology, critical to normal function at a peripheral nerve level is the integrity of the muscle in question, the neuromuscular junction, and afferent and efferent nerve fibres located in the peripheral nerve. The autonomic and somatic nerve cell bodies that supply the pelvic floor arise in the conus medullaris portion of the sacral spinal cord at S2–S4. Further descending control is mediated by the central nervous system, by way of corticospinal activity (38).

From cerebral cortex to muscle itself, all levels of the neurophysiology of the anorectal structures and pelvic floor are potentially measurable (39). In practice however, outpatient testing in the typical anorectal physiology laboratory is limited to the activity of the peripheral nerve, neuromuscular junction, and muscle.

Electromyography

Technique

Electromyography (EMG) assesses the functional integrity of the peripheral motor unit, comprising the anterior horn cells in the central nervous system, the peripheral nerves, and the muscle fibres (ie EAS and pelvic floor) themselves (38). Spontaneous and voluntary electrical activities (ie motor unit potentials) can be recorded. Both myopathic and neuropathic processes can be detected. Recording can be achieved with a needle electrode inserted directly into the muscle, or with a surface electrode placed on the skin/mucosa immediately adjacent to the muscle.

Two main needle EMG techniques are used. In concentric needle EMG of the EAS, the electrodes are typically inserted into four quadrants of the EAS. Multiple recordings are taken with the patient at rest and during different manoeuvres such as straining, coughing and squeezing. In the less widely practised single-fibre EMG, motor unit morphology or fibre density (ie the mean number of muscle fibres belonging to an individual motor unit) can be estimated. It is a sensitive indicator of collateral reinnervation after partial muscle denervation.

In normal subjects, the pelvic floor muscles display tonic activities in the resting state. The increased muscle recruitment during squeezing or coughing is reflected in an increase in the amplitude and duration of the motor unit potentials above these baseline activities. Conversely, muscle relaxation during straining will either result in electrical silence or a reduction in the number of motor unit potentials.

Although needle EMG remains the gold standard EMG technique, it does have the disadvantage of causing patient discomfort and requires an experienced clinician for its use. Surface electrodes are an alternative. They avoid the pain that is associated with needle insertion while still producing consistent results (40–41).

Utility

Prior to the advent of endoanal ultrasound (EAUS), EMG was of most use in the investigation of faecal incontinence. It is an electrodiagnostic means of characterizing the extent of neuromuscular injury, mapping out the location of normal muscle, and defining the location of muscle that has been replaced by scar tissue (38). St Mark's Hospital, London pioneered much of this research in the 1970s and 80s using single-fibre EMG, in particular in the setting of pudendal nerve injury and post-obstetric faecal incontinence(42–44). Much of this work involved the elucidation of normal neuromuscular activities of the pelvic floor, and this is perhaps the most important legacy of this progressive period, as the clinical applications of EMG have receded in recent years.

Since the arrival and refinement of EAUS (and latterly magnetic resonance imaging (MRI)), the role of EMG in describing anal sphincter anatomy has been superseded. However EMG can still provide useful information about a coexistent neuropathic aetiology in patients with a sonographic EAS defect and/or manometric evidence of EAS weakness (39).

A more relevant application of EMG currently is to disclose abnormal muscle activity, such as anismus/pelvic floor dyssynergia. During normal defaecation the tonic activities of the pelvic floor muscles are inhibited. Failure of this inhibition or para-doxical activation is a feature of anismus and manifests as OD (45). This should be interpreted in light of other examination and radiologic findings, as the EMG findings do not necessarily correlate with ability to evacuate or with the OD symptoms (46). Nonetheless this is perhaps where surface EMG is at its most useful, since EMG can be performed using the anal sponge electrode, demonstrating non-relaxation of the pub-orectalis muscle and/or anal canal (Fig. 3.4). This is especially useful for biofeedback therapy, as it is minimally invasive, can be easily applied and is well-tolerated by the patient (40,41).

Pudendal nerve terminal motor latencies

Technique

Pudendal nerve terminal motor latency (PNTML) refers to the time delay between an electrical stimulation of the pudendal nerve at the ischial spine and the resultant compound muscle action potential at the EAS. In the usual transanal approach, a disposable stimulator (the St Mark's electrode) is mounted on the examiner's finger and the tip placed over the ischial spine transanally (47). It consists of a flexible printed circuit with a stimulating electrode at the fingertip and a recording electrode at the finger base (Fig. 3.5). The device simultaneously stimulates the nerve with the finger-tip electrode and records the anal motor response with the recording electrode.

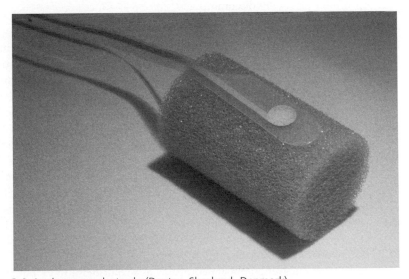

Fig. 3.4 Anal sponge electrode (Dantec, Skovlund, Denmark).

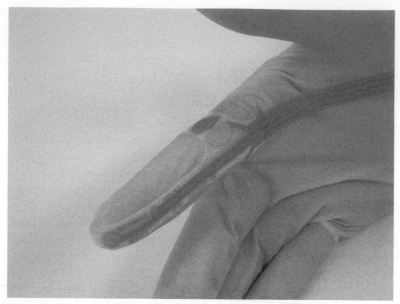

Fig. 3.5 St Mark's electrode (Dantec, Skovlund, Denmark).

Bilateral measurements are taken. The normal latency as measured with this technique is less than 2.2 milliseconds (ms) (47) although some centres will accept up to 2.5ms (38). An increased latency indicates pudendal neuropathy.

Utility

Following the first reported use of PNTML by Kiff and Swash at St Marks in 1984, there was much initial enthusiasm for its application in detecting pudendal neuropathy in FI and the descending perineum syndrome. A number of studies have since reported prolonged PNTML in up to 70% of patients with FI (48–52). In particular Snooks et al studied a cohort of women before and after childbirth and found significant prolongation of PNTML with obstetric-related neuropathic incontinence (48). Prolonged PNTML has not clearly been shown to be predictive of treatment outcome following EAS repair surgery (38).

Since its initial promise, the value of PNTML has now become questionable, with the emergence of new data. The technique is less sensitive than needle EMG studies for showing anal sphincter denervation, mainly because it is based on latency rather than on compound muscle action potential (CMAP) amplitude measurements (38,39). PNTML measures only the fastest conducting fibres in the pudendal nerve, therefore nerve latencies may be normal even if only a few normally conducting fibres remain (12). PNTML correlates poorly with manometry (39). Lastly, the operator-dependent nature of the test and the degree of patient discomfort have limited its reproducibility.

PNTML testing can uncover potential neuropathy as a contributor to FI, but in its current form using the St Mark's electrode, its interpretation is difficult and it is an uncomfortable test. Its routine use is currently not widely supported (53).

Endoanal ultrasound

Equipment and techniques

Endoanal ultrasound (EAUS) is a real-time structural evaluation of the anal sphincter. It is now an established component of the anorectal physiology laboratory. Several endoanal probes have been developed. These range from the older mechanical sectoral probes with limited field of view of 120–210 degrees, to radial probes with 360 degrees of view ('2D EAUS'), to the latest three-dimensional probes that allow digital reconstruction of volume information ('3D EAUS'). These probes range in frequency from 5–16 MHz. At least 10 MHz is preferred in the anal canal as it gives improved resolution of the anal sphincter given its shorter focal length.

Endosonographically the anal canal is visible as 4 layers, heading away from the EAUS cone (54):

- ◆ Subepithelium: moderate echogenicity. It lies immediately outside the EAUS cone.
- ◆ Internal anal sphincter: well-defined and hypoechoic.
- ◆ Longitudinal muscle layer: (hyperechoic). This presents a wide variability in thickness and is not always distinct along the entire anal.
- ◆ External anal sphincter: mixed echogenicity.

Images are obtained at the upper, middle and lower anal canal, each level showing specific components of the anal sphincter. The interpretation of these levels was problematic prior to the advent of 3D EAUS, with reported over-diagnosis of sphincter defects on 2D EAUS, particularly due to the anatomy of upper anal canal (55). 3D EAUS has confirmed a natural gap in the EAS below the puborectalis muscle in female patients, which in the past may have been interpreted as an EAS defect (55). Therefore in the normal female, the views at each of these levels will look as described in Figure 3.6.a–c.

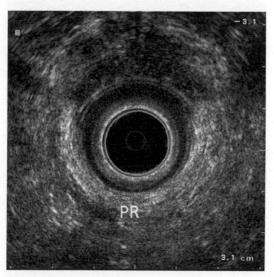

Fig. 3.6.a High anal canal:the sling of the puborectalis (PR) and the deep part of the EAS are fused posteriorly. EAS is absent anteriorly.

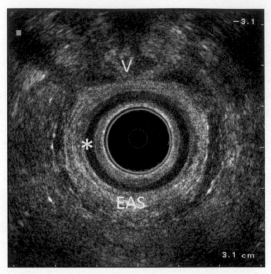

Fig. 3.6.b Mid anal canal: external anal sphincter (EAS), internal anal sphincter (*), and vagina (V).

As discussed below, EAUS has an essential role in the investigation of faecal incontinence and obstructed defaecation. It is also extensively used in other benign colorectal disorders such as perianal fistula and fistula-in-ano; these conditions are beyond the scope of this chapter. While 2D EAUS is the commonest modality in use today, 3D EAUS is emerging as its likely successor. It takes a series of two-dimensional

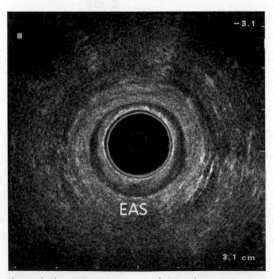

Fig. 3.6.c Low anal canal: the commencement of the subcutaneous part of the EAS and the caudad termination of the IAS.

images throughout the length of the anal canal that are then reconstructed as a three-dimensional 'cube' of data which is displayed on the monitor of the 3D EAUS machine. This cube can be rotated, tilted, and sliced in the coronal, sagittal and oblique planes and stored for later analysis (Fig. 3.7). It has already enhanced our knowledge of sphincter structure and length (55), and its variation with gender and age (56). It has also been used to study the normal endopelvic fascia and its defects in rectoceles (57). Visualisation of the EAS has always been problematic with 2D EAUS, with endoanal-MRI proving superior. 3D EAS seems to match the accuracy of endoanal-MRI in this regard (58). This is particularly relevant to detection of EAS atrophy. Evidence from endoanal-MRI studies has shown that EAS atrophy could underpin poor results of anal sphincter repair (59).

Utility in faecal incontinence

EAUS is the gold standard modality in demonstrating anal sphincter anatomy. The utility of EAUS in FI is well-established (60). IAS defects can be easily visualized as hyperechoic breaks in a normally hypoechoic ring in the mid anal canal where it is most prominent. With EAS defects, a break can be seen in the circumferential mixed hyperechoic band. Unlike the IAS however, images for EAS can sometimes be difficult to interpret due in part to the heterogeneity of its ultrasound characterstics (61).

In experienced hands, EAUS is reported to achieve a sensitivity and specificity of 100% for detecting EAS defects, and 100% and 96% respectively for IAS lesions (62). While it is operator-dependent, the inter-observer agreement is usually good (80%) (63).

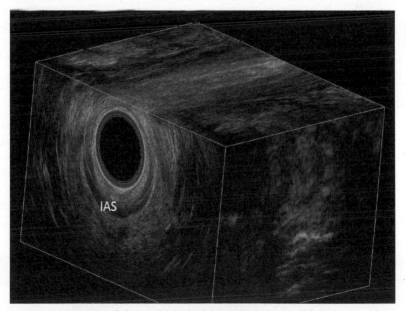

Fig. 3.7 3D EAUS image of the anal canal with an anterior IAS defect The superior surface of the image cube has been 'sliced' along the length of the EAS, just anterior to the deficient IAS.

In spite of this, it is important to realize that the finding of an anal sphincter defect does not necessarily mean that it is the cause of FI, and ultrasound findings should always be interpreted in association with other clinical and physiological findings.

Utility in obstructed defaecation

In patients presenting with OD, EAUS can provide valuable anal sphincter assessment. In a subgroup of patients with OD the IAS is hypertrophied. This has been reported in association with full thickness rectal prolapse, rectal intussusception and solitary rectal ulcer syndrome (54).

As a rare cause of OD, congenital IAS hypertrophy from a primary myopathy has been reported (64). This is shown on EAUS as an increased IAS thickness. It is inherited in an autosomal dominant manner and the smooth muscle cells in these patients demonstrate pathognomonic inclusion bodies on biopsy. Medical treatment with calcium-channel blockers and surgical treatment with partial thickness myectomy has been reported (65).

Emerging techniques

Dynamic transperineal ultrasonography

This technique (see chapter 20) images the organs of the anterior, middle and posterior pelvic compartments as they interact in straining and simulated defaecation (66). It utilizes a surface probe placed over the perineum to obtain images while the patient attempts to expel intrarectally-placed gel. The main role of dynamic transperineal ultrasonography is in the evaluation of evacuatory disorders in the setting of rectocele and enterocele (67) It has been shown that this technique correlates well with defaecating proctography in assessing rectoceles (68). It is an attractive modality as it avoids radiation and can be office-based. It is operator-dependent however, and its role in the management of OD is still evolving.

Colonic manometry

This emerging technique involves the colonoscopic placement of a manometric catheter to record colonic pressures along its length and across a defined timeframe. Conventional catheters have sixteen recording sites, at 7.5cm intervals. It has already markedly improved our knowledge of normal colonic function (69), and is fast gaining relevance in the evaluation of constipation (70). It is usually performed with the patient as a hospital inpatient however, so is not suited to the standard anorectal physiology lab at present.

Key points

- Anorectal ultrasound and physiology provides a useful objective documentation of sphincter structure and function
- Structural abnormalities should be correlated with functional findings.

Editor's summary

Anorectal physiology and anal ultrasound are considered by some a research tool, providing little additional information to clinical findings, varying too significantly between and within patients to be useful. To the extent to which they influence the surgical practice of such individuals, this may well be true.

However, for those who have a mature pelvic floor practice, this view could not be more misplaced. The tests provide very useful objective documentation of sphincter structure and function. The findings are most useful when they correlate with the clinical findings to enable a coherent 'picture' of the pelvic floor to be developed. Static studies rarely pick up short-lived abnormalities, and ambulatory studies, currently impractical, are likely to come into vogue as technologies improve.

References

1. Higgins PD, Johanson JF. Epidemiology of constipation in North America: a systematic review. *Am J Gastroenterol.* 2004;**99**(4):750–9.
2. Macmillan AK, Merrie AE, Marshall RJ, Parry BR. The prevalence of fecal incontinence in community-dwelling adults: a systematic review of the literature. *Dis Colon Rectum.* 2004;**47**(8):1341–9.
3. Hallan RI, Marzouk DE, Waldron DJ, Womack NR, Williams NS. Comparison of digital and manometric assessment of anal sphincter function. *Br J Surg.* 1989;**76**(9):973 5.
4. Eckardt VF, Kanzler G. How reliable is digital examination for the evaluation of anal sphincter tone? *Int J Colorectal Dis.* 1993;**8**(2):95–97.
5. Vaizey CJ, Carapeti E, Cahill JA, Kamm MA. Prospective comparison of faecal incontinence grading systems. *Gut.* 1999;**44**(1):77–80.
6. Altomare DF, Spazzafumo L, Rinaldi M, Dodi G, Ghiselli R, Piloni V. Set-up and statistical validation of a new scoring system for obstructed defaecation syndrome. *Colorectal Dis.* 2008;**10**(1):84–88.
7. Agachan F, Chen T, Pfeifer J, Reissman P, Wexner SD. A constipation scoring system to simplify evaluation and management of constipated patients. *Dis Colon Rectum.* 1996;**39**(6):681–5.
8. Rockwood TH, Church JM, Fleshman JW, Kane RL, Mavrantonis C, Thorson AG, et al. Fecal Incontinence Quality of Life Scale: quality of life instrument for patients with fecal incontinence. *Dis Colon Rectum.* 2000;**43**(1):9–16; discussion -17.
9. Sun WM, Rao SS. Manometric assessment of anorectal function. *Gastroenterol Clin North Am.* 2001;**30**(1):15–32.
10. Simpson RR, Kennedy ML, Nguyen MH, Dinning PG, Lubowski DZ. Anal manometry: a comparison of techniques. *Dis Colon Rectum.* 2006;**49**(7):1033–8.
11. Rao SS, Hatfield R, Soffer E, Rao S, Beaty J, Conklin JL. Manometric tests of anorectal function in healthy adults. *Am J Gastroenterol.* 1999;**94**(3):773–83.
12. Bharucha AE. Update of tests of colon and rectal structure and function. *J Clin Gastroenterol.* 2006;**40**(2):96–103.
13. Azpiroz F, Fernandez-Fraga X, Merletti R, Enck P. The puborectalis muscle. *Neurogastroenterol Motil.* 2005;**17** Suppl 1:68–72.

14. Sun WM, Read NW. Anorectal function in normal human subjects: effect of gender. *Int J Colorectal Dis*. 1989;**4**(3):188–96.
15. Park UC, Choi SK, Piccirillo MF, Verzaro R, Wexner SD. Patterns of anismus and the relation to biofeedback therapy. *Dis Colon Rectum*. 1996;**39**(7):768–73.
16. Telford KJ, Ali AS, Lymer K, Hosker GL, Kiff ES, Hill J. Fatigability of the external anal sphincter in anal incontinence. *Dis Colon Rectum*. 2004;**47**(5):746–52; discussion 52.
17. Bilali S, Pfeifer J. Anorectal manometry: are fatigue rate and fatigue rate index of any clinical importance? *Tech Coloproctol*. 2005;**9**(3):225–8.
18. Jones MP, Post J, Crowell MD. High-resolution manometry in the evaluation of anorectal disorders: a simultaneous comparison with water-perfused manometry. *Am J Gastroenterol*. 2007;**102**(4):850–5.
19. Miller R, Lewis GT, Bartolo DC, Cervero F, Mortensen NJ. Sensory discrimination and dynamic activity in the anorectum: evidence using a new ambulatory technique. *Br J Surg*. 1988;**75**(10):1003–7.
20. Ronholt C, Rasmussen OO, Christiansen J. Ambulatory manometric recording of anorectal activity. *Dis Colon Rectum*. 1999;**42**(12):1551–9.
21. Gladman MA, Scott SM, Chan CL, Williams NS, Lunniss PJ. Rectal hyposensitivity: prevalence and clinical impact in patients with intractable constipation and fecal incontinence. *Dis Colon Rectum*. 2003;**46**(2):238–46.
22. Chan CL, Scott SM, Williams NS, Lunniss PJ. Rectal hypersensitivity worsens stool frequency, urgency, and lifestyle in patients with urge fecal incontinence. *Dis Colon Rectum*. 2005;**48**(1):134–40.
23. Lane RH, Parks AG. Function of the anal sphincters following colo-anal anastomosis. *Br J Surg*. 1977;**64**(8):596–9.
24. Mertz H, Naliboff B, Munakata J, Niazi N, Mayer EA. Altered rectal perception is a biological marker of patients with irritable bowel syndrome. *Gastroenterology*. 1995;**109**(1):40–52.
25. Shouler P, Keighley MR. Changes in colorectal function in severe idiopathic chronic constipation. *Gastroenterology*. 1986;**90**(2):414–20.
26. Gosselink MJ, Schouten WR. Rectal sensory perception in females with obstructed defecation. *Dis Colon Rectum*. 2001;**44**(9):1337–44.
27. Rao SS, Welcher KD, Pelsang RE. Effects of biofeedback therapy on anorectal function in obstructive defecation. *Dig Dis Sci*. 1997;**42**(11):2197–205.
28. Diamant NE, Kamm MA, Wald A, Whitehead WE. AGA technical review on anorectal testing techniques. *Gastroenterology*. 1999;**116**(3):735–60.
29. Lowry AC, Simmang CL, Boulos P, Farmer KC, Finan PJ, Hyman N, et al. Consensus statement of definitions for anorectal physiology and rectal cancer. *ANZ J Surg*. 2001;**71**(10):603–5.
30. Ebert EC. Gastric and enteric involvement in progressive systemic sclerosis. *J Clin Gastroenterol*. 2008;**42**(1):5–12.
31. Roe AM, Bartolo DC, Mortensen NJ. New method for assessment of anal sensation in various anorectal disorders. *Br J Surg*. 1986;**73**(4):310–2.
32. Broens PM, Penninckx FM. Relation between anal electrosensitivity and rectal filling sensation and the influence of age. *Dis Colon Rectum*. 2005;**48**(1):127–33.
33. Beck DE. Simplified balloon expulsion test. *Dis Colon Rectum*. 1992;**35**(6):597–8.

34. Ternent CA, Bastawrous AL, Morin NA, Ellis CN, Hyman NH, Buie WD. Practice parameters for the evaluation and management of constipation. *Dis Colon Rectum.* 2007;**50**(12):2013–22.

35. van der Sijp JR, Kamm MA, Bartram CI, Lennard-Jones JE. The value of age of onset and rectal emptying in predicting the outcome of colectomy for severe idiopathic constipation. *Int J Colorectal Dis.* 1992;**7**(1):35–7.

36. Gladman MA, Dvorkin LS, Lunniss PJ, Williams NS, Scott SM. Rectal hyposensitivity: a disorder of the rectal wall or the afferent pathway? An assessment using the barostat. *Am J Gastroenterol.* 2005;**100**(1):106–14.

37. Gladman MA, Dvorkin LS, Scott SM, Lunniss PJ, Williams NS. A novel technique to identify patients with megarectum. *Dis Colon Rectum.* 2007;**50**(5):621–9.

38. Olsen AL, Rao SS. Clinical neurophysiology and electrodiagnostic testing of the pelvic floor. *Gastroenterol Clin North Am.* 2001;**30**(1):33–54, v-vi.

39. Lefaucheur JP. Neurophysiological testing in anorectal disorders. *Muscle Nerve.* 2006;**33**(3):324–33.

40. Lopez A, Nilsson BY, Mellgren A, Zetterstrom J, Holmstrom B. Electromyography of the external anal sphincter: comparison between needle and surface electrodes. *Dis Colon Rectum.* 1999;**42**(4):482–5.

41. Pfeifer J, Teoh TA, Salanga VD, Agachan F, Wexner SD. Comparative study between intra-anal sponge and needle electrode for electromyographic evaluation of constipated patients. *Dis Colon Rectum.* 1998;**41**(9):1153–7.

42. Snooks SJ, Setchell M, Swash M, Henry MM. Injury to innervation of pelvic floor sphincter musculature in childbirth. *Lancet.* 1984 8;2(8402):546–50.

43. Neill ME, Swash M. Increased motor unit fibre density in the external anal sphincter muscle in ano-rectal incontinence: a single fibre EMG study. *J Neurol Neurosurg Psychiatry.* 1980;**43**(4):343–7.

44. Henry MM. Neurophysiological assessment of the pelvic floor. *Gut.* 1988;**29**(1):1–4.

45. Fucini C, Ronchi O, Elbetti C. Electromyography of the pelvic floor musculature in the assessment of obstructed defecation symptoms. *Dis Colon Rectum.* 2001;**44**(8): 1168–75.

46. Miller R, Duthie GS, Bartolo DC, Roe AM, Locke-Edmunds J, Mortensen NJ. Anismus in patients with normal and slow transit constipation. *Br J Surg.* 1991;**78**(6):690–2.

47. Kiff ES, Swash M. Slowed conduction in the pudendal nerves in idiopathic (neurogenic) faecal incontinence. *Br J Surg.* 1984;**71**(8):614–6.

48. Snooks SJ, Swash M, Henry MM, Setchell M. Risk factors in childbirth causing damage to the pelvic floor innervation. *Int J Colorectal Dis.* 1986;**1**(1):20–24.

49. Cheong DM, Vaccaro CA, Salanga VD, Wexner SD, Phillips RC, Hanson MR, et al. Electrodiagnostic evaluation of fecal incontinence. *Muscle Nerve.* 1995;**18**(6):612–9.

50. Hill J, Mumtaz A, Kiff ES. Pudendal neuropathy in patients with idiopathic faecal incontinence progresses with time. *Br J Surg.* 1994;**81**(10):1494–5.

51. Kafka NJ, Coller JA, Barrett RC, Murray JJ, Roberts PL, Rusin LC, et al. Pudendal neuropathy is the only parameter differentiating leakage from solid stool incontinence. *Dis Colon Rectum.* 1997;**40**(10):1220–7.

52. Laurberg S, Swash M, Snooks SJ, Henry MM. Neurologic cause of idiopathic incontinence. *Arch Neurol.* 1988;**45**(11):1250–3.

53. Barnett JL, Hasler WL, Camilleri M. American Gastroenterological Association medical position statement on anorectal testing techniques. *Gastroenterology* 1999;**116**(3):732–5.

54. Santoro GA, Di Falco G. Benign anorectal diseases: diagnosis with endoanal and endorectal ultrasound and new treatment options. Berlin: Springer; 2006.

55. Bollard RC, Gardiner A, Lindow S, Phillips K, Duthie GS. Normal female anal sphincter: difficulties in interpretation explained. *Dis Colon Rectum*. 2002;**45**(2):171–5.

56. Knowles AM, Knowles CH, Scott SM, Lunniss PJ. Effects of age and gender on three-dimensional endoanal ultrasonography measurements: development of normal ranges. *Tech Coloproctol*. 2008;**12**(4):323–9.

57. Reisinger E, Stummvoll W. Visualization of the endopelvic fascia by transrectal three-dimensional ultrasound. *Int Urogynecol J Pelvic Floor Dysfunct*. 2006;**17**(2):165–9.

58. Williams AB, Bartram CI, Halligan S, Marshall MM, Nicholls RJ, Kmiot WA. Endosonographic anatomy of the normal anal canal compared with endocoil magnetic resonance imaging. *Dis Colon Rectum*. 2002;**45**(2):176–83.

59. Briel JW, Stoker J, Rociu E, Lameris JS, Hop WC, Schouten WR. External anal sphincter atrophy on endoanal magnetic resonance imaging adversely affects continence after sphincteroplasty. *Br J Surg*. 1999;**86**(10):1322–7.

60. Stoker J, Halligan S, Bartram CI. Pelvic floor imaging. *Radiology*. 2001;**218**(3):621–41.

61. Rociu E, Stoker J, Eijkemans MJ, Schouten WR, Lameris JS. Fecal incontinence: endoanal US versus endoanal MR imaging. *Radiology*. 1999;**212**(2):453–8.

62. Deen KI, Kumar D, Williams JG, Olliff J, Keighley MR. Anal sphincter defects. Correlation between endoanal ultrasound and surgery. *Ann Surg*. 1993;**218**(2):201–5.

63. Gold DM, Halligan S, Kmiot WA, Bartram CI. Intraobserver and interobserver agreement in anal endosonography. *Br J Surg*. 1999;**86**(3):371–5.

64. Guy RJ, Kamm MA, Martin JE. Internal anal sphincter myopathy causing proctalgia fugax and constipation: further clinical and radiological characterization in a patient. *Eur J Gastroenterol Hepatol*. 1997;**9**(2):221–4.

65. de la Portilla F, Borrero JJ, Rafel E. Hereditary vacuolar internal anal sphincter myopathy causing proctalgia fugax and constipation: a new case contribution. *Eur J Gastroenterol Hepatol*. 2005;**17**(3):359–61.

66. Dietz HP, Haylen BT, Broome J. Ultrasound in the quantification of female pelvic organ prolapse. *Ultrasound Obstet Gynecol*. 2001;**18**(5):511–4.

67. Dietz HP, Steensma AB. Posterior compartment prolapse on two-dimensional and three-dimensional pelvic floor ultrasound: the distinction between true rectocele, perineal hypermobility and enterocele. *Ultrasound Obstet Gynecol*. 2005;**26**(1):73–7.

68. Beer-Gabel M, Teshler M, Schechtman E, Zbar AP. Dynamic transperineal ultrasound vs. defecography in patients with evacuatory difficulty: a pilot study. *Int J Colorectal Dis*. 2004;**19**(1):60–7.

69. Dinning PG. Colonic manometry and sacral nerve stimulation in patients with severe constipation. *Pelviperineology*. 2007;**26**:113–6.

70. Dinning PG, Bampton PA, Andre J, Kennedy ML, Lubowski DZ, King DW, et al. Abnormal predefecatory colonic motor patterns define constipation in obstructed defecation. *Gastroenterology*. 2004;**127**(1):49–56.

Chapter 4

Faecal incontinence:
a pathophysiological approach

Ian Lindsey

The traditional sphincter-centric approach to faecal incontinence

Few treatments for incontinence result in perfection. Until quite recently the surgical management of faecal incontinence (FI) has, for almost 25 years, focussed on the repair of injuries sustained to the anal sphincter complex. The advent of anal ultrasound in the late 1980s allowed better case selection through improved recognition and characterization of anterior obstetric anal sphincter defects amenable to repair, an assessment that previously relied on clinical examination with or without needle electromyographic mapping.

However, the long-term results of sphincter repair remain at best modest (1). At 5 years, only 50% of patients maintain a benefit and very few are perfectly continent. This suggests either a longer-term failure of the procedure, the presence or development of unrecognized aetiological factors, or both. More recently, sacral nerve modulation (SNM) has emerged as a promising new technique in patients with an intact sphincter ring. It has also been successfully used in patients who continue with incontinence after an anatomically correct sphincter repair. Although its precise mode of action remains unclear, it is likely that a number of mechanisms are involved, all predominantly neural in basis. Centres with experience are now reporting successful neuromodulation despite the presence of an unrepaired anterior external sphincter defect.(2) Whilst no one can dispute that SNM has revolutionised the outlook for patients with incontinence, it too has its failures; although 75–80% experience an improvement of > 50%, only 50% have normal continence (3).

An alternative approach: the role of internal rectal prolapse

Internal rectal prolapse is a manifestation of pelvic floor weakness presenting typically as the syndrome of obstructed defaecation. However, it is not widely recognized that most patients (about 75%) also admit to faecal incontinence, and a not insignificant minority will present with faecal incontinence alone (4).

Several factors have led to the historical and still widely held view of internal rectal prolapse being a variant of normal. A small, but widely quoted proctography study in the 1980s suggested that 20% of asymptomatic normal volunteers had a high-grade internal rectal prolapse (an intussusception impinging on or entering into the anal canal) (5). Two large series using proctography in symptomatic patients showed that internal prolapse seldom progresses to external rectal prolapse (6,7). As a result of these studies, most surgeons still do not regard internal rectal prolapse as a true pathological-anatomical entity that can be surgically corrected. The poor functional results of using a traditional posterior rectopexy for correcting internal rectal prolapse have not helped (8). However, a Cochrane analysis (9) and a randomized controlled trial (RCT) (10) concluded that posterior rectal mobilization in external rectal prolapse leads to autonomic rectal-denervation and the development of a hindgut neuropathy; worse or new-onset obstructed defaecation (OD) is then seen in about 50% of patients (8). Unsurprisingly, posterior rectopexy by inducing a similar neural lesion results in a worsening of the obstructed defaecation that was the very indication for surgery, and became discredited as a method of treating internal rectal prolapse (8). The condition then became medicalized and was managed almost exclusively by biofeedback.

Rectopexy for faecal incontinence

Despite ongoing debate about the significance of internal rectal prolapse, several published series have already demonstrated improvement in faecal incontinence after rectopexy. Lazorthes found internal rectal prolapse in 27% of patients with idiopathic faecal incontinence referred for proctography (11). Significant improvement in faecal incontinence was seen after Orr-Loygue (anterior-posterior) rectopexy, with 6 patients achieving full continence at six months follow up. Similarly, Schultz et al reported significant improvement in faecal incontinence scores in 12 patients with internal rectal prolapse, and this was maintained at median follow up of 5.4 years (12). Although these two studies report on the use of posterior rectopexy, the improvement in faecal incontinence supports the proposed role of internal rectal prolapse in the multifactorial aetiology of faecal incontinence. Ventral rectopexy also improves faecal incontinence (in about 90%, Faecal Incontinence Severity Index preoperative 28 versus 12 months postoperative 8; p < 0.0001) (4,13) and interestingly with greater reliability than that seen with obstructed defaecation.

A reappraisal of the significance of internal rectal prolapse

More recently there has been a radiological re-evaluation of internal rectal prolapse in asymptomatic normal volunteers. Dvorkin et al. demonstrated that internal rectal prolapse is morphologically more advanced in symptomatic patients, with significantly more full-thickness and recto-anal intussusceptions rather than mucosal, shallower, rectorectal intussusceptions in asymptomatic individuals (14). Pomerri, who showed (15) that the rectal folding thickness and the ratio between intussuscipiens diameter and the intussusceptum lumen diameter were significantly greater in the symptomatic rather than asymptomatic volunteers, supports these findings (16).

Ventral rectopexy: a new nerve-sparing approach

D'Hoore (16) has popularized a ventral nerve-sparing approach, which avoids damage to rectal branches of the pelvic autonomic hypogastric plexus by abandoning the traditional dorso-lateral rectal mobilization, mainly for external prolapse, with excellent functional results. Similar results for external prolapse have been reported (13,17). Our results in using this novel ventral approach for high-grade internal prolapse (4) have mirrored those reported by the Bristol group. In their series of 80 patients undergoing ventral rectopexy (external prolapse 55%, internal prolapse 45%), improvement in faecal incontinence was seen in 39 of 43 patients (91%) (13).

The role of proctography in faecal incontinence

Not infrequently, patients undergoing standard workup for often quite severe faecal incontinence are demonstrated as having both normal or near-normal sphincter pressures on anorectal manometry and intact sphincters on ultrasound. Previously these patients were labelled as having idiopathic faecal incontinence. We recommend using routine proctography as part of standard faecal incontinence workup. Our data show that about two-thirds of patients undergoing selective proctography for otherwise unexplained faecal incontinence have high-grade internal prolapse (18). Dench has recently reported a high incidence of proctographic anatomical abnormalities (70%) (19) in their retrospective analysis of routine proctography undertaken for faecal incontinence.

Potential mechanisms of internal rectal prolapse causing incontinence

The exact mechanism of faecal incontinence in internal rectal prolapse remains unclear. One possibility is that an internal prolapse enters the anal canal and begins to stretch the internal anal sphincter. It has been demonstrated that internal sphincter pressures are not only diminished in external prolapse but improve if the prolapse is corrected. Our data show a significant correlation between advancing grade of internal prolapse and a progressive decrease in internal anal sphincter pressures (20), which we would anticipate to give rise to passive faecal incontinence. Another possibility is that the prolapse itself, in descending to the anorectal junction causes inappropriate firing of the recto-anal inhibitory reflex (RAIR), leading to temporary reversal of the usual pressure gradient between the rectum and anus and the development of urge faecal incontinence. This mechanism has also been shown to be a contributing factor in external prolapse (21) and it too recovers post rectopexy. A third possibility is simple post-defaecatory leakage from incomplete rectal emptying. In our experience, the pattern of faecal incontinence in internal prolapse is mixed, with patients complaining of each of these three types of FI, and often a combination of two or all three.

Clinical assessment

Assessment on history establishes the severity of symptoms (need for a pad, loss of solid stool, effect on social and general life), and the likely cause (obstetric issues, presence of middle compartment prolapse, pattern of faecal incontinence). Whilst recognizing their limitations, the use of questionnaires (St Mark's, Cleveland Clinic, Faecal Incontinence Severity Index (FISI)) is to be encouraged. They allow grading of severity, co-assessment of quality of life (FISI) and a more objective comparison against baseline scores for treatment interventions. Some specific questions (Do you stake out the lavatory in advance when going shopping? Can you hold on in a queue for 5 minutes? Do you take spare underpants with you when you go out?) are in themselves as useful as questionnaires in quantifying severity.

In females, with the three main aetiological groups in mind (posterior compartment prolapse, pudendal neuropathy and obstetric sphincter injury), an obstetric history is mandatory but not discriminatory, as all three are by and large related to pregnancy and mode of delivery. A long second stage might suggest neuropathy. Instrumental delivery marks a risk for any of these 3 causes; forceps delivery is associated with an external sphincter injury approaching 80%. Nulliparity could suggest a prolapse, as 20% of patients with prolapse are nulliparous (22) (half of these are men). In men, a history of anal surgery (fistulotomy, anal stretch, internal sphincterotomy, haemorrhoidectomy) should also be ascertained as about 25% of male patients with faecal incontinence have an iatrogenic internal sphincter injury (23). This is also relevant in females, but in general more sphincter-sparing anal surgery is being recommended and undertaken in women. Urge urinary incontinence is associated with anterior and middle compartment prolapse and improves with gynaecological anti-prolapse surgery. A gynaecological surgical history can be garnered through a perusal of the old notes: index interventions that suggest prolapse include transvaginal tape (TVT) sling for stress urinary incontinence, hysterectomy for uterine prolapse, anterior and posterior repairs for vaginal prolapse.

The pattern of faecal incontinence can be helpful in indicating a cause. External sphincter weakness has been associated with urge and internal sphincter, passive incontinence (24). It is probably more complex than that simple arrangement, because often symptoms are mixed and this also overlooks the complaint of post-defaecatory leakage. Whilst males invariably complain of passive incontinence, females with type III-V incontinence complain in equal measure of urge, passive incontinence or both. The presence of mixed symptoms of faecal incontinence and obstructed defaecation (as common as pure faecal incontinence) can point to underlying posterior compartment prolapse.

Examination must exclude organic pathology (rectal cancer, colitis) with digital rectal exam and rigid sigmoidoscopy. The pelvic floor is inspected for a descended (low-lying or effaced pelvic floor at rest) or descending perineum (new or further descent on straining). Limitations of assessment during straining include left lateral positioning and anxiety over an accident or passing wind in clinic. This may be overcome by straining during digital rectal exam, when an anal intussusception may be subtly felt, and confirmed at straining proctoscopy, usually anteriorly. Visualisation of a high take-off intussusception requires straining rigid sigmoidoscopy and is more difficult because insufflations impede caudal collapse of the rectum. The sphincters are assessed, first by inspection, for anal gape seen with low resting tone, and absence of voluntary contraction of the external sphincter seen with pudendal neuropathy.

The resting and squeeze pressures are assessed digitally. Finally external rectal prolapse is sought, if necessary with inspection after straining on a commode.

Diagnostic workup

The indication for diagnostic workup of patients with faecal incontinence depends on the symptom severity, response to initial conservative management, and ultimate fitness for surgery. Nevertheless, if the patient has significant symptoms we have a fairly low threshold for investigation because treatment needs to be tailored to the pathology, and many modern interventions are very safe (e.g. silicone anal bulking). Conventional workup has included anorectal physiology and anal ultrasound. This largely evaluates the structure and function of the anal sphincters, particularly with respect to anterior obstetric sphincter injury. However, other more subtle clues can be picked up on ultrasound. Classical features of an unrecognized external rectal prolapse, an eccentric sometimes thickened internal anal sphincter, often with gross circumferential thickening of the submucosa (25).

Defaecating proctography has not traditionally been recognized as a useful test for faecal incontinence and it does depend on the patient's ability to retain paste. For us it has become an essential diagnostic tool and is used more or less routinely. If it is used selectively, it is indicated when the conventional tests have failed to identify a clear cause (eg normal or near normal pressures and intact sphincter).

One of the shortcomings of pelvic floor workup has been an inability to discriminate between a neurological and structural cause for faecal incontinence (e.g. the presence or not of pudendal neuropathy alongside an external sphincter injury). Pudendal nerve terminal motor latency (PNTML) has not been a reliable discriminator for various reasons, and has in many centres been discarded. We have come to use peripheral nerve examination (PNE) or test phase of sacral neuromodulation (SNS) as a type of 'super PNTML test'. We perform this as an outpatient procedure under local anaesthetic; cost limits its usefulness as a routine test.

Oxford faecal incontinence classification

As patients pass through this modern diagnostic cascade, they fall into more or less discrete patient groups, depending on sex and accepting the general limitation of neurological assessment. These patient groups provide a new classification of faecal incontinence reshaped largely on recognition of pelvic floor weakness or posterior compartment prolapse as a major contributor to faecal incontinence (Fig. 4.1). The classification requires definitions (footnote Table 4.1) and inevitably patients will not necessarily fall neatly into a box. There are also miscellaneous patients who are not catered for (eg those with spinal injury, old age, and iatrogenic sphincter injury after anal surgery in females. Nevertheless, the classification is generally workable and practical, allowing a specific management plan to be developed for most patients, according to the underlying cause.

The limitation on assessment of neurological injury makes the classification less neat than it might be: eg in type II faecal incontinence, one is left wondering if the

A. Congenital
  Hirschprung's disease
  Anorectal agenesis
B. Acquired
  1. Trauma
        Perineal trauma
        Sphincter injury
              Postoperative
              Postpartum
  2. Rectovaginal fistula
        Trauma
        Inflammatory
        Malignant
  3. Inflammatory disease
        Crohn's disease
        Ulcerative colitis
  4. Functional disease
        Irritable bowel syndrome
        Rectal prolapse
        Megarectum
  5. Neoplastic disease
        Villous adenoma
        Colorectal carcinoma
  6. Postirradiation
        Proctitis
  7. Postoperative (after colorectal or anal surgery)
  8. Neurological disease
        Diabetic neuropathy
        Multiple sclerosis
        Inflammatory arachnoiditis
        Caudal equina lesions
              Spina bifida
              Central disc prolapse
              Trauma
              Postoperative
        Pudendal neuropathy
              Parturition injury
              Perineal descent
        Other peripheral and central lesions
        Neurofibromatosis
        Degenerative
              Stroke
              Dementia

Fig. 4.1 Aetiology of faecal incontinence.
Keighley MR, Williams NS. Faecal Incontinence (26)

outcome of sphincteroplasty will be impaired by the presence of pudendal neuropathy. Yet this has always been a relevant issue and prospective documentation of the type when proceeding with PNE or sphincteroplasty will help derive the optimal management pathway, and allow for better comparison between series.

Patient groups and treatment algorithm

Part of the rationale for workup for severe faecal incontinence in parallel rather than after a failed initial trial of conservative management, is that the results of conservative management using a modern diagnostic algorithm are unknown. Historical case series

Table 4.1 Oxford Faecal Incontinence Classification and Management Approach

DPG	ARP	AUS	Classificalion	Approach
Female				
Traditional				
No RAI	Low MSP	Normal EAS	type I (N)	SNS
No RAI	Low MSP	Defect EAS	type II (SIN)	SNS v Sphincteroplasty
Emerging.addition				
RAI	Normal MSP	Normal EAS	type III (P)	Ventral rectopexy
RAI	Low MSP	Normal EAS	type IV (PN)	SNS v Ventral rectopexy
RAI	Low MSP	Defect EAS	type V (PS/N)	SNS v Ventral rectopexy*
Male				
No RAI	Low MSP	Defect IAS	type I (s)	Silicone anal bulking
RAI	Low MSP	Normal or thick IAS	type II (P)	Ventral rectopexy

DPG=defaecating proctogram

ARP=anorectal physiology

AUS~anal ultrasound

RAI=rectoanal intussusceptions

MSP=maximum squeeze pressure

MRP~maximum resting pressure

EAS=external anal sphincter

IAS=internal anal sphincter

SNS=sacral neuromodulation

*+1-additional sphincteroplasty as needed

Definitions:

Low MSP:	<50mmHg squeeze increment
Normal EAS:	No surgically remediable gap
Defect EAS	Surgically remediable gap
Low MRP	<45mmHg
Normal IAS	No gap
Defect IAS	IAS gap
Thick IAS	>2.5mm

Female:

N	Pudendal Neuropathy
S/N	Sphincter Injury and/or Pudendal Neuropathy
P	Prolapse
PN	Prolapse + Pudendal Neuropathy
PS/N	Prolapse + Sphincter Injury and/or Pudendal Neuropathy
s	Iatrogenic IAS injury (male)

examining the results of biofeedback do not specify underlying pathophysiology nor define diagnostic subgroups that may especially benefit or not from an arduous and time-consuming six month pelvic floor rehabilitation programme. We commence conservative therapy from the initial consultation. This includes Loperamide syrup (5ml = 1mg, 2.5–5.0 ml 2–3 times daily) titrated to symptoms, Amitriptyline syrup (paediatric strength 5–10 mg nocte) and on occasion, rubber band ligation of mucosal prolapse. Biofeedback is not commenced until the patient has been worked up and undergone a trial of conservative medical therapy.

The classification outlined in Table 4.1 yields several patient groups. About 15% fall into the traditional patient group of either a pure pudendal neuropathy (type I or N) or a sphincter injury and/or pudendal neuropathy (type II or S/N). These patients undergo PNE and if successful, implantation of an SNS device. Indications for sphincteroplasty are limited to: failed PNE and cloacal deformity, mandating sphincter repair with perineoplasty. Almost 45% have pure high-grade prolapse (type III or P). If biofeedback fails they, in our opinion, become candidates for laparoscopic ventral rectopexy. Success rates for pure faecal incontinence are about 75%. Another 40% have a combination of posterior compartment prolapse plus either pudendal neuropathy (type IV or PN) or a sphincter injury or both (type V or PS/N). The options for these last two groups (type V is rather uncommon) lie between SNS and ventral rectopexy; choice depends on several factors including age, co-morbidity, the presence of mixed symptoms, sphincter pressures and local funding arrangements. A successful diagnostic PNE makes this decision. In our experience, outcomes for these 2 types fall into 3 subgroups: those responding only to ventral rectopexy (failure of PNE appears to predict a successful outcome with ventral rectopexy), those responding only to PNE and SNS, and a group who could be treated successfully with either modality. More prospective data needs to be collected to examine outcomes across these 3 subgroups.

Key points

- Although maintenance of continence is a complex physiological process, traditional approaches have focussed predominantly on the role of the anal sphincters
- As faecal incontinence has a multifactorial aetiology, so traditional approaches solely directed at external anal sphincter defects are unlikely to be broadly successful
- Results from ventral rectopexy strongly suggest that internal rectal prolapse is not a normal variant but represents a significant and correctable pathology
- It is poorly recognized that most patients with internal rectal prolapse will complain of faecal incontinence, either alone or with obstructed defaecation
- Defaecating proctography should be part of the routine work up of patients with faecal incontinence

Editor's summary

Maintenance of continence is a complex physiological process and faecal incontinence has a multifactorial aetiology, which is unlikely to be solved by therapies solely directed at external anal sphincter defects. Results from ventral rectopexy strongly suggest that internal rectal prolapse is not a normal variant but represents a significant and correctable pathology, and that most of these patients will complain of faecal incontinence, with or without obstructed defaecation. We recommend defaecating proctography as part of the routine work up of patients with faecal incontinence.

References

1. Malouf AJ, Norton CS, Engel AF, Nicholls RJ, Kamm MA. Long-term results of overlapping anterior anal sphincter repair for obstetric trauma. *Lancet* 2000; **355**: 260–5.

2. Chan MK, Tjandra JJ. Sacral nerve stimulation for fecal incontinence: external anal sphincter defect vs. intact anal sphincter. *Dis Colon Rectum* 2008; **51**(7): 1015–24; discussion 1024-5.

3. Jarrett ME, Mowan G, Glazener CM, Fraser C, Nicholls RJ, Grant AM et al. Systematic review of sacral nerve stimulation for faecal incontinence and constipation. *Br J Surg* 2004; **91**: 1559–69.

4. Collinson R, Wijffels N, Cunningham C and Lindsey I. Laparoscopic ventral rectopexy for internal rectal prolapse: short-term functional results. *Colorectal Dis* 2010; **12**: 97–104.

5. Shorvon PJ, McHugh S, Diamant NE, Somers S, Stevenson GW. Defecography in normal volunteers: results and implications. *Gut* 1989; **30**(12): 1737–49.

6. Mellgren A, Schultz I, Johansson C, Dolk A. Internal rectal intussusception seldom develops into total rectal prolapse. *Dis Colon Rectum* 1997; **40**: 817–20.

7. Choi JS, Hwang YH, Salum MR, Weiss EG, Pikarsky AJ, Nogueras JJ, Wexner SD. Outcome and management of patients with large rectoanal intussusception. *Am J Gastroenterol* 2001; **96**: 740–4.

8. Orrom WJ, Bartolo DC, Miller R, Mortensen NJ, Roe AM. Rectopexy is an ineffective treatment for obstructed defecation. *Dis Colon Rectum* 1991; **34**(1):41–6.

9. Bachoo P, Brazzelli M, Grant A. Surgery for complete rectal prolapse in adults. *Cochrane Database Syst Rev.* 2000; (2):CD001758. Review. Update in Cochrane Database Syst Rev. 2008; (4):CD001758.

10. Speakman CT, Madden MV, Nicholls RJ, Kamm MA. Lateral ligament division during rectopexy causes constipation but prevents recurrence: results of a prospective randomized study. *Br J Surg* 1991; **78**(12):1431–3.

11. Lazorthes F, Gamagami R, Cabarrot P, Muhammad S. Is rectal intussusception a cause of idiopathic incontinence? *Dis Colon Rectum* 1998; **41**(5):602–5.

12. Schultz I, Mellgren A, Dolk A, Johansson C, Holmstrom B. Continence is improved after the Ripstein rectopexy. Different mechanizms in rectal prolapse and rectal intussusception? *Dis Colon Rectum* 1996; **39**(3):300–6.

13. Slawik S, Soulsby R, Carter H, Payne H, Dixon AR. Laparoscopic ventral rectopexy, posterior colporrhaphy and vaginal sacrocolpopexy for the treatment of recto-genital prolapse and mechanical outlet obstruction. *Colorectal Dis* 2008; **10**(2):138–43.

14. Dvorkin LS, Gladman MA, Epstein J, Scott SM, Williams NS, Lunniss PJ. Rectal intussusception in symptomatic patients is different from that in asymptomatic volunteers. *Br J Surg* 2005; **92**(7):866–72.

15. Pomerri F, Zuliani M, Mazza C, Villarejo F, Scopece A. Defecographic measurements of rectal intussusception and prolapse in patients and in asymptomatic subjects. AJR *Am J Roentgenol* 2001; **176**(3):641–5.

16. D'Hoore A, Cadoni R, Penninckx F. Long-term outcome of laparoscopic ventral rectopexy for total rectal prolapse. *Br J Surg* 2004; **91**(11):1500–5.

17. Boons P, Collinson R, Cunningham C, Lindsey I. Laparoscopic anterior rectopexy for rectal prolapse improves constipation and avoids new-onset constipation. *Colorectal Dis* 2010; **12**:97–104.

18. Collinson R, Cunningham C, D'Costa H, Lindsey I. Rectal intussusception and unexplained faecal incontinence: findings of a proctographic study. *Colorectal Dis* 2009; **11**(1):77–83.

19. Dench J, Hickey F. Evacuation proctography - should it be a part of the assessment of all patients with faecal incontinence? [Abstract]. *Colorectal Dis* 2006; **8**(s2):723 [abst].

20. Harmston C, Cunningham C, Lindsey I. The relationship between internal rectal prolapse and internal anal sphincter function. *Colorectal Dis* 2009; **11**(Suppl 2): 4 [abst].

21. Farouk R, Duthie GS, Bartolo DC, MacGregor AB. Restoration of continence following rectopexy for rectal prolapse and recovery of the internal anal sphincter electromyogram. *Br J Surg* 1992; **79**(5):439–40.

22. Wijffels N, Collinson R, Cunningham C, Lindsey I. What is the natural history of internal rectal prolapse? *Colorectal Dis* 2010; **12**:822–30.

23. Harmston C, Cunningham C, Lindsey I. Patterns of male faecal incontinence. *Colorect Dis* 2009; **11** (suppl.2): x [abstract].

24. Engel AF, Kamm MA, Bartram CI, Nicholls RJ. Relationship of symptoms in faecal incontinence to specific sphincter abnormalities. *Int J Colorect Dis* 1995; **10**:152–5.

25. Dvorkin LS, Chan CL, Knowles CH, Williams NS, Lunniss PJ, Scott SM. Anal sphincter morphology in patients with full-thickness rectal prolapse. *Dis Colon Rectum* 2004; **47**: 198–203.

26. Keighley MR, Williams NS. Faecal Incontinence. In: Keighley MR, Williams NS (eds) *Surgery of the Anus, Rectum and Colon.* Second Edition. Edinburgh: WB Saunders; 2001. pp. 592–700.

Chapter 5

Obstructed defaecation: a pathophysiological approach

Tony Dixon

Physiology of normal defaecation

Defaecation requires normal colonic motility, intact anorectal sensation, coordinated expulsion forces, and relaxation/contraction of the pelvic floor; usually triggered by the gastrocolic reflex. Rectal distension is registered in the cerebral cortex, leading to reflex relaxation of the internal anal sphincter (IAS) (the recto-anal inhibitory reflex or RAIR). Sampling receptors in the upper anal canal determine the nature of the content, and if the time is appropriate, efferent impulses contract the left colon and rectum, and relax the external anal sphincter (EAS), puborectalis, and pelvic floor. This relaxation widens the anorectal angle and produces an unobstructed anal channel. Defaecation is suppressed by voluntary contraction of the EAS, pelvic floor, and puborectalis, which in-turn propels the luminal contents back up the rectum and the urge to defaecate ceases.

Classification of chronic constipation

Constipated patients have either impaired colonic transit (slow transit constipation–STC) and/or pelvic floor dysfunction (obstructed defecation–OD). Functional constipation is defined by Rome II criteria (Table 5.1). Depending on aetiology, constipation can be considered into two groups: surgical (mechanical, STC or OD) or medical constipation (endocrine or neurological disease, drugs, psychological factors etc).

In constipation due to OD, the urge to defaecate is preserved, but defaecation is difficult and requires effort and straining. OD-type constipation is observed in about 10% of the adult population and more than half of constipated patients; it occurs more frequently in peri- or post-menopausal females when progressive weakening of the normal supportive tissues occurs; it is more common after hysterectomy (1,2). The causes of OD are many but in practice can be considered as:

- Functional OD eg anismus
- Mechanical OD eg high-grade rectal intussusception or external rectal prolapse
- Dissipation of force vector eg isolated rectocele

In considering mechanical OD, traditional discussion has focused on physiology and largely disregarded the anatomical dimension and the deficiencies of the female

Table 5.1 Rome II classification of chronic constipation*

Excessive straining
Lumpy/hard stools
Sensation of incomplete evacuation
Sensation of obstruction
Digitation, vaginal, or perineal support to facilitate evacuation
< 3 defaecations/week
> 25% of defaecations over at least three months in the preceding two years

pelvic floor. No more is this more evident than in the traditional methods used for treating recto-enterocele and recto-genital prolapse, which are based on assumptions now increasingly seen as flawed (3). As a result, efforts in the recent past have been directed towards medical management and biofeedback. Operations that remain standard (posterior colporrhaphy, Delorme's, posterior rectopexy) are based on thinking that, on current best practice, is now seen to be outdated.

Erroneous assumptions from the past

The basis of pelvic organ support was a mystery to surgeons of 100 years ago who thought that it was all due to the stiffness of the vaginal walls held in place by the levator ani and perineal body. Little distinction was made between the individual components of recto-urogenital prolapse. Surgery comprised little more than the construction of a shelf in the lower vagina and constriction of the urogenital hiatus, achieving little more than hiding the problem above a levatorplasty (4).

This approach of high transverse levatorplasty fell out of favour in the 1960s because of the high incidence of dyspareunia and its inherent failure to address the enterocele. Surgical focus then drifted towards Denonvillier's fascia. Based on the assumption that rectoceles arose through fascial attenuation, surgeons began plicating the central portion of the rectovaginal septum using either transvaginal or trans-anal routes. There was limited understanding of the true underlying patho-anatomy: gynaecologists operated for 'bulge control', colorectal surgeons for OD. Both approaches delivered reasonable short-term symptom control but neither addressed the anatomical defect; both have largely been ineffective at restoring normal defaecatory mechanisms and each carries a significant risk of dyspareunia. Gynaecologists next turned to the concept of repairing tears in the rectovaginal septum. Whilst early reports were promising, randomised trials have shown them to be quite inefficient (5). If anything is to be achieved, surgical repair has to address the biomechanics of pelvic organ support and set aside any belief that rectoceles arise through fascial attenuation.

Biomechanics of pelvic support

Key to this understanding is the endopelvic fascia and in particular the peri-cervical ring, which does not stretch, but rather tears along lines of stress. This connective tissue of the posterio-apical compartment forms a thick, highly collagenized leash, running from sacrum to perineum–the 'vaginal suspensory axis' (6). Obstetric damage to this support almost always occurs in the mid-pelvis. If the endopelvic fascia tears during engagement of the head, the upper margin of the peri-cervical ring separates from the uterosacral ligaments; setting the scene for a 'cervix first' prolapse. Conversely, if the damage occurs whilst exiting the plane of least dimension (rotation and extension), the rectovaginal septum is likely to be shorn away from the inferior border of the peri-cervical ring. The foetal head then pushes the detached septum downwards and outwards.

This injury creates a low-pressure zone in the upper vagina, into which the pelvic contents herniate, driven by intra-abdominal pressure, defaecation, and our bipedal posture:

◆ Loss of the stiffening effect of an intact rectovaginal septum allows the rectal wall to bulge forwards (rectocele)

◆ Stool pockets in the bulge and disrupts the mechanism of defaecation

◆ With careful dissection, the apical edge of this detachment can usually be seen at laparoscopy in the lower vagina

◆ Fibrotic pre-peritoneal fat is invariably found above the line of septal avulsion–a sure sign of an accompanying enterocele or sigmoidocele.

So why has surgical repair been so difficult? Pelvic connective tissue alone is not structurally suited to chronic load bearing and requires the pelvic floor muscles (with their durability and contractility) to absorb most of the load. Myofibrils are susceptible to strain induced fatigue fracture. Ageing and childbirth disrupt collagen homeostasis and hence amplify the tendency of fascia to fail over time, and whilst muscle hypertrophies in response to tears and becomes stronger, this effect diminishes with increasing age (7). Slow twitch fibres maintain constant postural tone and elevate the levator plate like a dome, which in turn opposes and tendency of the pelvic viscera to prolapse. Fast twitch fibres provide reflex contraction to counteract Valsalva forces from overwhelming the sphincter pressures. The endo-pelvic fascia functions as an investing mesentery, rather than a suspensory system, and stabilizes the pelvic organs to the axial skeleton over the centre of the levator plate. Whilst able to resist short-term forces, it is prone to fail under sustained load, particularly if compounded by age and childbirth damage.

The pathogenesis of prolapse

Whilst the hormones of pregnancy soften the pelvic connective tissue, the key event is vaginal delivery whose prime insult is probably direct avulsion of the pelvic diaphragm from its origin on the levator tendon (8). Elongation of the 'fixed' pudendal nerve causes a stretch neuropathy, which can eventually lead to muscle fibre atrophy. In addition, the endo-pelvic fascia can tear, leading to fascial defects. The concave levator plate then sags and the urogenital hiatus widens. Valsalva pressures are now deflected downwards and outwards, creating a sliding stress on the pelvic organs. If the fascial mesentery is also torn, the pelvic viscera align over the widened hiatus and prolapse occurs.

These injuries may be compensated for some time by strong connective tissue in young women.

Nulliparous women and men comprise a substantial subset of patients with prolapse (20%) and OD (5%) and other co-factors must be sought (which may or may not be also present in multiparous women). These generally fall under the umbrella of congenital or non-obstetric acquired pelvic floor weakness, and in each case the underlying mechanism is likely to be a collagen deficiency: Ehlers Danlos syndrome or the common (20% of the population) phenotypical variation of benign joint hypermobility syndrome, rapid weight loss, anorexia nervosa in adolescence or weight gain (central obesity), chronic straining (promoter in a vicious cycle rather than direct cause), smoking, menopausal loss of oestrogen and ageing. Prolapse tissue biopsies have decreased collagen concentrations (9), lower collagen I: III ratios (10) and up to four times higher levels of lytic protease enzymes that remodel collagen (11).

Clearly, a hysterectomy will lead to further loss of rectal and pelvic floor support. The concept of advocating excision surgery for prolapse, hysterectomy rather than hysteropexy is illogical, and the recurrence risk fails to diminish with each re-operative attempt (12). Failures do not relate to tissue thinning, in fact the vaginal muscularis layer in these types of patients is thicker than normal (13).

Surgical options for repair place reliance on the pelvic fascia. The main concerns are dynamic bridging grafts (where tissue flexibility and low morbidity are the main concerns). If properly sized and shaped they can perform well as a suspensory strut, suspended from the sacral promontory, rather than the sacrospinal ligament (ventral mesh rectopexy). The causes of obstructed defaecation will now be discussed in more detail.

Failure to relax the pelvic floor: anismus

Anismus (anal dysynergia, spastic pelvic floor syndrome or paradox) is characterized by inappropriate or paradoxical contraction of the EAS and puborectalis during straining. This makes defaecation impossible since the anal canal is functionally closed off. Symptoms of difficult evacuation, incomplete evacuation and/or digitation are common. It is more common in women with a history of sexual abuse. As physiological testing is required for diagnosis, its true prevalence is unknown. Clinical examination is accurate in ruling it out (14). Anismus, however, is a common finding in healthy controls and patients with incontinence and prolapse. Ambulatory manometry demonstrates that 80% of patients suspected of anismus have appropriate sphincter relaxation on straining. Confronted with this problem of false positives, strict diagnostic criteria should be applied (see chapter 10).

Mechanical outlet obstruction

An intussusception of the anterior rectal wall or a rectal prolapse may cause a mechanical obstruction of the opening of the anal canal making it impossible to defaecate. Evacuation proctography identifies five grades of prolapse (15):

+ Grade I (descends no lower than the proximal limit of the rectocele)
+ Grade II (descends into the rectocele but not to the top of the anal canal)
+ Grade III (descends to the top of anal canal)

◆ Grade IV (descends into the anal canal)

◆ Grade V (protrudes from the anus).

This Oxford classification is similar to Shorvon's (16) except that mucosal only prolapse and non-circumferential intussusception are excluded. Large intussusceptions, however, may cause no symptoms at all. Extrinsic obstruction results from straining in the presence of an enterocele or sigmoidocele within a deep pouch of Douglas, when defaecation can become difficult to initiate and complete.

Inefficient (diminished) force vector

Although increased intra-abdominal pressure is used to expel rectal content, it requires a channelling of the force that increases intrarectal pressure, which in turn is dependent on a degree of resistance from the supporting structures of the rectum, uterus-cervix and pelvis. A 'loss of push' occurs if the force is dissipated by the rectum bulging forwards (rectocele), or downwards (intussusception, recto-genital prolapse and descending perineum).

Rectocele

Rectoceles are constituted by a 'herniation' of the anterior attenuated rectal wall through a defect in the posterior vaginal septum in the direction of the vagina. Straining results in bulging of the rectocele, at the expense of efficient evacuation, with stool directed into the rectocele rather than the anal canal. High rectoceles are often associated with loss of uterine support and genital prolapse. An intermediate level rectocele may be associated with a defect in the rectovaginal septum and bulging of the posterior vaginal wall. Low rectoceles can be associated with disruption of the perineal body and direct tears from an obstetric injury.

Rectoceles and descending/bulging perineums are seen in men whose examination under anaesthetic (EUA)/laparoscopic finding in common is that of a gynaeoid pelvis. As in women who present with the same problem, the symptoms and signs (pain, dragging discomfort) reflect a lack of pelvic floor support for the rectum and peri-rectal tissues. The majority, have an associated high-grade intussusception. The anatomical deficiency is almost certainly congenital; perhaps Denonvillier's fascia has failed to fuse behind the prostate?

Defaecography identifies three types:

◆ Type I (digit form rectocele or single hernia through the rectovaginal septum)

◆ Type II (large saculation, lax rectovaginal septum, anterior rectal mucosal wall prolapse, and deep pouch of Douglas, enterocele)

◆ Type III (in which a rectocele is associated with intussusception or even rectal prolapse).

Rectoceles may be asymptomatic or interfere with normal defaecation. Small rectoceles (< 2cm in depth) are identified in about 20% of normal subjects (17). Larger ones may result in impaired evacuation, constipation, pelvic pain and bleeding; patients often have the sensation of a vaginal mass or bulge and to defaecate they support their vaginal wall or perineum with their fingers; 1/3 have to digitate (2).

Defaecograpghy demonstrates incomplete evacuation of the rectocele and barium trapping.

Following the menopause when atrophy of the perineum progresses, rectoceles elongate and the sphincters stretch: this tends to result in the development of progressive incontinence, urgency, tenesmus, and impaired evacuation. Furthermore, repeated straining may result in increased pelvic floor descent and a traction pudendal neuropathy.

The traditional surgical approach to rectoceles has been:

- Type I (endo-anal excision of mucosa at apex of rectocele with longitudinal plication of the anterior rectal muscle and transverse plication of IAS or transvaginal/transperineal repair of fascial defects in the rectovaginal septum)
- Type II (posterior colporrhaphy and Douglasography with or without a sacrospinal fixation of any associated vault prolapse)
- Type III (combined abdominal and vaginal approaches).

Posterior colporrhaphy together with levator-ani plication has a 48–54% incidence of postoperative constipation and evacuatory dysfunction; 50% develop a degree of vaginal tightness and dyspareunia (18,19). Studies of the trans-anal repair (20) report better results with regard to improvements in constipation; 80% of a highly selected group of 35/143 women had complete resolution of their pre-operative symptoms. The improved efficacy of this approach probably related to surgical correction of the intussusception, which is not addressed by traditional posterior colporraphy.

Other techniques using synthetic mesh to reinforce the rectovaginal septum, either transperineally or laparoscopically (21) are successful in 80%; patient numbers however were small and follow-up short. Only one study of transperineal levatorplasty (22) has shown a subjective improvement in disordered defaecation in 74% of 35 patients with a rectocele. In all these studies the results in patients with faecal incontinence were less satisfactory.

Enterocele

Enterocele is defined as a herniation of the peritoneal sac between the vagina and rectum and may contain either sigmoid or ileum. Symptoms include pelvic discomfort, a feeling of prolapse, pelvic pressure, and ODS. It is commonly found in elderly, multiparous females; and of all patients attending a pelvic floor dysfunction clinic, 50% have an enterocele (23); 80% of these descend into the lower 1/3 of the vagina and perineum. In our colorectal practice (2,24) almost 2/3 of the women with a symptomatic enterocele had undergone a previous hysterectomy–usually vaginal. Various repairs have been advocated:

- Transvaginal repair (high recurrence rate and risk of dyspareunia)
- Rectovaginopexy and obliteration of pelvic inlet

Short-term follow up has shown that repair improves discomfort. However, 25% recur within two years (25); colpopexy alone is insufficient because it does not obliterate the lateral parts of the pouch of Douglas, especially on the left. Gosselink et al reported (26) that complete obliteration of the pelvic inlet with a U-shaped mesh was effective. Anteriorly the mesh was sutured to the apex of the vagina and posteriorly to the presacral fascia at the level of the promontory ie a sacrocolpopexy was performed as well as obliteration of the inlet. Although the technique was effective in terms of pelvic discomfort and evacuatory proctography showed an adequate repair, ODS persisted in almost all patients. Similar poor results (80% persistent OD) were reported following both modified 'Ripstein' rectopexies and novel transvaginal repairs using autologous fascia lata grafts.

These poor results are not surprising given that none of these approaches addresses the cause of the prolapse or the rectal intussusception. Autonomic nerve sparing ventral mesh rectopexy (24,27) obliterates the enterocele and intussusception as well as supporting the pelvic floor, vault and/or uterus and alleviates ODS in 80–84% of patients. Symptom control is maintained beyond the median term. STARR is contraindicated (2) in enterocele; more importantly it has no effect in terms of closing the potential space for the enterocele/sigmoidocele or in repairing the fascial defects.

Rectal intussusception

Rectal intussusception (RI) manifests primarily as obstructed defaecation (ODS) with incontinence reported in > 50% of patients. Surgery for occult or internal prolapse has not enjoyed a good reputation over the last 20 years. Controversy arose through Shorvon's study (16), which demonstrated internal prolapse in normal volunteers and infrequent progression to external prolapse (28). Whilst widely quoted these studies have many problems; most notably that only 47% of subjects were women, all were nulliparous, and only 20% had the more morphologically advanced or high-grade RI; a large number of normal patients with high-grade RI were excluded from the study and went on to have corrective surgery!

The London group again (29) readdressed the question of RI being a variant of normal. They compared proctograms in 30 patients whose sole abnormality was RI with 11 asymptomatic volunteers found to have RI. Full-thickness RI was rare in the control group (22 vs 2). The intussusceptum was seen to be thicker in patients than controls (median 8mm vs. 4mm) and was more likely to occlude the rectal lumen (20 vs 3). They concluded that asymptomatic RI in controls is more likely to be mucosal rather than the morphologically advanced full-thickness.

As said earlier, it is not surprising that posterior rectopexy, the mainstay of treatment of RI in the 1980s, was abandoned and biofeedback considered the mainstay of treatment, as the operation denervates the rectum and leads to severe constipation in 50%, particularly when the lateral ligaments are divided. In addition it offers no support to either the anterior rectum or middle compartment. In autonomic nerve sparing laparoscopic ventral rectopexy for external prolapse, constipation/evacuatory dysfunction is improved in 80–84%, with infrequent new-onset or worsening of constipation (24,27). Similar functional improvements are also seen in carefully selected patients with high-grade internal prolapse (RI) undergoing the same procedure (24,30) suggesting a similar pathophysiological mechanism for both internal and external prolapse. Stapled trans-anal rectal resection (STARR) treats internal prolapse by excising the intussusception alone (2). Both techniques elevate the perineal body and correct the rectocele. Ventral rectopexy also elevates the cervix and vaginal vault to its normal position and obliterates the potential space for enterocele development.

Rectal prolapse

Rectal prolapse causes IAS dysfunction through IAS dilatation and intermittent activation of the recto-anal inhibitory reflex (RAIR) by the prolapsed rectal bolus. Rectal prolapse waves and a reduced rectal reservoir also play their part. It is important to remember that intermittent relaxation of the IAS secondary to the RI will be missed when performing anorectal physiology with the patient in the left lateral position without evacuation proctography to reveal occult pelvic floor disorders. Like high-grade RI, external prolapse is frequently associated with urogynaecological prolapse (2,24) and joint hypermobility.

Management includes open and laparoscopic posterior rectopexy as well as Delorme's. The latter is frequently advocated in the elderly. Its major problem is its unacceptable high recurrence rate (20%) and poor restoration of continence (stretched sphincters and loss of rectal compliance). Laparoscopic posterior rectopexy is associated with faster recovery and earlier hospital discharge, lower recurrence (0 vs 5%), lower major morbidity (0 vs 21%) compared to its open counterpart (31). Recurrence rates of both posterior approaches and restoration of incontinence were comparable as were the resultant high levels of constipation; colonic inertia and constipation (worsening or new) was seen in almost half of patients.

Rectal prolapse is associated with reduced resting and squeeze anal pressures, with incontinence reported in up to 75% of patients, of whom approximately 90% are women aged > 60 years. After correcting the prolapse the majority of incontinent patients improve and about 2/3 will regain full continence. This figure rises to 90% when a nerve sparing ventral mesh rectopexy is performed (24,27). The improvement in IAS electromyography (EMG) frequency and mean resting pressures after transabdominal surgery suggests that the IAS has an important role in maintaining continence in rectal prolapse. IAS function recovery is better in younger patients. The improved resting and squeeze pressures seen after surgical correction indicate that the EAS also has a major role.

Bristol approach to obstructed defaecation

Some would argue that physical signs are unreliable and that examining the patient is a waste of time and would place a large emphasis on diagnostic tests. However, the key to making an accurate clinical assessment of the pelvic floor to help direct management is to gain the confidence of an embarrassed patient and obtain a thorough and careful history and clinical examination. If any of this is performed in a cursory manner the assessment becomes limited. Pelvic floor examination is a good example of a technique dependent manoeuvre. It is a skill to get the patient to relax; to position the legs appropriately; examine the anterior compartment in both supine and left lateral; observe the dynamics of the pelvic floor; look for signs of recto-urogenital prolapse; and perineal descent at both rest and strain. Many of these manoeuvres are

Table 5.2 The Bristol approach to OD and prolapse

Indications for ventral mesh rectopexy–vaginal sacrocolpopexy

Hysterectomy (vaginal > total abdominal hysterectomy), vault and/or vaginal prolapse

Large cystocele (additional laparoscopic colporraphy)

Grade IV/V rectal intussusception, grade III enterocele, descending perineum

Poor sphincter function

External prolapse

Young men with above and/or solitary rectal ulcer (SRU)

SRU (failed STARR), established & fibrotic SRU

Relapsing symptoms post STARR

Slow transit constipation & internal prolapse

Any of above (in women) plus urinary stress incontinence or stress incontinence post ventral mesh rectopexy (additional tension free vaginal tape (TVT))

Failed gynecological repairs, Delorme's, Altemeire, posterior rectopexy, poorly executed ventral rectopexy

Indications for STARR

Young women with well-supported uterus, or men with isolated grade III or low take-off grade IV rectal intussusception, or early SRU with no enterocele or perineal descent

'Pseudo-Anismus', failed biofeedback–prolapse found at EUA

Previous open abdominal surgery in the presence of obesity, elderly with grade IV intussusception unfit for long GA

Males (**no** perineal descent), grade IV haemorrhoids, or truncal obesity

Failed ventral mesh rectopexy with residual prolapse seen at EUA: posterior > lateral > anterior STARR

Indications for sacral neuromodulation (SNS) in ODS

Anatomy corrected–OD persists

Indications for additional procedure for prolapsed haemorrhoids (PPH)

Residual symptomatic everted anal canal & haemorrhoids post ventral rectopexy

Indications for EUA± laparoscopy

Conflicting special investigations, symptoms, clinical findings

Indications for laparoscopic colectomy and ileorectal

Slow transit constipation (STC) persists after correction of prolapse & evacuation

Indications Botulinum toxin

True anismus and failed biofeedback (no prolapse), proctalgia fugux and high resting pressure in puborectalis–no prolapse, high pressures & continuing symptoms post STARR/ ventral mesh rectopexy

Management of complications

Mesh erosion post rectopexy (transvaginal excision & repair), infected mesh (transvaginal or laparoscopic removal), dyspareunia (laparoscopic removal)

nuanced eg assessment of anismus, palpable rectocele/rectal shelf, enterocele, RI/prolapse, urogynaecological prolapse. Straining rigid sigmoidoscopy of an empty rectum (digitally evacuated by the surgeon if necessary), on withdrawal from the rectosigmoid junction, is key to making an assessment of prolapse.

Dynamic defaecography is important in our practice as an adjunct to the above. If there is any conflict of assessment, EUA with or without laparoscopy will clarify. Physiology is used selectively eg when anismus is suggested by any of the above, or when we employ biofeedback–usually after anatomical correction. Our choice of intervention is determined by what we assess the anatomical problem to be (Table 5.2).

Summary

An understanding of the anatomy of the pelvic floor and its endopelvic fascial support and physiology gives some insight not only into the possible mechanisms of system failure but also the underlying principles behind the success of modern approaches (and the failings of established approaches) in the surgical correction of OD. Restoration of normal anatomy, support and physiology is the ultimate goal if optimal function is to be achieved. Key to this operative selection is an accurate history and clinical examination.

Key points

- An accurate clinical assessment of the pelvic floor requires the confidence of an embarrassed patient and if this is performed in a cursory manner the assessment becomes limited
- Many of these manoeuvres are nuanced e.g. assessment of anismus, palpable rectocoele or enterocele or internal rectal prolapse (straining rigid sigmoidoscopy on withdrawal from the rectosigmoid junction is key to assessment)
- Dynamic defaecography is important in our practice as an adjunct to the above. If there is any conflict of assessment, EUA ± laparoscopy will clarify
- Physiology is used selectively eg when anismus is suggested by any of the above, or when we employ biofeedback–usually after anatomical correction
- Choice of intervention is determined by what we assess the anatomical problem to be (Table 5.2).

Editor's summary

The approach to obstructed defaecation is largely an anatomical one. Though physiological disturbance can be present as well, or even dominate, in the great majority of patients the major problem is anatomical. The challenge is to recognise when an anatomical/surgical approach is unlikely to succeed (or indeed has failed), and to develop an alternative strategy in this cohort of patients.

References

1. Irvine EJ, Ferrazzi S, Parc P, Thompson WG, Rance I. Health-related quality of life in functional GI disorders: focus on constipation and resource utilization. *Am J Gastroenterol* 2002;**97**: 186–93.

2. Titu L, Riyad K, Carter H, Dixon. Staple Trans Anal rectal Resection for obstructed defecation: a cautionary tail. *Dis. Colon Rectum* 2009;**52**: 1716–22.

3. Orrom WJ, Bartolo DC, Miller R, Mortenson NJ, Roe AM. Rectopexy is an ineffective treatment for obstructed defecation. *Dis Colon Rectum* 1991;**34**: 41–6.

4. Howkins J. *Shaw's Textbook of Operative Gynaecology*. Third edition. Edinburgh and London: E&S Livingstone Ltd; 1968.

5. Parasio MF, Barber MD, Muir TW, Walters MD. Rectocele repair: a randomized trial of three surgical techniques including graft augmentation. *Am.J.Obstet Gynaecology*. 2006;**195**: 1762–71.

6. Zimmerman CW. Surgical correction of defects in pelvic support. In *TE Linde's Operative Gynaecology*. Eds: Rock JA, Jones HW III, 9th edition; Philadelphia: Lippincott, Wiilliams and Wilkins, 2003: 927–48.

7. Marzetti E, Leeuwenburgh C. Skeletal muscle apoptosis, sarcopenia and frailty in old age. *Exp Gerontol* 2006;**41**: 1234–8.

8. De Lancy JO, Kearney R, Chou Q et al. The appearance of levator ani muscle abnormalities in magnetic resonance imaging after vaginal delivery. *Obstet Gynaecol* 2003;**101**. 46–53.

9. Soderberg MW, Falconer C, Bystrom B, Malmstrom A, Ekman G. Young women with genital prolapse have a low collagen concentration. *Acta Obstet Gynaecol Scand* 2004; **83**: 1193–8.

10. Jackson S, Avery NC, Tarlton JF et al. Changes in metabolism of collagen in genitourinary prolapse. *Lancet* 1996;**347**: 1658 61.

11. Moalli PA, Shand SH, Zyczynski HM, Gordy SC, Men LA. Remodelling of vaginal connective tissue in patients with prolapse. *Obstet.Gynaecol* 2005;**106**: 593–63.

12. Clark AL, Gregory T, Smith VJ, Edwards R. Epidemiological evaluation of reoperation for surgically treated pelvic organ prolapse and urinary incontinence. *Am J Obstet Gynaecol* 2003;**189**: 1261–7.

13. Tulikangas PK, Walterd MD, Brainard JA, Webber AM. Enterocele: is there a histological effect? *Obstet Gynaecol* 2001;**98**: 634–7.

14. Chausade S, Khyari A, Roache H et al. Determination of total and segmental colonic transit time in constipated patients. *Dig Dis Sci* 1989;**34**: 1168–72.

15. Collinson R, Cunningham C, D'Costa H, Lindsey I. Rectal intussusception and unexplained faecal incontinence. *Dis Colon Rectum* 2008;**11**: 77–83.

16. Shorvon PJ, McHugh S, Diamant NE, Somers S, Stevenson GW. Defecography in normal volunteers: results and implications. *Gut* 1989;**30**: 1737–49.

17. Yoshioka K, Matsui Y, Yamada O et al. Physiologic and anatomic assessment of patients with rectocele. *Dis Colon Rectum* 1991;**34**: 704–8.

18. Kahn MA, Stanton SL. Posterior colporrhaphy: its effects on bowel and sexual function. *Br J Obstet Gynaecol* 1997;**104**: 882–6.

19. Mellgren A, Anzen B, Nilsson BY et al., Results of rectocele repair. A prospective study. *Dis Colon Rectum* 1995;**38**: 7–13.

20. Murthy VK, Orkin BA, Smith LE, Glassman LM. Excellent outcome using selective criteria for rectocele repair. *Dis Colon Rectum* 1996;**39**: 374–8.

21. Lyons TL, Winner WK. Laparoscopic rectocele repair using polyglactin mesh. *J Am Assoc Gynecol Laparosc* 1997;**4**: 381–4.

22. Ommer A, Kohler A, Athanasiadis S. Results of transperineal levatorplasty in treatment of symptomatic rectocele. *Chirurg* 1998;**69**: 966–72.

23. Cronje HS, De Beer JA, Bam R. The pathophysiology of an enterocele and its management. *J Obstet Gynaecol*. 2004;**24**: 408–13.

24. Slawik S, Soulsby R, Carter H, Payne H, Dixon AR. Laparoscopic ventral rectopexy, posterior colporrhaphy and vaginal sacrocolpopexy for the treatment of recto-genital prolapse and mechanical outlet obstruction. *Colorectal Dis*. 2008;**10**: 138–43.

25. Jean F, Tanneau Y, Le Blanc-Louvry I, Leroi AM, Denis P, Michot F. Treatment of enterocele by abdominal colpo- rectsacropexy–efficacy on pelvic pressure. *Colorectal Dis* 2002;**4**: 321–5.

26. Gosselink MJ, van Dam JH, Huisman WM, Ginai AZ, Schouten WR. Treatment of enterocele by obliteration of the pelvic inlet. *Dis Colon Rectum* 1999;**42**: 940–4.

27. D'Hoore A, Cadoni R, Penninckx F. Long-term outcome of laparoscopic ventral rectopexy for total rectal prolapse. *Br J Surg* 2004;**91**: 1500–5.

28. Mellgren A, Schultz I, Johansson C, Dolk A. Internal rectal intussusception seldom develops into total rectal prolapse. *Dis Colon Rectum* 1997;**40**: 817–20.

29. Dvorkin LS, Gladman MA, Epstein J, Scott SM, Williams NS, Lunnis PJ. Rectal intussusception in symptomatic volunteers is different from that in asymptomatic volunteers. *Br J Surg* 2005;**92**: 866–72.

30. Collinson R, Vandjuivendiuk P, Cunningham C, Lindsay I. Laparoscopic anterior rectopexy improves obstructed defecation in patients with rectal intussusception. *Colorectal Dis* 2007;**9** (Suppl 1): 31–104.

31. Solomon MJ, Young CJ, Eyers AA, Roberts RA. Randomized clinical trial of laparoscopic versus open abdominal rectopexy for rectal prolapse. *Br J Surg* 2002;**89**: 35–9.

Chapter 6

Chronic anorectal pain: a pathophysiological approach

Roel Hompes and Ian Lindsey

Traditional approach and shortcomings

Chronic idiopathic perineal pain (CIPP) is a term used to try to describe several subgroups of patients with chronic anorectal pain. The most common pain syndromes are chronic proctalgia (called levator ani syndrome in the US), proctalgia fugax and coccydynia. These pain syndromes have generally been poorly understood and managed, this is reflected in the space dedicated to their care in current colorectal reference textbooks (7.5 of 4000 pages (1,2)). There is probably considerable overlap in the symptomatology of these subgroups and they may in fact represent variations of the same general disorder (1). In general they are distinguished on the basis of duration of painful episodes, frequency, and other characteristics.

Proctalgia fugax

This syndrome of sudden, short-lived, severe, self-limiting bursts of anorectal pain was first described by Thaysen in 1953 (3). Although pain may occasionally last for up to 30 minutes, only 10% of patients report that the pain lasts longer than 5 minutes. Attacks appear irregularly and at different intervals, although usually < 5 times per year in 51% of patients. The lifetime prevalence ranges from 8% to 18%, and both men and women are equally affected. Symptoms rarely begin before puberty. It is usually anal in distribution (90%), precipitated in 1/3 by defaecation, and often occurs at night (30%). Associated mucous per rectum and abdominal distension have been described (4). Unlike levator ani syndrome, patients are asymptomatic during rectal examination and no characteristic clinical findings can be found to support the diagnosis.

Chronic idiopathic anal pain (CIAP) or levator ani syndrome

This syndrome has been even more obscure. Todd reported symptoms of a 'bearing down pain', like a 'ball obstructing the rectum' (5). Tenesmus has also been reported. The pain is often worse with sitting than with standing or lying down. Prevalence ranges from 6% to 7%, and seems to decline after the age of 45 years. Women are thought to be affected more than men. Major psychological overlay is described, including emotional lability (6) and compensation-seeking behaviour (1). A frequent clinical finding is tenderness on palpation of the puborectalis muscle, as the examining finger moves from the coccyx posterior to the pubis anteriorly. Often this tenderness is asymmetric, predominantly on the left side.

Coccydynia

This describes severe rectal, perineal and sacrococcygeal pain, mainly in women (85%) and first reported by Simpson in 1859. The hallmark feature is worsening on sitting down and relief with standing. It is often described as a burning pain and is continuous, radiating into the buttocks and thighs. Regardless of cause, the key to diagnosis is the reproduction of pain when the coccyx is manipulated (7); this distinguishes coccydynia from levator ani syndrome. Most treatments have been unsatisfactory, particularly surgical attempts at cure with coccygectomy.

New approaches: proctographic data from Oxford

We have collected prospective data on a series of patients presenting with CIPP with or without obstructed defaecation (OD) to a dedicated colorectal pelvic floor clinic. Fifty-nine patients were identified (females 80%, mean age 53, range 22–84 years), 33 (56%) with CIPP alone (mean Wexner score 5.9), and 26 (44%) with CIPP plus OD (mean Wexner score 15.3). Proctographic diagnosis was as follows: high-grade internal rectal prolapse (47%), low-grade internal rectal prolapse (29%), anismus (19%), mucosal prolapse (5%). Examination under anaesthesia was necessary in 16 patients (27%) because proctography was non-diagnostic despite clinical findings or treatment of anismus by botox injection which had failed (8); this led to a revision of the proctographic diagnosis in several patients. The most common final diagnosis (59%) was high-grade internal rectal prolapse (CIPP plus OD 73% versus CIPP alone 48%, $p < 0.05$). Other final diagnoses included anismus (5%), mucosal prolapse (3%) and familial internal sphincter myopathy (2%). Most of these patients had persistent pain symptoms and were not typical of a nerve entrapment syndrome, and thus were probably best classified as chronic idiopathic anal pain.

Of 543 controls, 422 with high-grade internal rectal prolapse (IRP) and 121 with external rectal prolapse (ERP), anorectal pain was present to some degree (some, most or all of the time) in 50%. Maximum resting pressure was similar (mean 88.3 versus 84.5 mmHg) and maximum squeeze pressure higher (mean 119 versus 104 mmHg) in patients with CIPP alone versus CIPP plus OD. Mean maximum resting pressure was significantly different between patients with CIPP (86.0 mmHg) and controls with IRP and OD (58.9 mmHg, $p<0.0001$), IRP and mixed OD/FI (47.5 mmHg, $p<0.0001$), IRP and FI (41.2 mmHg, $p<0.04$) and ERP (31.4 mmHg, $p=0.005$).

These data highlight several issues in CIPP. Firstly, complaints of anorectal pain, from modest to more severe, are common, occurring in half of patients presenting primarily with disturbance of bowel function and high-grade prolapse, at least some of the time, in the absence of a circumscribed chronic perineal pain syndrome. Secondly, they appear to indicate that prolapse is a disease commonly associated with

CIPP and may be the commonest underlying cause. Finally, proctography had a strong tendency to undercall prolapse disease in the setting of CIPP. There may some particular reasons for this, apart from the usual explanations of embarrassment and the un-physiological and unnatural circumstances of the investigation. The presence of both pain during attempts at defaecation and the resisting force of a relatively high anal closing pressure may be related and lead to resistance of adequate descent of the prolapse during proctography to allow a diagnosis of high-grade prolapse to be made.

Clinical assessment

It is important to exclude more straightforward organic causes of pain such as a chronic intersphincteric abscess or chronic anal fissure. These should be suggested on clinical examination. Retrorectal tumours such as chordoma should be specifically examined for digitally.

The characteristics of the pattern of the pain are important and can be useful. Eliciting a relationship of the pain to sitting or standing can be very helpful. As a general rule, in nerve entrapment syndromes such as pudendal pain syndrome, the pain is induced by sitting and relieved by standing, whereas with pain associated with prolapse syndromes, the converse is true. For details of distribution of pain in specific subtypes of nerve entrapment syndromes, the reader is referred to chapter 15 (Pudendal pain syndrome).

Diagnostic workup

The workup of patients with chronic idiopathic perineal pain involves two components. The colorectal surgeon should initiate an exploration for and assessment of an underlying pelvic floor disorder. In parallel, a chronic pain specialist with an interest/expertise in pelvic floor disorders should be engaged early for an assessment of any possible pain syndrome.

Tests of diagnostic exclusion

Depending on the patient's age, at least a flexible sigmoidoscopy and frequently colonoscopy should be arranged to exclude organic luminal disease. MRI should be employed liberally to exclude unusual but important causes of chronic pain such as retrorectal tumours, spinal pathology and occult anorectal sepsis.

Anorectal physiology and anal ultrasound

Anal sphincter assessment using anorectal physiology (ARP) and anal ultrasound (AUS) should be organized as standard. Simple proctological diagnoses, such as an intersphincteric abscess, can be easily excluded on AUS. A hypertensive and extremely thickened (> 5 mm) internal anal sphincter (IAS) on ARP and AUS, respectively, suggests a rare inherited IAS myopathy. This should prompt IAS biopsy for inclusion bodies demonstrable on electron microscopy. A hypotensive, thickened (particularly anteriorly and in the upper anal canal) IAS suggests high-grade (anal) internal rectal prolapse (recto-anal intussusception).

Defaecating proctography

Proctography is perhaps the most helpful of the investigations when an underlying prolapse syndrome is suspected. In the presence of obstructed defaecation and CIPP, we would expect to ultimately demonstrate a significant prolapse of the posterior compartment in about 75% of cases. Where a pure CIPP presentation manifested, a prolapse syndrome may underlay this in about 50% of cases. Having said that, it is particularly in the situation of CIPP that proctography has a tendency to undercall the actual posterior prolapse grade. This probably explains the previously reported relative lack of usefulness of proctography in pain syndromes in circumstances where prolapse was highly suggested on history. The reasons for the diagnostic shortfall are not entirely clear but it is possible that induction of pain limits the ability or willingness of the patient to strain adequately. It is also emerging that the nature of internal sphincter function is related to the way in which patients with high-grade internal rectal prolapse present. It is not possible to determine which is the chicken and egg, but those with external rectal prolapse and faecal incontinence have significantly lower resting pressures than patients presenting with obstructed defaecation or pain. It is possible that the response of the internal sphincter to the repeated trauma of prolapse into the anal canal is different in these two general subsets of patients. Pain may be a manifestation of the resistance of the internal sphincter to prolapse, perhaps by development of hypertrophy which might conceivably lead to anal canal hypoperfusion and ischaemia. Patients with CIPP seem to have especially high resting pressures.

Rectal examination under anaesthetic

Whatever the explanation, it is of special importance in patients with CIPP to pursue potential prolapse syndromes where suggested clinically but where proctography has proved non-diagnostic. This is also necessary when an enterocele has been demonstrated at proctography. This can in itself give rise to symptoms of pelvic pressure and pain, but also suggests a more profound degree of posterior compartment prolapse. In such situations a rectal examination under anaesthetic is very helpful; a general anaesthetic overcomes patient pain and apprehension, and the true grade of prolapse can be observed. The correct instrumentation must be used. An Eisenhammer speculum, with its bivalve design and long blades tends to obscure the proper view of prolapse disease and splint the prolapse in place. A preferable technique is the use of a circular anal dilator (CAD) device (Frankenman International Ltd, Hong Kong). This allows a prolapse to circumferentially fall into the proctoscope and gives a superior assessment of the presence and grade of prolapse.

Chronic pain management

Having made a diagnosis of high-grade prolapse, a difficult management problem then arises. The patient is usually greatly relieved to have a diagnosis established.

There has frequently been a long delay in recognition that there may be a physical basis for the pain and making the diagnosis. Not uncommonly, up till then the patient may have been, openly or inadvertently, made to feel that they are imagining things and that no physical explanation has been found. The pressure to offer an immediate surgical remedy is thus very high. This must be resisted and the correct treatment formula determined.

It is critical to have an established clinical relationship with a chronic pain specialist, ideally one with interest and experience in pelvic floor disorders and CIPP. Patients will benefit from early referral to and engagement with a pain specialist. This will enable the development of a chronic pain care package for the patient, which might include pharmacological, physical, rehabilitational and psychological approaches. For details of specific pain management techniques, the reader is referred to chapter 15.

The treatment hierarchy: prolapse or pain?

Nerve entrapment syndromes

If there is a recognisable nerve entrapment syndrome, referral to a pain specialist with expertise in the specific management of these syndromes is vital. The pain specialist should have an appreciation of and access to the plethora of diagnostic approaches including radiological-guided nerve blocks, steroid injections, nerve stimulation techniques and a relationship with peripheral nerve surgeons capable of nerve-release or transposition techniques.

In our experience, the most recognisable of these, pudendal nerve entrapment, is relatively uncommon in colorectal practice. It is perhaps responsible for about 5–10% of our patients presenting with CIPP (who make up 5% of all colorectal patients with a pelvic floor disorder). It usually occurs in parallel with obstructed defaecation and is seen especially in the subgroup of patients with extreme pelvic floor descent (usually > 6cm). In this group of patients, the pain syndrome symptoms usually overwhelm the bowel dysfunction and thus in the treatment hierarchy the priority must be the pain itself.

Prolapse syndromes

As a general rule, treatment of the chronic pain takes precedence over treatment of prolapse where it exists. This is particularly so for severe well-established pain because in these circumstances, although the prolapse syndrome may underlie and be driving the pain syndrome, unwinding of the pain will not necessary follow correction of the prolapse. Indeed, the trauma of surgery may well exacerbate the pain. It is our practice to refer the patient to a chronic pain specialist but detail the pelvic floor disorder and identify a requirement at some stage to correct the underlying prolapse. In some cases, some modest pain management plans are put in place and the patient is sent back for surgery, in others a formal rehabilitation program is commenced and a surgical 'window' for treatment identified as the patient's pain is brought under control.

Key Points

◆ CIPP is an uncommon extreme manifestation (severe pain) of a more common component complaint (mild to moderate pain) in the spectrum of prolapse syndromes

◆ Proctography is frequently unreliable; but despite historic literature to the contrary, a thorough diagnostic evaluation will commonly throw up a structural abnormality, usually posterior compartment prolapse, particularly if associated obstructed defaecation is present

◆ Early referral to a chronic pain specialist is essential, and if anti-prolapse surgery is contemplated, it should be in concert with, and generally after, a chronic pain therapy programme has been initiated and probably only conducted in a tertiary care setting.

References

1. Keighley MR, Williams NS. Chronic Idiopathic Perineal Pain. In: Keighley MR, Williams NS (eds). *Surgery of the Anus, Rectum and Colon.* pp 878–84. Second Edition 2001. Edinburgh: WB Saunders.

2. Gordon P. Miscellaneous Entities. In: Gordon P, Nivatvongs S (eds). *Surgery of the Colon, Rectum and Anus.* Second Edition. St Louis: Quality Medical Publishing; 1999. pp. 1389–90.

3. Thaysen ThEH. Proctalgia fugax: a little known form of pain in the rectum. *Lancet* 1953; **ii**:243–6.

4. Thompson WG. Proctalgia fugax in patients with the irritable bowel, peptic ulcer or inflammatory bowel disease. *Am J Gastroenterol* 1984;**79**:450–2.

5. Todd IP. Clinical evaluation of the pelvic floor. In Henry MM and Swash M (eds) *Coloproctology and the Pelvic Floor* 1985. pp 187–8. London: Butterworth.

6. Neill ME, Swash M. Chronic perineal pain: an unsolved problem. *J R Soc Med* 1982; **75**:96–101.

7. Thiele GH. Coccydynia: the mechanism of its production and its relationship to anorectal disease. *Am J Surg* 1950;**79**:110–6.

8. Hompes R, Jones OM, Cunningham C, Lindsey I. What causes chronic idiopathic perineal pain? *Colorectal Dis* 2010;**12**:(Suppl. 1)24 [abst].

Chapter 7

Conservative treatment of pelvic floor disorders

Karen Nugent

Conservative management of obstructive defaecation or rectal evacuatory disorders

Obstructive defaecation and evacuatory difficulties occur in a large number of the population. Although they may occur in isolation, these problems are often part of a mixed pattern of pelvic floor dysfunction. Patients presenting with obstructive defaecation often find it difficult to discuss their problem with other people and may have a puzzling number of other symptoms which make diagnosis confusing. They may complain of constipation; this refers not to a single problem or a disease nor is it a specific diagnosis but a group of symptoms. In a large population based series (1) it was estimated that up to 20% of middle aged people have functional constipation and 10% have symptoms of obstructive defaecation. Symptoms may include bloating and abdominal distension, both of which are more often associated with slow transit constipation as well as difficulty in emptying the bowel. Symptoms often overlap and the pattern of constipation may be slow transit (STC), obstructive defaecation (ODS) or a mixture of both. Many of the studies relating to treatment of constipation are therefore difficult to interpret. An essential part of the treatment of these patients is to understand the pathophysiology behind their diagnosis (STC, ODS or both). When separating out obstructive defaecation from other types of constipation there may be both functional and structural problems causing the evacuatory difficulty or once again a mixed role.

Initial management

It is important to understand the patient's expectation and perception of their problem before initiating treatment. Some patients, simply by understanding their defaecatory problem, are able to manage their symptoms better and live with their problem in a more positive light. Simple conservative methods should start with dietary and fluid advice. Patients should be encouraged to drink adequate amounts of non caffeinated fluids, preferably water, although a lot of this fluid will be absorbed in the colon. However, stool consistency relies on an adequate degree of hydration. Dietary advice should begin with looking at the patient's normal diet. Although fibre and its osmotic effect may be useful, in some patients with irritable bowel syndrome or symptoms of bloating and wind, it may be counterproductive (as wheat fibre has increased propensity to cause increased flatus and bloating). It is probable that soluble fibre is better than insoluble fibre in limiting the bloating side effects, however it is also known that in patients with severe constipation fibre may be worse than useless. In patients with bloating it is often advisable to limit the wheat fibre and replace this with oat fibre or even limit fibre completely in order to reduce their symptoms.

Laxatives

The use of laxatives in the Western world is extremely common with up to 40% of the population taking occasional or regular laxatives. Increased usage is seen with increasing age corresponding to an increase in symptoms of ODS from 10% in middle-aged people to 20% in those over 65 years of age (2). Although both men and women are known to use laxatives, women tend to take them for a longer length of time and constipation is three times more common in women than men (3). It is preferable for people to avoid stimulant laxatives, as patients can develop a dependence on these for their bowel to act at all. One of the commonest used laxatives is (Fybogel) or ispaghula husk. These act by increasing the bulk of the stool and are a reasonable adjunct to behavioural therapy in patients with mild symptoms or hard stool. They probably have little additional benefit than fibre in the diet and as with dietary fibre they can cause bloating and wind. An alternative to fibre supplements is stool softeners such as magnesium hydroxide or sodium docusate. These are useful in patients who have hard stools.

Many patients arrive to see the doctor already on some form of stimulant laxatives. These act by increasing colonic motility and are often senna based. These stimulant laxatives are often associated with melanosis coli in long term use. This is a darkening of the mucosa of the colon and is an indicator of chronic laxative abuse, although there do not appear to be any functional or structural problems associated with the colon due to the melanosis coli (4).

An alternative to these and more recently used in increasing prominence are the osmotic laxatives. One of the commonest of these is lactulose. This is poorly absorbed in the gut and causes retention of fluid within the lumen of the bowel. Lactulose can be associated with bloating and increased wind; this is probably due to its reaction within the colon where it is altered into short chain fatty acids and has a further osmotic effect. Polyethylene glycol based polymers eg Macrogol have been shown to work extremely well in patients with chronic constipation. They have fewer problems with colicky pain than the stimulant laxatives however there is a small chance of water retention in the elderly.

In patients with obstructive defaecation syndrome or rectal defaecatory disorders, glycerine suppositories may be of benefit. These are stimulant only within the rectum. An alternative rectal laxative is either sodium citrate enemas (Peristeen pump®) or phosphate enemas in those with emptying problems.

Rectal irrigation

Following the benefit seen in some patients with severe constipation by using an ante-grade colonic enema (ACE) approach (5), it seemed logical to try forms of retrograde colonic or rectal irrigation. This would have the benefit of not requiring any form of surgery for those with a rectal evacuatory problem attempting to empty the rectum using simple warm water. A system using a cone and pump has been available since the late 90s and more recently since April 2007 the Peristeen pump® (Coloplast Ltd) has been available by prescription.

Patients electing to trial this equipment for either constipation or incontinence require input from a specialist nurse (either in hospital or the community). The amount of irrigation fluid required and the time to irrigate varies between patients. The warm water should be instilled gently and the process should be comfortable. The patient should sit comfortably on the toilet and insert the lubricated cone or tubing. It is usual to start with 3–500 ml of tap water. The patient then removes the tubing after 1–2 mins and evacuates water and stool. The process can be undertaken a few times and patients may then experience an urge to defaecate 10–15 mins after finishing the process (6).

Results depend on patient motivation and their attitude to the process. In a retrospective review article looking at 48 patients treated with irrigation (33 with incontinence and 15 with constipation) 50% felt that the treatment was successful in relieving their symptoms (6). Over half irrigated daily and the others had tailored the timings to suit their symptoms.

It is a useful adjunct in patients who have failed other medical and surgical therapies. Antegrade irrigation is usually more successful than retrograde irrigation but is more invasive.

Behavioural therapy

Many of patients with constipation have developed 'bad habits' and are not responding to the normal pathophysiology of bowel emptying. They should be encouraged to go to the toilet at the same time every day in order to retrain their bowels; preferably in the morning or at times when the gastrocolic reflex will kick in, e.g. just after the end of a meal. Weight loss and physical activity are also thought to improve gut movement and exercise combined with re-toileting times may improve bowel emptying. A specialist pelvic floor nurse is ideal to help deliver this treatment.

Biofeedback

The need to defaecate and the process of defaecation is an extremely complex and co-ordinated process some of which is under voluntary control but the rest of which is under autonomic feedback loops. Biofeedback is a technique used to try and retrain this complex process using a variety of different forms. It can be done using visual, auditory or even sensory feedback and particularly useful if there is a degree of pelvic floor discoordination or anismus. Initial parts of the biofeedback treatment are to establish a link with the patient and to advise them on the position required to defaecate and the use of other muscles in a coordinated fashion. Patients should be shown how to sit on the toilet with their feet raised off the ground usually on some form of step stool in order to open the anorectal angle further and to prevent straining and tensed position.

Good results have been seen in patients with poor rectal emptying (7) but also in patients with slow transit constipation (8). Both short and long term benefit is evident in over 60% of unselected patients attending for biofeedback (8,9). The benefit is on gut function, reduction in laxative usage and also in quality of life scores.

In summary rectal evacuatory problems are common in women with increasing age. Lifestyle and dietary advice as well as biofeedback may improve their symptoms greatly. Laxatives can help but wind forming ones should be avoided and rectal suppositories, enemas, or irrigation systems are useful adjuncts to treatment.

Irritable bowel syndrome

The symptoms associated with irritable bowel syndrome (IBS) overlap and often exacerbate the other symptoms of pelvic floor dysfunction in patients both with constipation and incontinence. The most common functional gastrointestinal disorder, accounting for 25% of outpatient visits, is IBS (10). Patients usually present with abdominal pain, altered bowel habits, bloating and the sensation of incomplete emptying. They are more often female, young and from higher socio-economic status. Based on the pattern of bowel alteration IBS can be described as diarrhoea- or constipation-predominant. The National Institute for Health and Clinical Excellence published a helpful review emphasising the need to establish a positive diagnosis; identify worrying symptoms which require prompt referral to hospital; and work with the patient to manage their symptoms (11). The positive diagnostic criteria for IBS are: the presence of symptoms for at least 6 months; abdominal pain or discomfort that is relived by defaecation or associated with altered bowel frequency or stool form; and at least two of the following: altered stool passage; abdominal bloating; symptoms made worse by eating; and passage of mucus. The only tests required to exclude other pathology (except when cancer or more serious pathology is expected) are a full blood count, c-reactive protein, plasma viscosity, and antibody for celiac disease.

Treatment for IBS

The main thrust of advice is reassurance and warning about the recurrent nature of attacks for life. General dietary advice around regular meals and fluid intake; restriction of caffeine based products and fizzy drinks; limiting high fibre and resistant starch often helps relieve bloating symptoms. Antispasmodic agents are sometimes helpful when offered with advice on life style changes. For those patients with diarrhoea predominant IBS–loperamide should be used as the anti-motility of agent of choice–aiming for a Bristol stool chart consistency of 4 (Fig 7.1).

Sometimes laxatives (not lactulose) are helpful in constipation predominant IBS, however fibre is not beneficial and may cause an increase in symptoms (12). Tricyclic antidepressants are useful at a low dose (5–10mg increasing to a maximum of 30mg) for their analgesic effects (13). If tricyclics are ineffective then a selective serotonin inhibitor may help.

A study by Creed (14) suggests that one of the most cost effective treatments long term is cognitive behavioural therapy showing a significant health care cost reduction

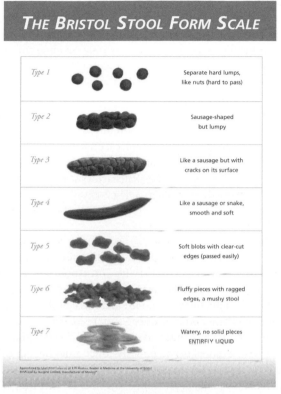

Fig. 7.1 The Bristol Stool form Scale. Reproduced by kind permission of Dr KW Heaton, Reader in Medicine at the University of Bristol. © 2000 Norgine Pharmaceuticals Ltd.

a year after treatment. Patients undergoing hypnotherapy also show long term improvement in symptom relief. In a series of 204 patients, 71% showed initial improvement with hypnotherapy and 81% maintained their improvement over time (15).

In summary, patients with IBS should not be over-investigated and should be treated with dietary and lifestyle alterations and reassurance. Further treatment may include constipating agents, laxatives, tricyclics at low dose and psychological therapy or hypnotherapy.

Conservative treatment for incontinence

Faecal incontinence is a sign or symptom but not a diagnosis. A full history and examination is required to gain an understanding of the causes, mechanism of incontinence and what investigations or treatment may be required. The treatment of faecal incontinence depends on its cause and underlying pathology. Reversible factors should be addressed before attempting medical and then surgical treatment.

Although incontinence may affect 1–10% of adults, probably 1% have such signifi-cant symptoms that it adversely affects their quality of life. The recent NICE guidelines have emphasised the social stigmatisation of these symptoms and placed significant emphasis on managing the psychological aspects and providing emotional support, as well as helping to maintain dignity for these patients (16). Simple help with skin care and access to disabled toilets can transform the patient's ability to manage their problem.

Before addressing the problem of incontinence, underlying conditions should be addressed. These include faecal loading, potentially treatable causes of diarrhoea (eg inflammatory bowel disease), cancer or polyps, prolapse, rectocele or haemorrhoids.

Once pathology has been identified and treated, residual incontinence should be treated by aiming to help the patient pass a satisfactory stool at a predictable time with ideal stool consistency (Bristol stool chart 4. Fig 7.1).

Dietary changes

Whilst ensuring a well balanced diet, patients with poor sphincter tone often have incontinence to flatus as well as stools (with soft stools being worse than firm). Excluding stimulants such as, caffeine, artificial sweeteners, nicotine and alcohol may improve continence by reducing the amount and force of the stool arriving into the rectum. A low fibre diet will aim to produce a more formed stool and also limit the amount of wind; this should be combined with a reasonable fluid intake. Patients with incontinence may have a global pelvic floor dysfunction following childbirth trauma and sometimes find that they are unable to defaecate or empty the rectum with a hard stool. These patients may still benefit from a low fibre diet creating a hard stool with which they no longer leak and some form of rectal emptying aid once a day to empty their rectum (see above).

Medication

Some medications may be associated with more loose stools (eg metformin) and an alternative drug may help limit the change in consistency and prevent faecal incontinence.

After dietary and medication changes the next approach to stool consistency mani-pulation is to prescribe an anti-diarrhoeal drug. Patients who have urge incontinence with soft stools or even with normal type stools often do very well with a very low dose of loperamide hydrochloride. This comes in a syrup form, which allows patients to titrate closely the amount of loperamide (2 teaspoons = 1 tablet). Occasionally patients develop abdominal pain with this and these patients should be offered Codeine Phosphate or Co-phenotrope instead. Patients should not be offered loperamide if they have an acute flare of ulcerative colitis, hard or infrequent stools, or diarrhoea without a diagnosed cause. It should also be avoided in pregnancy and whilst breast feeding. It is usually beneficial to start the loperamide at 1 tsp or less and to advise patients to use the loperamide to manipulate their bowel movements and consistency (aiming for Bristol stool chart 4) rather than allowing their bowel movements to control their lifestyle. Occasionally patients may benefit from a combination of a bulking agent (eg Fybogel™) and a constipating agent when they need a reasonable amount of stool in order to be able to defaecate.

Many of these patients have injuries or problems post-childbirth; they have poor pelvic floor muscles and a reduced recto-anal angle which contributes to their incontinence. These patients should be referred for physiotherapy, electrical stimulation and management within the continence advisory service. This gives them access to a group of professionals who are readily available to help manage their needs for both pads and anal plugs, and who can then provide a link back into the secondary health care when appropriate.

Patients who continue to have episodes of faecal incontinence after this initial management, may need to be referred to a specialist continence service where they can undertake pelvic floor retraining, bowel retraining, biofeedback, electrical stimulation, or rectal irrigation (see above).

Patients with poor internal sphincter function will tend to suffer from passive leakage (with or without urge incontinence–as a consequence of concomitant external sphincter damage). These patients are often unaware of the leakage until they feel a dampness in their underwear or have stained underwear. They need an empty rectum in order to try to limit the leakage, alternatively they need firm stools remaining in their rectum. In these patients a combination of a constipating agent (loperamide) and a rectal evacuatory aid (suppository or irrigation system) may help to limit the leakage.

Post defaecatory leakage is often lessened with the help of a rectal evacuatory aid in the case of a non emptying rectum or a rectocele. Patients who do not wish for more definitive treatment for mucosal or haemorrhoidal prolapse may have less post defaecatory leakage with simple cleaning measures post defaecation using E45 cream on the toilet paper or showering after defaecation.

Biofeedback

The Cochrane review of biofeedback and/or sphincter exercises for the treatment of faecal incontinence (17) found a paucity of well designed studies to examine these treatments for faecal incontinence. Only three studies were methodologically sound and no study reported a major difference in outcome between any method of biofeedback or exercises when compared to other conservative treatment. Indeed the paper from St Marks (18) found that conservative treatment improved continence, quality of life and psychological well-being in the short and medium term but neither pelvic floor exercises nor biofeedback gave any additional benefit.

What may be of benefit is pelvic floor muscle training during pregnancy and after birth for reducing both urinary and faecal incontinence (19). Women receiving pelvic floor muscle training were about half as likely to report faecal incontinence post childbirth.

If these simple managements have failed or further treatment is required it is suggested by NICE that patients should be referred to a specialist continence service (16) for consideration for further investigations and surgery where appropriate.

Key points

- Patients with faecal incontinence should have simple dietary advice and medication in order to manipulate their stool consistency into a manageable firm stool
- Advice with regard to anal hygiene, pads and lifestyle often helps in managing from day to day
- Further assessment by specialist services will be needed in order to decide if other surgical treatments are necessary.

Editor's summary

It is generally good practice to manage pelvic floor patients initially by conservative means: those responding will avoid invasive intervention. Yet for some this approach will simply delay optimal surgical treatment. The challenge is to try and select patients who are unlikely to benefit from a conservative approach and offer early surgery. Unfortunately, for most of the last 15 years, a conservative approach was the mainstay of care, particularly for those with chronic constipation. As a result, surgeons lost interest in making specific pelvic floor diagnoses: why differentiate conditions when it did not influence treatment? It remains unclear from biofeedback data if patient subsets do particularly well or badly. We generally recommend that biofeedback, which is very labour-intensive, is used empirically only if patients have mild symptoms or are less fit for surgery. All others should be fully worked up including proctography. This will ensure that in the future patients are better stratified, and patients with clear-cut indications for surgery and relative contra-indications for biofeedback (eg unrecognized external rectal prolapse) are not overlooked.

References

1. Talley NJ, Weaver AL, Zinsmeister AR, Melton LJ, 3rd. Functional constipation and outlet delay: a population-based study. *Gastroenterology*. 1993;**105**:781–90.
2. Talley NJ, Fleming KC, Evans JM, O'Keefe EA, Weaver AL, et al. Constipation in an elderly community: a study of prevalence and potential risk factors. *Am J Gastroenterol*. 1996;**91**:19–25.
3. Johanson JF, Sonnenberg A, Koch TR. Clinical epidemiology of chronic constipation. *J Clin Gastroenterol*. 1989;**11**:525–36.
4. Chatoor D, Emmnauel A. Constipation and evacuation disorders. *Best Pract Res Clin Gastroenterol*. 2009;**23**:517–30.
5. Williams NS, Hughes SF, Stuchfield B. Continent colonic conduit for rectal evacuation in severe constipation. *Lancet*. 1994;**343**:1321–4.
6. Crawshaw AP, Pigott L, Potter MA, Bartolo DC. A retrospective evaluation of rectal irrigation in the treatment of disorders of faecal continence. *Colorectal Dis*. 2004;**6**:185–90.

7. Heymen S, Scarlett Y, Jones K, Ringel Y, Drossman D, et al. Randomized, controlled trial shows biofeedback to be superior to alternative treatments for patients with pelvic floor dyssynergia-type constipation. *Dis Colon Rectum*. 2007;**50**:428–41.

8. Chiotakakou-Faliakou E, Kamm MA, Roy AJ, Storrie JB, Turner IC. Biofeedback provides long-term benefit for patients with intractable, slow and normal transit constipation. *Gut*. 1998;**42**:517–21.

9. Brown SR, Donati D, Seow-Choen F, Ho YH. Biofeedback avoids surgery in patients with slow-transit constipation: report of four cases. *Dis Colon Rectum*. 2001;**44**:737–9; discussion 9–40.

10. Drossman DA, Camilleri M, Mayer EA, Whitehead WE. AGA technical review on irritable bowel syndrome. *Gastroenterology*. 2002;**123**:2108–31.

11. National Institute for Health and Clinical Excellence. Irritable bowel syndrome in adults: Diagnosis and management of irritable bowel syndrome in primary care. CG61. London: National Institute for Health and Clinical Excellence; 2008.

12. Snook J, Shepherd HA. Bran supplementation in the treatment of irritable bowel syndrome. *Aliment Pharmacol Ther*. 1994;**8**:511–4.

13. Jackson JL, O'Malley PG, Tomkins G, Balden E, Santoro J, et al. Treatment of functional gastrointestinal disorders with antidepressant medications: a meta-analysis. *Am J Med*. 2000;**108**:65–72.

14. Creed F, Fernandes L, Guthrie E, Palmer S, Ratcliffe J, et al. The cost-effectiveness of psychotherapy and paroxetine for severe irritable bowel syndrome. *Gastroenterology*. 2003;**124**:303–17.

15. Gonsalkorale WM, Miller V, Afzal A, Whorwell PJ. Long term benefits of hypnotherapy for irritable bowel syndrome. *Gut*. 2003;**52**:1623–9.

16. National Institute for Health and Clinical Excellence. Faecal incontinence: the management of faecal incontinence in adults. CG49. London: National Institute for Health and Clinical Excellence; 2007.

17. Norton C, Cody JD, Hosker G. Biofeedback and/or sphincter exercises for the treatment of faecal incontinence in adults. *Cochrane Database Syst Rev*. 2006;**3**:CD002111.

18. Norton C, Chelvanayagam S, Wilson-Barnett J, Redfern S, Kamm MA. Randomized controlled trial of biofeedback for fecal incontinence. *Gastroenterology*. 2003;**125**:1320–9.

19. Hay-Smith J, Morkved S, Fairbrother KA, Herbison GP. Pelvic floor muscle training for prevention and treatment of urinary and faecal incontinence in antenatal and postnatal women. *Cochrane Database Syst Rev*. 2008;**4**:CD007471.

Chapter 8

Three compartments–working with a multidisciplinary team

Karen Nugent

Background

It is hardly surprising, considering the mechanisms of injury resulting in pelvic floor problems in the colorectal patient, that many of these patients have co-existing urological and gynaecological problems. The anatomy of the pelvic floor, both muscular and neurological, suggests that damage to one part of the anatomy may well result in damage to a closely related organ. Traditionally the pelvic floor has been divided into compartments; anterior, middle, and posterior; with each part being looked after by a separate group of surgeons (urologists, gynaecologists and coloproctologists). This has often led to multiple procedures at different times and the patient's problems rarely being addressed as a whole, but as separate parts. This is despite the fact, that over many years the co-existence of problems has been recognized.

There have been many studies examining the relationship of faecal incontinence (FI) and urinary incontinence (UI) over many years, some from the gynaecological point of view and others from the coloproctologists. In a study from the Cleveland Clinic Florida (1) replies were received from 51 patients operated on for FI and 32 patients operated on for rectal prolapse (and also a control group). Over 50% of both groups of colorectal patients had UI. Genital prolapse was present in 17% of those with FI and 34% of those who had been operated on for rectal prolapse.

A recent gynaecological study looked at 800 consecutive patients assessing them for symptoms of both UI and FI. Overall, 29% had UI and 13% FI. 57% of patients with FI also had UI, whereas 26% of UI patients also complained of FI. Parity and episiotomy were associated with UI as well as FI (2). This suggests that the mechanism of delivery can damage anterior, middle, and posterior compartments.

Pelvic floor anatomy

The pelvic floor is made up of a gutter-shaped sheet of muscles, the pelvic diaphragm (3) through which the urethra, vagina, and anus exit in the midline. The muscles of the pelvic diaphragm arise from the ischium (ischio-coccygeus), the pubis and arcus tendinus (leavtor ani muscle). The fibres then coalesce into the ano-coccygeal raphe and onto the coccyx. The perineal branch of the fourth sacral nerve and branches from the inferior rectal nerve innervate the muscles. The function of the pelvic floor is divided into postural and contractile.

Pelvic floor function

When standing upright the weight of the viscera falls onto the pubic bones anteriorly, and posteriorly onto the perineal body. Damage to the perineal body during childbirth may result in excess movement in this region during standing. Abdominal pressure increases are accompanied by contraction of the abdominal wall, diaphragm and parts of the pelvic floor muscles. This occurs in coughing and sneezing as well as micturition and defaecation, although parts of the pelvic floor musculature also have to relax to allow the process to take place. This complex contraction and relaxation process helps to maintain continence during exercise and also prevents prolapse from occurring.

Pelvic floor dysfunction

Weakness, structurally or functionally, to the pelvic floor complex of muscles may result in loss of function to one or more of the structures running through the muscles. Dysfunction occurs as a result of direct muscle damage, or stretching, or neurological damage (eg prolonged labour or forceps delivery). It is said that any stretch of a somatic nerve of more than 12% can lead to permanent damage to that nerve (4). Damage to the fibro-muscular layers between organs can lead to herniation between compartments. Rectoceles, cystoceles and enteroceles, which result from these herniations, may present with structural or functional symptoms. An understanding of the problems which may ensue in other compartments than the primary one for a particular specialist, as well as knowledge of the treatments available, allows the patient to be treated as a whole person rather than a series of separate problems.

A pelvic floor multidisciplinary team

The concept of a multidisciplinary team (MDT) approach for patient care has been popularised within the cancer field. The theory behind involving different disciplines early on the management of these types of patients, is to optimise patient care and make the patient journey as seamless as possible. The complexity of pelvic floor disorders lends itself well to a multidisciplinary approach and although algorithms to assist management of these patients exist (5), patients often present with a mixture of symptoms across all three compartments requiring expertise from members of many departments. Different approaches to bring the specialties together have been used in different hospitals.

Multidisciplinary clinics

Joint colorectal-urogynaecology clinics

Letters of referral, which include details of mixed compartment problems, lend themselves to the patient being seen in a joint clinic. The group at St George's Hospital in London set up a monthly joint clinic in 1994 to assess complex patients (6). The patients were seen with the results of investigations and a treatment plan formulated; 35% were managed conservatively, 25% underwent a colorectal procedure, 18% a uro-gynaecological procedure, and 20% a joint operation. The Mayday Hospital

(Croydon, UK) joint clinic examined the outcomes in 113 cases. The median number of clinic visits was two (7). There was a mean of three symptoms per patient and 25% ended-up undergoing a combined procedure. Patient satisfaction was high (85%); perceived advantages included: savings in the number of hospital visits, a joint examination and management plan as well as financial benefit (parking, transport, childcare and time off work).

The advantage of this type of approach is that it allows patients to have a single consultation and examination by both specialists. However it requires good, well-written letters of referral, which highlight the potential for multiple disciplines to be involved. Patients may need to be seen at the hospital, sometimes several times, and undergo multiple tests. Unfortunately, many patients do not disclose the full nature of their pelvic floor problems at a consultation with their general practitioner and it is only when seen at a secondary care clinic and when targeted questions are asked that the problems with multiple compartments are uncovered.

Many patients will undergo conservative treatment as a whole or part of their treatment for their pelvic floor problem. Physiotherapy and biofeedback may augment surgical results and should be started early. The model for some hospitals (eg The Royal London) is that patients are initially seen in a consultant nurse-led clinic and triaged for urological and colorectal pelvic floor problems. Investigations and initial treatment can then be organized and only those requiring assessment for consideration of a surgical procedure return to a joint or individual doctor led clinic. The Cleveland Clinic also runs a similar nurse-led initial triage history taking service. The nurse then schedules the appropriate investigations and further consultations (8).

The advantages of this type of system are that patients have a full history taken of all compartments and all initial treatment and investigations are ordered before triaging the patient to either a urogynaecology, colorectal, or combined clinic. The system takes time to set up and needs a well qualified nurse lead/consultant who has had training in the assessment of all compartments as well as the ability to order tests and instigate initial treatment. It is otherwise highly efficient for patients and doctors.

In Southampton we run a 'one-stop pelvic floor clinic' staffed by a colorectal consultant, biofeedback sister and pelvic floor practitioner. Patients with complex disorders and those travelling from long distances are seen and assessed within this specialist clinic. Patient questionnaires on incontinence, constipation and quality of life are administered on arrival. The patient then has a full urological, gynaecological and colorectal history taken. The patient is examined on a gynaecological couch. Uterine descent is assessed as well as the presence and size of rectocele and cystocele both at rest and under straining. The rectum is examined using a sigmoidoscope and proctoscope. The pelvic floor tone is assessed vaginally, as well as the resting and squeeze anal tone.

The patient then undergoes perineal, transvaginal and transanal ultrasound (see chapter 20). If anorectal physiology and/or biofeedback are required, the patient has these tests performed. The treatment plan is outlined and any initial treatment started. The pelvic floor practitioner then arranges to contact the patient at four weeks to assess treatment progression. Any combined or individual surgeon procedures are discussed and the patient is listed for surgery. As there is no urogynaecologist present, the listing of patients for urogynaecology interventions requires trust between colleagues.

Surgery

It is well recognized that surgical repair of one pelvic floor compartment sometimes leads to deterioration in another. This is especially true after Burch colposuspension, when there seems to be an accelerated deterioration in genital prolapse. It is not possible however, to predict the patients in whom this may occur (9).

Patients who have undergone a multidisciplinary approach to their diagnosis may quite rightly expect to have any procedures done simultaneously. It is important to know whether there is relatively more or less morbidity before undertaking procedures jointly. A study from the Cleveland Clinic looked at 44 patients undergoing an anterior sphincter repair for incontinence (20 as a single procedure and 24 in combination with procedures for pelvic organ prolapse (10). Outcomes were similar in both groups and 22 were pleased to have had both procedures done concomitantly. The operative time and hospital costs were significantly more in the combined group but there was no significant difference in length of stay. A combined approach offers the benefit of an overall decrease in hospital stay and time off work (when compared to two separate admissions) as well as a reduced exposure to anaesthetics. The outcome in these patients did not appear to be compromised.

Complex pelvic floor prolapse is a common problem with 50% of parous women over the age of 50 years old having a degree of pelvic organ prolapse (11). Recurrent prolapse also occurs in a significant number of women who have already undergone surgery and it is essential to assess all three compartments before deciding on the appropriate treatment options. In a recent study from the Cleveland Clinic (12) the operative time for combined surgery was almost double as was the blood loss, but recurrence rates were low.

The type of surgery will be based on the expertise of the local units but our unit favours the approach used in Leeds of combining rectopexy with sacrocolpopexy (13). A novel ventral approach pioneered in Leuven (14) and employed in Bristol (15) and Oxford (16) combines these procedures into one. Laparoscopic ventral rectopexy with concomitant sacrocolpopexy and posterior colporraphy is employed for the co-treatment of middle and posterior compartment prolapse. The results from all three centres confirm this approach to be safe, effective, and reproducible. The downside of the more traditional joint operating is the requirement to have two surgeons available for a list where only half of the surgery is being done by one of them at any point in time. We have addressed this in Southampton by running two lists alongside each other.

Functioning of the MDT

The MDT should encompass all specialists required to treat these complex patients. The team should meet to discuss not only difficult cases but also to develop an understanding of each other's roles, expertise and outcomes from differing treatments. Developing good relationships across the variety of disciplines allows for more rapid transfer of patients through the necessary treatment and investigations. The frequency of meetings will depend on the patient load and referral practice in each unit (5).

The Southampton MDT model is to meet once a month to discuss cases and concepts. Pivotal to the group is a pelvic floor radiologist who can interpret and undertake quality magnetic resonance (MR) proctograms and defaecating proctograms as well as pelvic floor ultrasound. Pelvic floor physiotherapists, biofeedback nurses, and physiologists are all essential members of the team. We are also fortunate in having a motility gastroenterologist, a pain specialist and a liaison psychiatrist attend these meetings. All patient discussions are recorded on an MDT page within the hospital intranet. The meetings are coordinated by the pelvic floor practitioner.

Treatment options and understanding of the problems of the whole pelvic floor are expanding. Understanding the role of newer procedures requires keeping up to date with the literature and attending training courses where appropriate. It is important to remember that surgery to patients with a benign disease, albeit, causing a poor quality of life, may cause morbidity and even occasionally mortality. Many units only have one colorectal surgeon specializing in pelvic floor disorders and may remain isolated; from this arose the concept of a regional pelvic floor MDT.

The longest established one in the UK is the Southern Pelvic Floor MDT. This meets every three months and colorectal surgeons from a wide area (Truro to Ashford) meet to discuss cases with each other and when possible, an interested radiologist and urogynaecologist also attend. Minutes of discussions are taken and decisions with regard to procedures are made. The surgeon is then asked to report back with the results. The group of surgeons are encouraged to attend an operating day the following day at the hosting hospital to learn procedures and techniques from each other.

- ◆ Colorectal pelvic floor disorders often occur as a result of widespread pelvic floor damage to either nerves or muscles

- ◆ Other organs in the anterior and middle compartment may also be compromised either structurally or functionally, and a thorough understanding of the nature of vaginal and urinary problems should be fostered through working in a multidisciplinary approach

- ◆ Several models of outpatient management have been used, and from the patient's perspective, combined working means fewer visits and less costs in making the diagnoses and planning further treatment

- ◆ Combined surgery does not seem to compromise outcomes (though data are sparse), but theatre time is prolonged and the availability of two surgeons is required

- ◆ It must be remembered that surgery in one compartment may unpredictably improve or worsen symptoms in other compartments, suggesting a more cautious step-wise approach is sometimes warranted.

References

1. Gonzalez-Argente FX, Jain A, Nogueras JJ, Davila GW, Weiss EG, et al . Prevalence and severity of urinary incontinence and pelvic genital prolapse in females with anal incontinence or rectal prolapse. *Dis Colon Rectum* 2001;**44**:920–6.

2. Ekin M, Kupelioglu LC, Yasar L, Savan K, Akcig Z, et al. The coexistence of anal incontinence in women with urinary incontinence. *Arch Gynecol Obstet* 2009;**280**:971–4.

3. Last RJ. Anatomy-regional and applied. 6th edn. ed. [S.l.]: Edinburgh; Churchill; 1978.

4. Davila GW. Concept of the Pelvic Floor as a Unit. In: Davila GW, Ghoniem GM, Wexner SD, editors. *Pelvic floor dysfunction: a multidisciplinary approach*. New York; London: Springer; 2006. p. 3–6.

5. Chatoor D, Soligo M, Emmanuel A. Organising a clinical service for patients with pelvic floor disorders. *Best Pract Res Clin Gastroenterol*. 2009;**23**:611–20.

6. Nager CW, Kumar D, Kahn MA, Stanton SL. Management of pelvic floor dysfunction. *Lancet*. 1997;**350**:1751.

7. Kapoor DS, Sultan AH, Thakar R, Abulafi MA, Swift RI, et al. Management of complex pelvic floor disorders in a multidisciplinary pelvic floor clinic. *Colorectal Dis* 2008;**10**:118–23.

8. Davila GW, Ghoniem GM, Wexner SD . Pelvic floor dysfunction: a multidisciplinary approach. London: Springer; 2008.

9. Kjolhede P, Noren B, Ryden G. Prediction of genital prolapse after Burch colposuspension. *Acta Obstet Gynecol Scand* 1996;**75**:849–54.

10. Halverson AL, Hull TL, Paraiso MF, Floruta C. Outcome of sphincteroplasty combined with surgery for urinary incontinence and pelvic organ prolapse. *Dis Colon Rectum* 2001;**44**:1421–6.

11. Subak LL, Waetjen LE, van den Eeden S, Thom DH, Vittinghoff E, et al. Cost of pelvic organ prolapse surgery in the United States. *Obstet Gynecol* 2001;**98**:646–51.

12. Riansuwan W, Hull TL, Bast J, Hammel JP. Combined Surgery in Pelvic Organ Prolapse is Safe and Effective. *Colorectal Dis* 2009;**12**(3):188–92

13. Lim M, Sagar PM, Gonsalves S, Thekkinkattil D, Landon C. Surgical management of pelvic organ prolapse in females: functional outcome of mesh sacrocolpopexy and rectopexy as a combined procedure. *Dis Colon Rectum*. 2007;**50**:1412–21.

14. D'Hoore A, Cadoni R, Penninckx F. Long-term outcome of laparoscopic ventral rectopexy for total rectal prolapse. *Br J Surg* 2004;**91**(11):1500–5.

15. Slawik S, Soulsby R, Carter H, Payne H, Dixon AR. Laparoscopic ventral rectopexy, posterior colporrhaphy and vaginal sacrocolpopexy for the treatment of recto-genital prolapse and mechanical outlet obstruction. *Colorectal Dis* 2008;**10**(2): 138–43.

16. Collinson R, Wijffels N, Cunningham C and Lindsey I. Laparoscopic ventral rectopexy for internal rectal prolapse: short-term functional results. *Colorectal Dis* 2010;**12**:97–104.

Part B

Clinical Syndromes

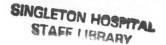
Chapter 9

Internal rectal prolapse

Ian Lindsey

Introduction

Internal rectal prolapse (IRP) is an invagination of the rectum into itself (Fig. 9.1). It is also known as occult rectal prolapse or rectal intussusception, and perhaps the variable nomenclature has contributed to the doubts surrounding its proper treatment. It is condition with a chequered surgical career. Its first cousin, external rectal prolapse, has always been regarded as a clear-cut surgical condition. Yet for various reasons, when a rectal prolapse invaginates and does not quite protrude from the anal verge, it has been regarded as quite a different condition: seen as a variant of normal and not appropriate for surgical remedy. Yet just external prolapse must represent an advanced stage of rectal prolapse disease, so IRP must be a precursor to more advanced prolapse: it is unimaginable that the day before someone develops an external prolapse, their pelvic floor was normal and they did not have a high-grade IRP. The conditions must be related and exist on a spectrum of prolapse disease. Findings at pelvic laparoscopy alone would attest to this.

IRP is part of the descending perineum syndrome, a term first coined by Parks. It included such demonstrable pathoanatomical entities as rectocele (with or without enterocele) and pelvic floor descent. Our understanding in Oxford is that IRP is the central component of this commonly co-existing triad including rectocele and descent. Therefore it is the main focus of our therapeutic intentions. Other centres have focussed on rectocele, for example the unit in Auckland will offer transanal rectocele repair by anterior Delorme's as a first operation (1) (see chapter 11). If symptoms are not improved, IRP is suspected and more substantial surgery may then be employed. Our understanding is that rectocele is uncommonly isolated (10%), and usually coexists with IRP (80%), though IRP may occasionally be seen without rectocele (10%).

Proctographic evidence: past and present

Several factors have led to a historical, widely-held and still largely prevailing view of IRP as a variant of normal. The small, widely-quoted proctographic study by Shorvon in the late 1980s demonstrated that 20% of asymptomatic normal volunteers were noted to have a high-grade IRP (an intussusception impinging on or entering into the anal canal) (2). Two large proctographic series of symptomatic patients showed that IRP seldom progressed to external rectal prolapse (3, 4).

More recently there has been a radiological re-evaluation of IRP in asymptomatic normal volunteers. Dvorkin showed that IRP is morphologically more advanced

Internal rectal prolapse

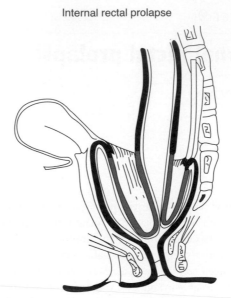

Fig. 9.1 Internal rectal prolapse.

in symptomatic patients, with significantly more full-thickness and anal intussusceptions rather than mucosal, shallower, rectal intussusceptions in asymptomatic individuals (5). These findings are supported by Pomerri who showed that the rectal folding thickness and the ratio between intussuscipiens diameter and the intussusceptum lumen diameter were significantly greater in the symptomatic rather than asymptomatic volunteers (6). The proctographic series could also be criticized. In one series, the most advanced prolapses were operated upon, leaving the lesser prolapses for follow up (3). It is unsurprising that this second group, highly selected and biased, rarely progressed to external prolapse. These studies were also limited in their follow up of patients. A study of the natural history of IRP suggests that progression to external prolapse is variable and slow (7) (Fig. 9.2). The time-line of progression of IRP to external prolapse is beyond the duration of most surgical studies to capture it. Males and nulliparous women appear to develop symptoms at a younger age and progress to higher grades of prolapse faster than parous females.

Classification of IRP

There have been several classifications of IRP but few have become established. The key to classifications becoming popular is simplicity and utility. The more complicated, the less inclination there is to use it, and the classification must lend itself to practical application.

The Oxford Prolapse Grading system divides IRP into 4 grades according to the most caudal descent of the lead point of the intussusceptum relative to the rectocele and anal sphincter (Table 9.1 and Fig. 9.3) (8). This breaks down into high and low rectal and anal intussusceptions. Grade 5 prolapse is external rectal prolapse. Generally speaking patients with grades 3–5 prolapse are suitable for surgery. Other grading

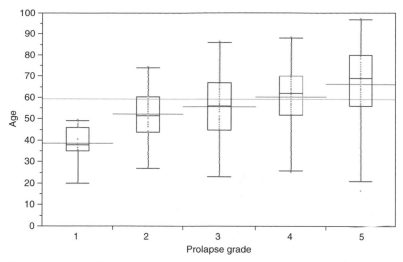

Fig. 9.2 Age (mean) versus prolapse grade.

systems used include that used by Shorvon (7 grades) (2), Pescatori, and the system used in Leuven, Belgium (grades I-III).

Symptoms

Previous proctographic studies have overestimated this group but undoubtedly some patients have high-grade prolapse without functional disturbance. When these patients do progress to develop an external rectal prolapse they do so without a functional prodrome. The proportion of external rectal patients who present without a functional prodrome is about 20% (unpublished personal series) (9).

It is not clear why some patients with IRP remain asymptomatic. One theory is that some patients are particularly susceptible to developing symptoms associated with

Table 9.1 Oxford Rectal Prolapse Grade

		Grade of Rectal Prolapse	Radiological characteristics of Rectal Prolapse
Internal (RI)	Rectal-rectal Intussusception (RRI)	I (high rectal)	Descends no lower than proximal limit of the rectocele
		II (low rectal)	Descends into the level of the rectocele, but not onto sphincter/anal canal
	Rectal–anal Intussusception (RAI)	III (high anal)	Descends onto sphincter/anal canal
		IV (low anal)	Descends into sphincter/anal canal
External (ERP)	External rectal prolapse (ERP)	V (overt rectal prolapse)	Protrudes from anus

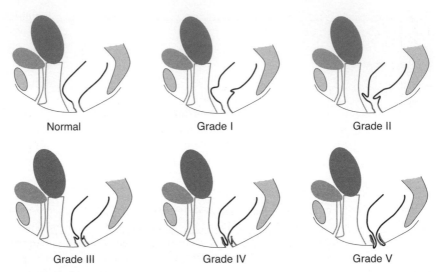

Fig. 9.3 Oxford Rectal Prolapse Grade.
Dark grey = Box-and-whisker plots.
Light grey lines = average age per prolapse grade.
Grey line = overall average age.

structural anatomical abnormalities. Patients with so-called 'visceral hypersensitivity' are commonly seen with functional disorders (10). Such patients have been noted to frequently have a heavy burden of psychological symptoms. This has given rise to a temptation to provide a psychological explanation for such symptoms, and would explain the significant apparent psychological overlay in many of these patients (11).

When IRP gives rise to symptoms, patients can present in several different ways with different symptoms and symptom combinations. The classically recognized symptom is obstructed defaecation (frequent ineffective evacuatory attempts), although sometimes stool infrequency in a pattern more usually attributed to slow transit constipation, or a variable pattern between both not uncommonly exists. Faecal incontinence is undoubtedly under-recognized as a symptom of IRP. It coexists with obstructed defaecation in about 60% of patients with high-grade internal prolapse coming to surgery (12). The remaining complain of either isolated obstructed defaecation (20%) or isolated faecal incontinence (20%). There is a high incidence of high-grade internal prolapse found on proctography in patients presenting with faecal incontinence with no significant structural or functional disturbance found on anorectal physiology and anal ultrasound (see chapter 3) (8). These patients were previously labelled as idiopathic faecal incontinence.

Other presentations include chronic idiopathic perineal pain (13) (see chapter 6) and solitary rectal ulcer syndrome (14) (see chapter 12). It is becoming apparent that in some patients IRP underlies more common proctological complaints, particularly recalcitrant problems, including chronic anal fissure and haemorrhoids (see chapter 14). It appears that there is a relationship between internal anal sphincter function and mode of presentation in IRP: those with poorer function and lower maximal resting pressures tend to present with faecal incontinence (or external prolapse); those with higher pressure, obstructed defaecation or solitary rectal ulcer, and those with highest, chronic idiopathic perineal pain (13).

Assessment

Clinical assessment

IRP can be suggested by clinical assessment during straining including digital rectal exam, rigid sigmoidoscopy (high take-off) and proctoscopy (low take-off). It is most evident anteriorly, and is distinguishable from mucosal prolapse by the smoothing out of the wrinkled mucosa as the prolapse descends into the anal canal.

Radiological assessment

The gold standard for diagnosing IRP remains proctography. It provides a very important hard-copy record of the degree of IRP that can be referred back to in order to justify surgical intervention. The intussusception can be seen as a space-occupying lesion in the contrast-filled rectum or anal canal. Most intussusceptions have their origin anteriorly (15) and this is best appreciated at proctoscopy. It is thought that the original lesion in the evolution of IRP is anterior mucosal prolapse (16). Despite their anterior origin, we are beginning to appreciate that some IRP are posterior-predominant and this may influence treatment approach.

Magnetic resonance imaging (MRI) and dynamic perineal ultrasound (see chapter 20) have been used to assess patients with descending perineum syndrome, but characterization of IRP has generally been inferior to that by proctography.

EUA rectum (operative assessment)

Ultimately, examination of the rectum under anaesthetic (EUA rectum) is a very accurate way of demonstrating an IRP and assessing its grade. It overcomes the limitations of proctography, though at the inconvenience of a general anaesthetic. It is of particular use when a significant IRP is suspected but cannot be confirmed on proctography. It is important that typical instrumentation such as an Eisenhammer retractor is not used as the long blades tend to splint the IRP in place and prevent it from descending to allow proper assessment. A circular anal dilator (CAD) device is used (Frankenman International Ltd, Hong Kong) which allows the prolapse to descend as far as it is able. Anterior or posterior predominance is noted.

Diagnostic laparoscopy

Occasionally the diagnosis of IRP proves extremely elusive and cannot be demonstrated at proctography or EUA. In these rare circumstances (always high take-off IRP), diagnostic laparoscopy and assessment of the shape of the pelvis and depth of the Douglas pouch will enable a diagnosis to be made or refuted.

Treatment

Conservative measures including biofeedback

Generally speaking a conservative approach is recommended at the outset. This would include laxatives, dietary advice and biofeedback/pelvic floor retraining (see chapter 7).

We would encourage a diagnostic workup before committing to a full six month course of biofeedback/pelvic floor retraining. This is because there is some early evidence from biofeedback data in our unit that a conservative approach is more likely to be successful with less advanced prolapse grades (Oxford grades 1 and 2). In addition, proctography may reveal an external rectal prolapse not demonstrated on clinical assessment, which is a clear indication for surgical intervention.

It is unclear how successful biofeedback is for IRP because patients have generally been not worked up and well stratified in the past. This was because 10–15 years ago, there were limited surgical options and surgical interest. Biofeedback was used as a rubbish bin for all undifferentiated patients with chronic constipation. Often no formal investigations were undertaken. We know that biofeedback works less well for chronic constipation than faecal incontinence (17). Beyond that, little else is known.

Surgery

The principles of surgery for IRP are by and large eliminating the intussusception either by fixation from above (rectopexy) or excision from below (stapled transanal rectal resection (STARR procedure)). However, despite ignorance about the precise physiological mechanisms involved, sacral neuromodulation may have a significant future role.

Posterior rectopexy (with or without resection)

A Cochrane analysis (18) including randomized, controlled studies concluded that posterior rectal mobilization in external rectal prolapse leads to autonomic rectal denervation and a hindgut neuropathy, with worse or new-onset constipation in about 50% of patients. Unsurprisingly posterior rectopexy has largely become discredited in IRP (19) because inducing a similar neural lesion and worsening constipation that was the very indication for surgery is not acceptable.

Some of these drawbacks can be offset by a resection-rectopexy and published results demonstrate reasonably good functional outcomes (20). However resected denervated hindgut makes a virtue out of a necessity, risks an anastomosis, and provides no direct co-treatment of middle compartment prolapse. Given that there is a nerve-sparing alternative not requiring an anastomosis, we believe a posterior approach, even with resection, cannot be recommended.

Laparoscopic ventral rectopexy

Laparoscopic ventral rectopexy for external prolapse was pioneered by D'Hoore and Penninckx (21) from Leuven, Belgium (see chapter 18). Recurrence rates are low (< 5%), constipation (75–80%) and faecal incontinence usually improve (85–90%) and rarely worsen. Exclusive to a ventral approach, middle compartment prolapse is effortlessly treated concurrently. Mortality (0%), morbidity (5–10%, mostly minor), and hospital stay (median 2 days) are extremely low and reassuringly the results are reproducible (22,23).

The features of laparoscopic ventral rectopexy that make it attractive for IRP are autonomic nerve-sparing and co-treatment of a range of prolapse-related pathoanatomical entities (rectocele, middle compartment prolapse and enterocele) (24).

The functional results of ventral rectopexy for IRP seem to generally mirror those for external prolapse, with an improvement in about 75–80% of patients with obstructed defaecation (25). This underlines the concept of it as a true autonomic nerve-sparing anti-prolapse procedure. It also supports the notion that IRP and external prolapse share many properties and exist on a spectrum of rectal prolapse disease. This idea has never truly been accepted in the past.

What about patients with colonic slow transit and outlet obstruction? About 30% of all patients attending the clinic at the Oxford Pelvic Floor Centre with chronic constipation will have slow transit constipation on a pellet study (26). About 85% of such patients will have a significant associated outlet obstruction (high-grade IRP) while 15% (about 5% of all patients) will have classical isolated slow transit constipation, with a normal proctogram. Therefore about one third of patients with outlet obstruction and high-grade IRP will have additional colonic slow transit (often in the second or third segments of the colorectum), and two thirds will have normal colonic transit. It was our initial policy to regard outlet obstruction with slow transit as a contraindication to IRP surgery. However, with the good results of ventral rectopexy in IRP with normal transit plus the pressure of referrals mainly from gastroenterology, these criteria were gradually relaxed. We expected these more complex patients to benefit less, and counselled them accordingly. However when their outcomes were reviewed, rather counter-intuitively, they appeared to benefit as much as those with normal colonic transit. In other words additional colonic slow transit did not adversely impact the results of surgery for IRP (27). D'Hoore et al. have shown that laparoscopic ventral rectopexy improves colonic transit time in the distal segment (distal third or rectosigmoid) of the colorectum (28).

Interestingly, faecal incontinence in IRP, the mechanism for which is unclear, improves more reliably than constipation (25). It is probable that internal rectal prolapse underlies many cases of faecal incontinence and may account for much of so-called idiopathic faecal incontinence. In Oxford proctography is routine in the work up for faecal incontinence (8), which is now an indication (with or out obstructed defaection) for ventral rectopexy (see chapter 4).

Failed ventral rectopexy, the concept of posterior residual prolapse and posterior STARR

In Oxford we use STARR mainly in the setting of a failed ventral rectopexy. About 75–80% of patients with obstructed defaecation secondary to IRP are successfully improved, leaving a cohort of 20–25% of patients who do not respond. Initially it was imagined that these patients had more underlying neural than mechanical aetiology in the mix and that perhaps sacral neuromodulation might be useful for this cohort. Postoperative proctography can sometimes be useful and disclose residual or recurrent posterior IRP. More often, however, it is unhelpful and we have found rectal EUA (with a CAD device) the assessment of choice after failed ventral rectopexy.

Why this cohort behaves differently to the 80% of patients in whom presumably both anterior and posterior IRP components, reduce and stay reduced, remains unclear. This is currently the subject of research, and it is our unconfirmed anecdotal impression that some patients have a posterior-predominant IRP from the beginning. In most patients (80%) ventral mesh will support posterior prolapse, but in the posterior-predominant IRP group it probably will not. In this setting, a posterior

STARR can be performed either at diagnostic EUA, or later if informed consent had not been given preoperatively. This approach of secondary complimentary posterior STARR improves about two-thirds of patient with persistent symptoms and posterior prolapse (unpublished data). Again it is our impression that patients suffer less urgency, typical of STARR, when just a posterior hemi-circumferential staple line is made.

Orr-Loygue rectopexy

The original description of Orr-Loygue rectopexy describes a full anterior and posterior rectal mobilization and support. Unfortunately high rates of constipation ensued. This would be predicted with our current understanding of posterior rectal mobilization and autonomic rectal denervation and the procedure fell out of favour except perhaps in France. However, the approach recognises the ventral origin of IRP, and with a modified restricted central posterior dissection Lazorthes recently appears to have achieved good functional results (29). It may well be that this modified incarnation of Orr-Loygue comes back into vogue outside of France.

STARR and Transtar

Stapled transanal rectal resection (STARR) is the other major new surgical treatment for IRP; it treats IRP by excision rather than reduction of the intussusception (see chapter 19). Although the success rates are generally similar (30), it has some advantages over laparoscopic ventral rectopexy. It is a perineal procedure and can be undertaken with spinal anaesthesia. It is also simpler to learn and perform.

There are disadvantages as well. It undoubtedly takes longer to obtain a good functional outcome compared to ventral rectopexy. Most patients complain of urgency, sometimes debilitating, and this may persist for several months. After ventral rectopexy, once patients are weaned from their postoperative laxative regime, they notice a significant functional benefit by four weeks if the procedure is successful. The STARR procedure is destructive, and the potential for complications is greater, though the risk of bleeding, anastomotic leak, sepsis and rectovaginal fistula appears to be quite small in well-trained hands. The PPH-01 stapler removes a fixed, standardized amount of prolapse, so the prolapse must not be too big to be completely excised by the stapler. Because of this limitation, a Contoured Transtar stapling technique has been used for a second generation procedure and this can remove variable-sized IRP and even external prolapse. Another disadvantage is that it is not suitable for high take-off IRP, though most IRP appears to be of the low take-off variety. It is also less suitable for the globally failing pelvic floor. Complex combinations of pelvic floor descent, IRP and enterocele are probably better off with an abdominal approach.

Sacral neural modulation (SNS)

The role of sacral neuromodulation for obstructed defaecation caused by IRP is unclear (see chapter 21). Data are most available for faecal incontinence, but there are some limited data for chronic constipation (31). Unfortunately causes for chronic constipation are largely lumped together and so therapeutic outcomes for subgroups including internal prolapse are unknown. Is in unclear exactly how SNS would improve function in obstructed defaecation but presumably some hindgut neural mechanism is involved. Currently in the UK, constipation is not an indication recognized by NICE guidance for SNS.

Key points

◆ IRP is the central pathoanatomical lesion in the legion of presentations and manifestations of pelvic floor disorders

◆ Defaecating proctography, while useful as a permanent documentary record of IRP, has its limitations and rectal EUA is the final arbiter of the presence or not of low take-off IRP

◆ Conservative management is generally favoured as initial treatment but subsets in whom this is unlikely to be successful need to be identified to allow early surgery

◆ Laparoscopic ventral rectopexy is the procedure that suits most contingencies; although LVR and STARR are generally complimentary rather than competing procedures

◆ A future challenge is to identify predictors of persistent posterior IRP after ventral rectopexy and develop preventative therapeutic modifications.

References

1. Abbas SM, Bissett IP, Neill ME et al. Long-term results of the anterior Delorme's operation in the management of symptomatic rectocele. *Dis Colon Rectum* 2005;**48**:317–22.

2. Shorvon PJ, McHugh S, Diamant NE, Somers S, Stevenson GW. Defecography in normal volunteers: results and implications. *Gut* 1989;**30**(12):1737–49.

3. Mellgren A, Schultz I, Johansson C, Dolk A. Internal rectal intussusception seldom develops into total rectal prolapse. *Dis Colon Rectum* 1997;**40**:817–20.

4. Choi JS, Hwang YH, Salum MR, Weiss EG, Pikarsky AJ, Nogueras JJ, Wexner SD. Outcome and management of patients with large rectoanal intussusception. *Am J Gastroenterol* 2001;**96**:740–4.

5. Dvorkin LS, Gladman MA, Epstein J, Scott SM, Williams NS, Lunniss PJ. Rectal intussusception in symptomatic patients is different from that in asymptomatic volunteers. *Br J Surg* 2005;**92**(7):866–72.

6. Pomerri F, Zuliani M, Mazza C, Villarejo F, Scopece A. Defecographic measurements of rectal intussusception and prolapse in patients and in asymptomatic subjects. *Am J Roentgenol* 2001;**176**(3):641–5.

7. Wijffels NA, Collinson R, Cunningham C, Lindsey I. What is the natural history of internal rectal prolapse. *Colorectal Dis* 2010;**12**:822–30.

8. Collinson R, Cunningham C, D'Costa H, Lindsey I. Rectal intussusception and unexplained faecal incontinence: findings of a proctographic study. *Colorectal Dis* 2009;**11**(1)77–83.

9. Franchelli L, Jones OM, Cunningham C, Lindsey I. (2009) No difference in patients with external rectal prolapse with and without bowel functional disturbance. (unpublished).

10. Walter S, Bodemar G, Hallbook O, Thorell LH. Sympathetic (electrodermal) activity during repeated maximal rectal distensions in patients with irritable bowel syndrome and constipation. *Neurogastroenterol Motil* 2008;**20**:43–52.

11. Miliacca C, Gagliardi G, Pescatori M. The 'draw-the-family test' in the preoperative assessment of anorectal diseases and psychological distress: a prospective controlled study. *Colorectal Dis* 2010;**12**:792–8.

12. Wijffels NA, Collinson R, Cunningham C, Lindsey I. Internal rectal prolapse: occult by name, occult by nature *Colorectal Dis* 2008;**10**(Suppl. 2)16. [abstr].

13. Hompes R, Jones OM, Cunningham C, Lindsey I. What causes chronic idiopathic perineal pain? *Colorectal Dis* 2010; **12**(Suppl. 1)16. [abstr].

14. Evans CE, Jones OM, Cunningham C, Lindsey I. Managing solitary rectal ulcer syndrome: Ignore the ulcer, treat the underlying posterior compartment prolapse *Colorectal Dis* 2010;**12**(Suppl. 1) 16. [abstr].

15. Broden B, Snellman B. Procidentia of the rectum studied with cineradiography. A contribution to the discussion of causative mechanism. *Dis Colon Rectum* 1968:**11**:330–47.

16. Sun WM, Read NW, Donnelly TC, Bannister JJ, Shorthouse AJ. A common pathophysiology for full thickness rectal prolapse, anterior mucosal prolapse and solitary rectal ulcer. *Br J Surg* 1989:**76**:290–5.

17. Koh CE, Young CJ, Young JM, Solomon MJ. Systematic review of randomized controlled trials of the effectiveness of biofeedback for pelvic floor dysfunction. *Br J Surg* 2008:**95**:1075–87.

18. Bachoo P, Brazzelli M, Grant A. Surgery for complete rectal prolapse in adults. *Cochrane Database Syst Rev* 2000; (2):CD001758. Review. Update in Cochrane Database Syst Rev. 2008; (4):CD001758.

19. Orrom WJ, Bartolo DC, Miller R, Mortensen NJ, Roe AM. Rectopexy is an ineffective treatment for obstructed defecation. *Dis Colon Rectum* 1991;**34**(1):41–6.

20. Tsiaoussis J, Chrysos E, Athanasakis E et al. Rectoanal intussusception: presentation of the disorder and late results of resection rectopexy. *Dis Colon Rectum* 2005;**48**:838–44.

21. D'Hoore A, Cadoni R, Penninckx F. Long-term outcome of laparoscopic ventral rectopexy for total rectal prolapse. *Br J Surg* 2004;**91**(11):1500–5.

22. Boons P, Collinson R, Cunningham C, Lindsey I. Laparoscopic anterior rectopexy for rectal prolapse improves constipation and avoids new-onset constipation. *Colorectal Dis* 2010;**12**:526–32.

23. Slawik S, Soulsby R, Carter H, Payne H, Dixon AR. Laparoscopic ventral rectopexy, posterior colporrhaphy and vaginal sacrocolpopexy for the treatment of recto-genital prolapse and mechanical outlet obstruction. *Colorectal Dis* 2008;**10**:138–43.

24. Samaranayake CB, Luo C, Plank AW, Merrie AE, Plank LD, Bissett IP. Systematic review on ventral rectopexy for rectal prolapse and intussception. *Colorectal Dis* 2010;**12**:504–12.

25. Collinson R, Wijffels N, Cunningham C and Lindsey I. Laparoscopic ventral rectopexy for internal rectal prolapse: short-term functional results. *Colorectal Dis* 2010;**12**:97–104.

26. Smyth E, McDonald R, Jones OM, Cunningham C, Lindsey I. Isolated slow transit constipation is a rare cause of chronic contipation. *Colorectal Dis* 2010;**12**(Suppl. 1):16. [abstr].

27. Harmston C, Wijffels NA, Cunningham C, Lindsey I. Colonic slow transit has no impact on the results of laparoscopic anterior rectopexy for internal rectal prolapse. *Colorectal Dis* 2009;**11**(Suppl. 1):7 [abstr].

28. D'Hoore A. New surgical techniques to correct rectal prolapse syndromes. PhD thesis, Chapter 7. *Laparoscopic Ventral Rectopexy in Symptomatic Patients with Rectal Intussusception.* Leuven University Press; 2007. pp. 107–28.

29. Portier G, Iovino F, Lazorthes F. Surgery for rectal prolapse: Orr-Loygue ventral rectopexy with limited dissection prevents postoperative-induced constipation without increasing recurrence. *Dis Colon Rectum* 2006;**49**:1136–40.

30. Boccasanta P, Venturi M, Stuto A, et al. Stapled transanal rectal resection for outlet obstruction: a prospective, multicenter trial. *Dis Colon Rectum* 2004:**47**:1285–9.

31. Holzer B, Rosen HR, Novi G et al. Sacral nerve stimulation in patients with severe constipation. *Dis Colon Rectum* 2008;**51**:524–29.

Chapter 10

Anismus

Chris Harmston

Background

Anismus has been described in the surgical literature as early as 1964, but it was Lennard-Jones who coined the phrase 'anismus', in comparison to the well described condition of vaginismus, in 1985 (1,2). It is best described as a functional disorder in which uncoordinated relaxation of the voluntary striated anal sphincter muscle occurs during attempted evacuation, resulting in outlet obstruction constipation. It is variously named spastic pelvic floor syndrome, dyssynergia or puborectalis syndrome. For the the sake of continuity it will be referred to as anismus in this text (3).

The incidence of anismus in the general population is not known, but in various series the incidence in constipated patients referred to secondary or tertiary care has been between 20% and 70%. We do know that it is more common in women, and in younger and middle aged individuals, although the demographics of patients with anismus are not completely understood. In the experience in Oxford about 15–20% of patients have a proctographic diagnosis of anismus, but about one quarter to one third of these (5%) will ultimately be classified as having true anismus.

Since its original description much has been spoken and written about the diagnosis, treatment, and indeed validity of anismus. This chapter aims to provide the reader with a modern, critical review and provide a practical algorithm for the management of patients with this condition (Fig. 10.1).

Diagnosis

Defining anismus

Early defining criteria for anismus hinged around the inability to expel a water filled rectal catheter and electromyography (EMG) confirmation of non relaxation of striated pelvic floor muscles in patients with constipation. This phenomenon does not normally occur in non-constipated controls, where either a rapid inhibition of puborectalis and the external sphincter complex, or a transient increase in recruitment followed by inhibition on continued straining occurs. These original criteria have formed the basis of a gold standard diagnosis of anismus. They do not, however, consider the presence or absence of propulsive forces present in the rectum on evacuation,

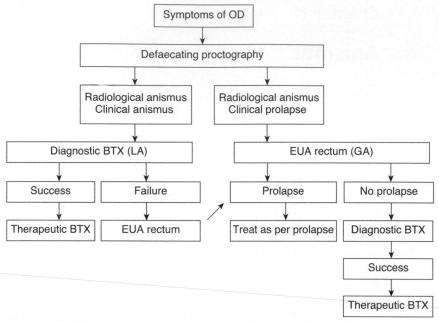

Fig. 10.1 Algorithm for the diagnosis and treatment of anismus.

and this led Roberts and co-workers to suggest a definition of anismus based on three criteria:

1. Demonstration of puborectalis EMG recuitment of more than 50%
2. Evidence of an adequate level of intrarectal pressure on straining (more than 50cm of water)
3. Presence of defective evacuation.

Whilst these definitions are adequate, presumptions are made regarding definition of defective evacuation, variably defined across most studies relating to anismus. It is reasonable therefore that the Rome III criteria for diagnosis of functional constipation is considered a prerequisite for a stringent diagnosis of anismus (table 10.1). A functional defaecatory disorder can then be diagnosed by the following criteria:

During repeated attempts to defaecate at least two of the following must also be present:

a) Evidence of impaired evacuation on balloon expulsion test or imaging
b) Inappropriate contraction of the pelvic floor muscles (ie anal sphincter or puborectalis) or less than 20% relaxation of basal resting pressure by manometry imaging or EMG
c) Inadequate propulsive forces assessed by manometry or imaging

Table 10.1 Rome III diagnostic criteria for functional constipation*

1. Two of the following must be present:

2. Straining during at least 25% of defaecations

3. Lumpy or hard stools on at least 25% of defaecations

4. Sensation of incomplete evacuation for at least 25% of defaecations

5. Manual manouvres to faciliatate at least 25% of defaecations

6. Fewer than three defaecations per week

7. Loose stools are rarely present without the use of laxatives

8. Insufficient criteria for irritable bowel syndrome

* for the previous three months with symptom onset at least 6 months prior to diagnosis

Which are further split into:

a) Dyssynergia (anismus) - which is the above with adequate propulsive forces

b) Inadequate defaecatory propulsion–which is the above with inadequate propulsive forces

It is obvious that this diagnostic pathway, although useful, is difficult to apply exactly for most practicing surgeons. It is likely that almost all surgical units do not have direct access to EMG, which has become a research tool, and are not able to effectively measure rectal propulsive forces. It is therefore more practical to determine what screening tools can be used to identify patients with anismus, or otherwise, so that effective treatment strategies can be proposed.

Symptoms

Patients with anismus are usually referred to secondary care with symptoms of chronic constipation, although patients my also present primarily with pain or anorectal disorders associated with straining. The majority of patients report an excessive need to strain, have a feeling of incomplete evacuation, and abdominal bloating; and around 50% of females (and 25% of males) are likely to use digitation to aid defaecation. It is likely that quality of life will be significantly affected, particulary in females. These are non-specific symptoms of chronic constipation, one must be aware that the symptoms of constipation are varied, and do not predict cause. Indicators considered pathognomonic by some, such as digitation, are highly specific but lack sensitivity.

Patients with anismus have higher levels of functional bowel disorders, depression and dypareunia as well as having a higher incidence of a range of upper gastrointestinal functional problems, such as globus, heartburn and functional chest pain. The patient may associate the onset of symptoms with a previous illness and in some it is associated with previous surgery such as appendicectomy, hysterectomy or gynaecological surgery. It is more common in women who have been sexually abused, an association that is stronger than that seen if one considers all patients with functional gastrointestinal disorders. The levels of abuse seen in different studies varies but has been reported as up to 20%. It is difficult to know if direct questioning to elicit this history should be employed routinely, and certainly the benefit of such a policy has never been tested. It does however make sense to treat patients with anismus in the same manner, regardless of past history.

Physical signs

A structured approach to the examination of patients with defaecatory disorders has been described in earlier chapters. The physical signs are highly predictive of anismus and may correlate with the radiological and manometric findings in patients with anismus. The key diagnostic feature on examination is the non relaxation of the puborectalis or external sphincter on straining. It is imperative to give a sound explanation of what is required of the patient. Sometimes in an apprehensive patient clinical findings of anismus may be elicited in the clinic, before the patient comprehends the instructions to bear down and relax their pelvic floor, rather than contract it, or overcomes their apprehension. It is important to repeat the instructions several times to see if clinical evidence of anismus is repeated or not.

Investigations

Defaecography

In 1995 Halligan and co-workers in a retrospective study showed that non evacuation at 30 seconds on proctography was 90% accurate in predicting anismus, compared to balloon expulsion and EMG (4) as gold standard. Importantly all controls evacuated contrast within 30 seconds, whereas 75% of patients with anismus did not evacuate more than 60% of contrast in this time. This yields a very simple radiographic end point–ability to evacuate 60% of contrast within thirty seconds. It is this simple rule that allowed us to more practically identify the majority of patients with anismus and exclude those without it: Halligan's diagnostic criteria became a simple, widely available surrogate for the more complex pre-existing gold standard, and has rendered EMG in a clinical setting obsolete.

Although sensitive, it has become apparent that these criteria are highly non-specific. We have data to show that inability to evacuate may also be associated with obstructed defaecation secondary to a mechanical rather than functional cause (discussed in more detail below). It is important therefore to be aware that treatment failure in suspected anismus may indicate a different pathology and prompt examination under anaesthetic (EUA).

As non-emptying on MRI is easily seen, along with contraction of puborectalis and non descent of the perineum, it seems logical that the same diagnostic principles can be applied to MRI defaecography. It would also seem logical that upright imaging in an open magnet system is mandatory. Despite all of this there are those who believe that imaging adds little to clinical examination when compared with physiology and/or balloon expulsion, as well as those that feel that over-diagnosis occurs regularly.

Electromyography

Measurement of the electrical activity in the external sphincter and puborectalis muscle, at rest and when active, can be recorded by insertion of fine wire electrodes into the sphincter complex, coupled to a standard electromyograph. It can be performed as either a laboratory or ambulatory investigation and has been considered as part of the gold standard of diagnosis of anismus. It is frequently used as a reference point to assess the specificity and sensitivity of other investigations. It is not, however, readily available, and although scientifically important is not likely to be used by clinicians in the day to day management of patients with anismus.

Anal manometry

Anal manometry, coupled with balloon expulsion, is commonly used as a diagnostic adjunct in patients with both constipation and incontinence, but its usefulness in clinical practice has been questioned. Anal pressure on evacuation can be estimated using manometric measurements on straining, confirmed by pelvic descent or passage of stool/flatus. A ratio in comparison with either mean resting pressure or maximum squeeze increment can then be calculated, some suggesting that this index correlates better with other diagnostic methods than absolute pressures (5). Otherwise an increase in pressure during straining is suggestive of anismus and a decrease in pressure on straining is likely to be normal. Patients in whom there is no pressure change may be deemed equivocal and warrant further investigation. In patients with anismus diagnosed on balloon expulsion tests and EMG, subjects had lower rectal pressures and higher anal canal pressures compared with other constipated patients (6)[6]. The correlation with other diagnostic modalities is variable, and it is likely that manometric diagnosis of anismus has a lower positive predictive value than most of the other investigations discussed, but in keeping with the others has a high negative predictive value.

Anal ultrasound

Ultrasound imaging of the anal sphincter complex is also readily available, easy to perform and reliable. Differences in the sphincter morphology on straining have been seen between patients with anismus when compared with other asymptomatic controls, those with anismus having a shorter and thicker puborectalis on straining. Its use as a diagnostic tool in patients with anismus has not however been investigated (7). It may provide useful information in those patients who fail treatment, with submucosal thickening and a thickened internal sphincter being associated with another common cause of outlet obstruction, internal rectal prolapse. The emerging technique of dynamic perineal ultrasound in pelvic floor disorders is interesting (see chapter 20) but as yet unvalidated, and may offer more power in the diagnosis of anismus.

EUA rectum

In the presence of radiographic findings of anismus with unusual symptomatology, or treatment failure, examination under anaesthetic to rule out internal rectal prolapse is an important diagnostic step and should be performed in all patients fulfilling these criteria (see below). We use a circular anal dilator (CAD) device

(Frankenman International Ltd, Hong Kong) that allows any prolapse to be seen to prolapse to or into the anal canal. Use of an Eisenhammer speculum tends to reduce and splint prolapse.

Response to Botulinum toxin

We now consider a therapeutic response to a 'diagnostic' first dose of Botulinum toxin to be the basis for a definitive diagnosis of anismus (see below).

Treatment

Botulinum toxin

Botulinum is a toxin that has been used worldwide in many disorders of voluntary muscle. It has a proven low risk and side effect profile. It was first used to treat anismus by injection into the external sphincter and puborectalis in 1988, and has superseded the use of biofeedback as a first line treatment in some units (8).

Botulinum toxin is produced intracellularly and cleaved inside the bacterium. The result is a two chain polypeptide linked by a disulphide bond. This is then cleaved by the target cell, resulting in a free light chain that destroys the SNAP-25 protein and therefore inhibits acetylcholine (ACh) release. This paralyses the muscle fibre. New axonal sprouts emerge over the course of 2–6 months and therefore the process is reversed.

Initial experience of botulinum toxin in seven patients saw symptom improvement, a reduction in resting and squeeze pressures, and an increase in the anorectal angle on straining. The dose used was based on previous experience with botulinum toxin in disorders of the extra-ocular and sternomastoid muscles. It was clear even at this stage that response was dose dependent, and that symptoms recurred. However this report led to its uptake in several units, and in larger studies the success rate has been shown to be around 50% (Table 10.2) (8–12).

Table 10.2 Results of Botulinum toxin in anismus

Author	N	Response	Dose*	Localisation	Repeated	Follow-up (months)
Hallan	7	57% improved	3ng	EMG	no	12
Sik Joo	4	50% improved	12U	EMG	no	12
Maria	4	100% short-term 75% long-term	30U	none	yes	24
Ron	25	38% satisfaction	30U	none	yes	6
Maria	24	71% improved	60U	AUS	yes	39
Harmston	25	44% initial 92% revised	500U**	none	yes	n/s

* BOTOX unless otherwise stated
** Dysport

Emerging new concepts in anismus

In a series of anismus patients from Oxford, the success rate for Botulinum toxin injection used in patients with proctographically diagnosed anismus was 44%. However as per protocol the 11 who failed Botulinum toxin underwent EUA of the rectum. Ten (91%) were found to have an alternative diagnosis to explain their symptoms (1 biopsy-proven internal anal sphincter myopathy, 1 external rectal prolapse, 8 high-grade (anal) internal rectal prolapse). One would not expect Botulinum toxin to be helpful in these patients. The revised success rate with Botulinum toxin (excluding these patients) was 92%.

Patients who responded did so in a classical temporary Botulinum toxin pattern, with onset of improvement in symptoms after 2–3 days, and a gradual relapse after 6–12 weeks. A repeat injection at the same dose led to an improvement in symptoms again but on a permanent basis. It seems that the second dose of Botulinum toxin may lead to some kind of down-regulation phenomenon. This is very useful because it means that the first dose can be given as a diagnostic 'test' dose: if it works, the second dose becomes therapeutic; if it fails, it wears off and an alternative diagnosis can be sought.

These data suggest several new and important concepts. Firstly, they suggest that Botulinum toxin is an ideal treatment for what is a disorder of voluntary pelvic floor musculature. The variable responses in the literature probably reflect variable diagnostic criteria for anismus: presumably some patients with prolapse disease were inadvertently included. Secondly it suggests that current proctographic surrogate diagnostic criteria for anismus (failure to empty more than 60% of paste at 30 seconds) are very non-specific. According to our data, 15–20% of patients undergoing proctography fulfil these criteria yet only 5% respond to Botulinum toxin. This means between 66% and 75% of patients are over-diagnosed by these traditional criteria. We have demonstrated a diagnostic explanation for this and call the proctographic findings in these patients with ultimately an alternative diagnosis 'radiological pseudoanismus'. Thirdly, they show that prolapse disease is probably under-diagnosed by current proctographic methods, and that EUA is a very useful ultimate diagnostic test.

Technique of Botulinum injection

No consensus exists on dosage or method of injection. One study has suggested that injection sites either laterally or posteriorly give similar results (11). The same study reported a 70% incidence of non severe anorectal pain following injection, but no major complications other than transient incontinence was reported. In our experience in Oxford, Botulinum toxin is well tolerated in an outpatient setting under a local anaesthetic anal block.

Anal blockade

In the left lateral position a mixture of 20 ml of 0.5% bupivacaine and 10 ml of 1% lignocaine are injected immediately at the lateral edge of the external sphincter using a 21 gauge needle. The needle is directed posteriorly and midline towards the coccyx, and cranially. The local anaesthetic is injected bilaterally into the ischiorectal spaces to block the anal branches of the pudendal nerve.

Botulinum toxin injection

One hundred units of OnabotulinumtoxinA or 500 units of AbobotulinumtoxinA is administered to the puborectalis and external sphincter under anal blockade and is a cost effective method. The ratio between the two different agents is said to be 1 unit OnabotulinumtoxinA: 3 units AbobotulinumtoxinA. The Botulinum toxin is then injected into the puborectalis and external sphincter at 3 and 9 o'clock using a 21 gauge needle in small aliquots along the muscle. Patients are followed up at six weeks and the presence of a classic temporal symptom response is noted. Patients with a successful response are treated with further Botulinum injections for recurrent symptoms that re-emerge between 6 and 12 weeks. Failure of treatment is followed by rectal EUA with a CAD device.

Biofeedback

Before the introduction of Botulinum toxin, biofeedback was the mainstay of treatment in patients with anismus, and continues to be used in many units. Various methods have been employed including sensory (balloon expulsion), EMG and manometric based methods. Much has been published on biofeedback use in constipation and outlet obstruction, but most studies have populations with mixed aetiology. This chapter only considers evidence directly describing biofeedback in anismus.

Bleijenberg and Kuijpers described biofeedback for anismus in 1984 with an EMG based technique being employed in 10 patients with anismsus, enjoying a 70% success rate. Following this publication several studies in adults appeared in the literature (Table 10.3)(13–26). The power of those studies to conclude whether biofeedback is superior to other treatments, or indeed placebo, is unknown as no randomized controlled trials have been performed. It should also be recognized that the numbers included are generally small, the time investment relatively high, and the follow up usually short. The method of biofeedback also varies. There are however several consistencies: all studies performed biofeedback in an outpatient setting, had minimal complications, and the results were mostly analysed on an intention-to-treat basis. In the larger series around a 30% drop-out rate is observed, in keeping with our experience.

Comparisons between EMG based biofeedback and manometric based biofeedback have either shown no difference or favoured EMG, although numbers were small in both studies (21,27). One study investigating factors associated with poor outcome suggested that previous pelvic floor damage with deranged physiology was associated with failure. Wexner in a large recent study suggested that outcome is unaffected by concurrent pelvic floor abnormalities such as rectocele or intussusception. The conclusion to this study, that patient compliance is the strongest predictor of outcome,

Table 10.3 Results of biofeedback in anismus

Author	N	Method of biofeedback	Outcome
Kawimbe	15	balloon expulsion	significant improvement in constipation score
Wexner	18	EMG	89% improved
Fleshman	9	manometric	100% improved
Turnbull	7	manometric	71% improved
Parks	68	EMG	58% improved
Ho	62	manometric	90% improved
Glia	26	manometric/EMG	58% improved
Karlbom	19	EMG	43% improved
McKee	30	manometric	30% improved
Rhee	45	EMG	69% improved
Lau	108	EMG	55% improved
Battaglia	14	EMG	50% improved

is an important consideration: success rates are considerably higher in those who complete treatment, though this is a self-fulfilling argument. Patients who do not improve are probably less likely to persevere. One study has reported on longer term outcomes and shown a 50% response rate at one year. It seems reasonable on this evidence to offer biofeedback to patients with anismus, based on local expertise and protocols, with an expected success rate of around 50%. The focus should be on patient compliance, rather than on any particular method.

Surgery

The treatment of anismus with surgery is of historical interest only. Keighley performed posterior division of the puborectalis in nine patients, but the results were poor with resolution of symptoms in only two and some form of incontinence reported in 5 patients (28). Myomectomy has also been performed in 29 patients with 'outlet obstruction'. Improvement in symptoms was seen in 62% and was associated with a reduction in maximum resting pressures; those not responding had no change. Squeeze pressures and sensation did not change (29). One group has employed progressive anal dilation and shown reasonable results with improvement in the number of spontaneous bowel movements and a reduction in the anal canal resting pressures, this treatment was suggested by the authors as an adjunct to biofeedback (30). The use of surgical intervention for true anismus has however largely and reasonably been abandoned, mainly due to the success of more conservative treatments.

Key points

◆ Anismus is a disorder of the striated pelvic floor musculature causing functional outlet obstruction constipation

◆ Its diagnosis should be considered in all cases of chronic constipation, and is frequently suggested on physical examination

◆ Proctography is sensitive but non-specific and cannot be relied upon to diagnose anismus

◆ Botulinum toxin is highly effective in carefully selected patients. The effect of an initial dose of Botulinum toxin is temporary, the response to which can be considered a 'diagnostic' test for anismus: if it fails, the diagnosis is almost certainly prolapse (demonstrable at EUA) and any side effects reversible

◆ Repeat treatment seems to be more or less permanent and can therefore be considered as 'therapeutic'.

Editor's summary

Anismus is a functional cause of outlet obstruction constipation, due to disordered striated pelvic floor muscle function, that can be treated effectively by pharmacological methods. It should be suggested on physical examination. Proctography is sensitive but non-specific and cannot be relied upon to diagnose anismus. Botulinum toxin is highly effective in carefully selected patients. It has the advantage of reversibility of the initial treatment, but a repeat treatment seems to be permanent. This means that the first dose can be considered a 'diagnostic' test for anismus; if it fails, the diagnosis is almost certainly demonstrable at EUA, and any side effects in this situation reversible. The second dose can be considered therapeutic.

References

1. Wasserman IF. Puborectalis Syndrome (Rectal Stenosis Due to Anorectal Spasm). *Dis Colon Rectum* 1964;**7**:87–98.

2. Preston DM, Lennard-Jones JE. Anismus in chronic constipation. *Dig Dis Sci* 1985;**30**(5):413–8.

3. Park UC, Choi SK, Piccirillo MF, Verzaro R, Wexner SD. Patterns of anismus and the relation to biofeedback therapy. *Dis Colon Rectum* 1996;**39**(7):768–73.

4. Halligan S, Thomas J, Bartram C. Intrarectal pressures and balloon expulsion related to evacuation proctography. *Gut* 1995;**37**(1):100–4.

5. Karlbom U, Edebol Eeg-Olofsson K, Graf W, Nilsson S, Pahlman L. Paradoxical puborectalis contraction is associated with impaired rectal evacuation. *Int J Colorectal Dis* 1998;**13**(3):141–7.

6. Rao SS, Welcher KD, Leistikow JS. Obstructive defecation: a failure of rectoanal coordination. *Am J Gastroenterol* 1998;**93**(7):1042–50.

7. Van Outryve SM, Van Outryve MJ, De Winter BY, Pelckmans PA. Is anorectal endosonography valuable in dyschesia? *Gut* 2002;**51**(5):695–700.

8. Hallan RI, Williams NS, Melling J, Waldron DJ, Womack NR, Morrison JF. Treatment of anismus in intractable constipation with botulinum A toxin. *Lancet* 1988;**2**(8613):714–7.

9. Joo JS, Agachan F, Wolff B, Nogueras JJ, Wexner SD. Initial North American experience with botulinum toxin type A for treatment of anismus. *Dis Colon Rectum* 1996;**39**(10):1107–11.

10. Maria G, Brisinda G, Bentivoglio AR, Cassetta E, Albanese A. Botulinum toxin in the treatment of outlet obstruction constipation caused by puborectalis syndrome. *Dis Colon Rectum* 2000;**43**(3):376–80.

11. Ron Y, Avni Y, Lukovetski A, Wardi J, Geva D, Birkenfeld S, et al. Botulinum toxin type-A in therapy of patients with anismus. *Dis Colon Rectum* 2001;**44**(12):1821–6.

12. Maria G, Cadeddu F, Brandara F, Marniga G, Brisinda G. Experience with type A botulinum toxin for treatment of outlet-type constipation. *Am J Gastroenterol* 2006;**101**(11):2570–5.

13. Bleijenberg G, Kuijpers HC. Treatment of the spastic pelvic floor syndrome with biofeedback. *Dis Colon Rectum* 1987;**30**(2):108–11.

14. Lestar B, Penninckx F, Kerremans R. Biofeedback defaecation training for anismus. *Int J Colorectal Dis* 1991;**6**(4):202–7.

15. Kawimbe BM, Papachrysostomou M, Binnie NR, Clare N, Smith AN. Outlet obstruction constipation (anismus) managed by biofeedback. *Gut* 1991;**32**(10):1175–9.

16. Wexner SD, Cheape JD, Jorge JM, Heymen S, Jagelman DG. Prospective assessment of biofeedback for the treatment of paradoxical puborectalis contraction. *Dis Colon Rectum* 1992;**35**(?):145–50.

17. Fleshman JW, Dreznik Z, Meyer K, Fry RD, Carney R, Kodner IJ. Outpatient protocol for biofeedback therapy of pelvic floor outlet obstruction. *Dis Colon Rectum* 1992;**35**(1):1–7.

18. Turnbull GK, Ritvo PG. Anal sphincter biofeedback relaxation treatment for women with intractable constipation symptoms. *Dis Colon Rectum* 1992;**35**(6):530–6.

19. Parks AG, Porter NH, Melzak J. Experimental study of the reflex mechanism controlling the muscle of the pelvic floor. *Dis Colon Rectum* 1962;**5**:407–14.

20. Ho YH, Tan M, Goh HS. Clinical and physiologic effects of biofeedback in outlet obstruction constipation. *Dis Colon Rectum* 1996;**39**(5):520–4.

21. Glia A, Gylin M, Gullberg K, Lindberg G. Biofeedback retraining in patients with functional constipation and paradoxical puborectalis contraction: comparison of anal manometry and sphincter electromyography for feedback. *Dis Colon Rectum* 1997;**40**(8):889–95.

22. Karlbom U, Hallden M, Eeg-Olofsson KE, Pahlman L, Graf W. Results of biofeedback in constipated patients: a prospective study. *Dis Colon Rectum* 1997;**40**(10):1149–55.

23. McKee RF, McEnroe L, Anderson JH, Finlay IG. Identification of patients likely to benefit from biofeedback for outlet obstruction constipation. *Br J Surg* 1999;**86**(3):355–9.

24. Rhee PL, Choi MS, Kim YH, Son HJ, Kim JJ, Koh KC, et al. An increased rectal maximum tolerable volume and long anal canal are associated with poor short-term response to biofeedback therapy for patients with anismus with decreased bowel frequency and normal colonic transit time. *Dis Colon Rectum* 2000;**43**(10):1405–11.

25. Lau CW, Heymen S, Alabaz O, Iroatulam AJ, Wexner SD. Prognostic significance of rectocele, intussusception, and abnormal perineal descent in biofeedback treatment for constipated patients with paradoxical puborectalis contraction. *Dis Colon Rectum* 2000;**43**(4):478–82.

26. Battaglia E, Serra AM, Buonafede G, Dughera L, Chistolini F, Morelli A, et al. Long-term study on the effects of visual biofeedback and muscle training as a therapeutic modality in pelvic floor dyssynergia and slow-transit constipation. *Dis Colon Rectum* 2004;**47**(1):90–5.

27. Bleijenberg G, Kuijpers HC. Biofeedback treatment of constipation: a comparison of two methods. *Am J Gastroenterol* 1994;**89**(7):1021–6.

28. Barnes PR, Hawley PR, Preston DM, Lennard-Jones JE. Experience of posterior division of the puborectalis muscle in the management of chronic constipation. *Br J Surg* 1985;**72**(6):475–7.

29. Yoshioka K, Keighley MR. Anorectal myectomy for outlet obstruction. *Br J Surg* 1987;**74**(5):373–6.

30. Maria G, Anastasio G, Brisinda G, Civello IM. Treatment of puborectalis syndrome with progressive anal dilation. *Dis Colon Rectum* 1997;**40**(1):89–92.

Chapter 11

Rectocele

Rowan Collinson

A rectocele is defined as a herniation or bulging of the anterior rectal wall and posterior vaginal wall into the vagina. Others extend the definition to encompass the pathophysiology, a defective rectovaginal septum.

Pathophysiology

Although the events that lead to development of a rectocele are poorly understood it is likely that the critical event is a deficiency of, or damage to, the supportive layer of fascia lying between the rectum and vagina. Some consider this fascia analogous to Denonvillier's fascia in the male, a fusion of the peritoneal lining of the embryonic rectogenital pouch (1). Others describe it as a specialized condensation of the visceral endopelvic fascia (2). There is also some support for a Mullerian origin (3). Regardless of its origin, the balance of evidence favours the existence of a 'surgically useful fascia'. It must be emphasised however that the layer does not exist in isolation but as a component of a more confluent connective tissue package that envelops the pelvic organs (endopelvic fascia) and is therefore intimately related to their mobility and support.

A contemporary model of the rectovaginal fascia is as a diaphragm-like structure or sheet, which has several points of fixity (Fig. 11.1) (3–5). Histologically it is a fibro-muscular elastic layer, consisting of dense collagen, smooth muscle, and coarse elastic fibres, with associated small blood vessels (1,3–5). In a cranio-caudal direction, DeLancey divides it into thirds (4); the upper third (Level I) blends with the peritoneum of the cul-de-sac, the uterosacral ligaments and the base of the cardinal ligaments. This is the least robust component of the layer on histological sections. In the distal third of the vagina/rectum (Level III), it blends with the perineal body that has an important role in supporting the perineum via its fascial attachments to the ischiopubic rami and, to a lesser extent, the urogenital diaphragm. In its middle third (Level II), the rectovaginal fascia extends laterally out to the fascia overlying the levator ani muscles: specifically the arcus tendineus fascia. Here it is a component of the endopelvic fascia that provides lateral support to the Level II structures; most of the lateral support comes from endopelvic fascia attaching directly into the posterolateral vaginal wall.

The existence of this discrete layer continues to be debated. Many anatomical studies are limited by too few dissections (3) of unknown parity and age (5), as well as varying methods of cadaver preparation. On balance, the layer probably exists, but is highly variable. For instance it is known to be more robust and demonstrable in DeLancey's

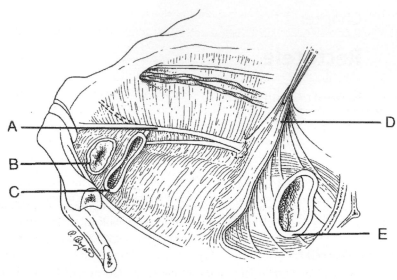

Fig. 11.1 Rectovaginal fascia viewed from above with bladder, uterus and vagina removed A. arcus tendineus fascia pelvis B. bladder neck C. vagina D. rectovaginal fascia. E. rectum. Reproduced with permission from Richardson AC. The rectovaginal septum revisited: its relationship to rectocele and its importance in rectocele repair. *Clin Obstet Gynecol*. 1993 Dec;**36**(4):976–83.

level II and level III (5), where it blends with the perineal body. Its integrity is also influenced by factors which influence all connective tissue: age, parity, hormonal status and genetic variation. Taking this all into account it is hardly surprising that it is not the same in all patients.

Richardson proposed a predictable pattern of fascial injury in the aetiology of rectocele (3), a description used by proponents to support the concept of defect-specific repair. The commonest injury described is a transverse break in the fascia just above its attachment to the perineal body. Almost as common was a midline vertical defect, which may not only involve DeLancey's Level III, but can extend up as high as Level I. Rarely there may be a lateral separation, running in the sagittal plane similar to the vertical midline defect. Finally there can be U or L-shaped variants, representing a combination of two or more of the above defects. As will be discussed later, rectocele repair can be defect-specific (directed at one of the above lesions) or non-specific.

Aetiology and demographics

A symptomatic rectocele rarely exists in isolation, being part of a much broader spectrum of failure of pelvic organ support systems, and as such often coexists with varying degrees of cystocele, uterovaginal prolapse, enterocele, excessive perineal descent and rectal intussusception (6,7). Hence the major risk factors in its development are those causing pelvic organ prolapse (POP). The condition can exist in both parous and nulliparous patients and in males, although parous females constitute the most affected group.

The major risk factor (8,9) is vaginal child birth which causes a multi-component injury to the musculo-aponeurotic pelvic floor and endopelvic connective tissue, as well as the pudendal and levator ani nerves. This varies in severity according to duration of labour, use of epidural anaesthesia, forceps and the size of the baby (9). The end result is attenuation or tearing of the rectovaginal fascia. Widening of the genital hiatus affects vaginal closure, meaning that the posterior vaginal wall is subjected to a high-pressure gradient from transmitted intra-abdominal pressure (4). Caesarean delivery is not necessarily protective (10).

Age is also associated with rectocele development, although rather than being a single risk factor, this is probably representative of a complex interplay of age-related connective tissue degeneration, post-menopausal hypo-oestrogenism, expression of the patient's collagen phenotype, and the onset of organic diseases (11). There is clearly an association with menopause and the resulting hypo-oestrogenism, although it is not clear whether this is solely a change in collagen metabolism, or fibroblast function or both (11). Genetic factors relating to collagen and elastin metabolism, and fibroblast activity are a growing focus of research as they may underpin some of the uncommon presentations of POP eg nulliparous females, male patients, and those with inherited disorders of collagen (11). A body mass index (BMI) of > 25 correlates with a higher stage of POP (12) and weight loss improves symptoms, specifically urinary incontinence (13), but not necessarily anatomical regression of the stage of prolapse (14). A first-degree relative with POP confers a 3-fold relative risk increase (11). There is also a racial influence (11). (Table 11.1)

However, a small rectocele in a female patient is a common finding and should not be regarded as abnormal. In Shorvon's widely reported study (15) of 46 nulliparous volunteers under 35 years of age with no defaecatory symptoms, small rectoceles (< 2cm) were found in 81% of female and 13% of male volunteers; only one had a rectocele > 2cm. An alternative interpretation of this is that rectoceles > 2cm are uncommon in otherwise asymptomatic young nulliparous women.

Table 11.1 Risk factors for rectocele development

Female gender
Vaginal childbirth
Pregnancy
Aging
Menopause/Hypo-oestrogenism
Genetic factors
Obesity
Chronically raised intra-abdominal pressure
Family history of pelvic organ prolapse
Chronic diseases/Musculoskeletal diseases
Race

Rectoceles are frequently found in patients presenting to pelvic floor clinics with a variety of symptoms. In the Swedish Uppsala and Ostersund observational population study, POP was diagnosed in over 50% of all women over 50 years of age, with an overall incidence of approximately 31% in women aged from 20 to 60 years (16). Rectocele was diagnosed in over 30% of the patients diagnosed with any stage of POP. However, most was morphologically at an early stage. In the US, one in 10 women will have surgery for symptomatic POP, with up to a third of operations being revisions (17); 76% undergoing surgery for documented POP had a rectocele. In the cost analysis study of Subak, 22% of USA women undergoing surgery for POP also underwent a rectocele repair (18). With an active, aging population, it is estimated that the rate of women seeking care for pelvic floor disorders will double over the next 30 years (19).

Symptoms, signs and investigations

Patients present with varying combinations of gynaecological and bowel symptoms: constipation, obstructed defaecation (ODS), incomplete evacuation, faecal incontinence, post-defaecatory soiling, pruritis ani, dyspareunia, pelvic pressure, and the presence of a palpable bulge. In reality, very few of these symptoms can be directly attributed to the rectocele. This is important for two reasons–firstly it is a reminder that symptomatic rectocele is often the tip of the 'iceberg' of a more global pelvic floor dysfunction (6), and secondly, it is symptoms which direct treatment. In terms of the bowel, the most reliable symptoms are the need to self-digitate, or a sense of incomplete evacuation (20). A 'rectocele-specific' symptom scoring system has recently been reported (21), which has potential for use as a clinical research tool. As yet it is un-validated, and it remains to be seen whether it offers any advantage over an established but less specific scoring system, such as the Obstructed Defaecation Score (22).

Physical examination characterizes not only the rectocele, but also the coexistent pelvic floor findings. The perineum may be descended at rest–at or below the ischial tuberosities–or may be obviously 'ballooned' outwards in the left lateral position. Further excessive descent (> 3 cm) may be noticed on straining. Note should be made of any evidence of cystocele or vaginal vault prolapse. Asking the patient to bear down during digital rectal examination may unmask a non-relaxing puborectalis. The same manoeuvre may reveal uterine prolapse or a rectal intussusception. The integrity of the perineal body and anal sphincter can also be assessed. Proctoscopy may demonstrate mucosal prolapse overlying the rectocele. The key differential diagnosis is enterocele, which also presents as a posterior vaginal protrusion. Simultaneous per rectum and vaginal palpation while the patient performs a Valsalva manoeuvre may clarify this. The negative predictive value of clinical examination is low, and ultimately the diagnosis may need to be excluded radiologically (23). Mellgren observed that patients with enterocele rarely have a coexistent rectocele, and hypothesised that the two may be mutually exclusive (24). In this study enterocele was strongly associated with rectal intussusception and rectal prolapse.

Colorectal surgeons sometimes describe rectocele size in terms of the amount of forward protrusion into the vaginal lumen, beyond the expected normal contour of the rectum at this point. This is similar to the radiological method of measuring the rectocele size on defaecating proctography (15). A recognized and reproducible clinical classification of rectoceles is that of the International Continence Society, the American Urogynecological Society and the Society of Gynecological Surgeons, proposed in 1996 (25). This is also known as the 'POP-Q' system of assessment of the anatomic grade of gynaecological prolapse, including rectocele. The rectocele severity is expressed as stages I to IV depending on its maximal protrusion inferiorly with reference to the hymenal ring when the patient is examined in the semi-upright lithotomy position during Valsalva manoeuvre, or standing. Adjunctive investigations are generally used to clarify the presence and significance of other related conditions, such as other features of POP, or abnormal pelvic floor muscle activity.

Defaecating proctography

Defaecating proctography techniques and relevance to outcome are described elsewhere (see Chapter 2). At its simplest, rectal contrast material alone can provide useful radiologic information. The size of the rectocele can be measured, although the reference point varies in the literature; some use a line parallel to the anterior wall of the anal canal while others use the extent of protrusion anteriorly beyond the expected normal contour of the rectum at that point (Fig. 11.2). Extent of perineal descent at rest or straining can be quantitated and anismus confirmed if present. Coexistent mucosal

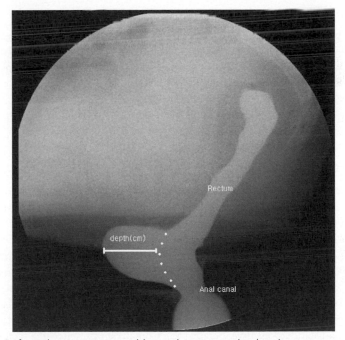

Fig. 11.2 Defaecating proctogram with rectal contrast only, showing measurement of rectocele size, using the extent of protrusion beyond the (dotted) line of the estimated anterior rectal wall contour.

or internal rectal prolapse will also be evident. Contrast trapping is thought to occur due to a low-pressure zone occurring within the rectocele on straining. Although trapping has been reported to be associated with larger rectoceles and the symptom of vaginal digitation, it does not appear to be predictive of treatment outcomes. In a variation on standard proctography, it has been proposed that a further radiograph taken after the patient has made a private visit to the lavatory may be a more valid representation of the degree of rectocele emptying *in vivo* (26).

Magnetic resonance imaging (MRI) defaecography

MRI defaecography is a new and attractive modality due to its lack of ionising radiation and the ability to visualise all the pelvic viscera. Two main methods exist–supine closed-configuration magnet, and the newer open-configuration magnet. A criticism of the former is that the patient position is unphysiological, and that asking the patient to bear down in the supine position is likely to underestimate the degree of POP. A solution to this problem is to use intra-rectal contrast (usually sonographic transmission gel) that the patient is required to evacuate. Using this technique, Kelvin et al. found that MRI compared favourably with triphasic fluoroscopic cysto-colpo-proctography in estimating rectocele size, but that it underestimated the extent of cystoceles and enteroceles (27). A distinct disadvantage is that it requires rectal evacuation on the MRI table, which may be distressing for the patient and radiology staff alike.

Dynamic perineal ultrasound

Dynamic perineal ultrasound is an exciting and emerging technique, and is extensively reviewed elsewhere (see chapter 20). Using the trans-labial technique, Perniola et al found a positive predictive value for rectocele of 0.82 when blindly compared with standard fluoroscopy, but a low negative predictive value (28). The authors concluded that as a screening test it may be useful, but a negative result may necessitate further investigation with fluoroscopic proctography. Beer-Gabel et al. reported promising results from a similar study, in which the patient evacuated intra-rectal gel (29).

Management and surgery

Although there is scant evidence examining the role of fibre in relation to rectocele it would seem sensible that patients be encouraged to optimise their diet prior to any escalation of treatment.

A discussion of the role of biofeedback is really a recognition of the frequent coexistence of anismus (pelvic floor dyssynergia) with a rectocele. In a defaecographic and electromyographic study of 112 patients with obstructed defaecation syndrome (ODS), Mellgren et al found that 60% of patients with rectocele had paradoxical anal sphincter activity, compared with 24% of those without rectocele (30). Biofeedback is an effective therapy of pelvic floor dyssynergia (31), with a recent study showing it to be more effective than standard laxative therapy (32). Concurrent presence of a rectocele does not affect the likelihood of success.

Patients with symptomatic rectocele in the presence of anismus should have a trial of biofeedback therapy before all operative options are pursued. However, whether failure of biofeedback is a contraindication to later proceeding to repair of the rectocele is not clear. Two case series report a worse subjective outcome in patients with untreated anismus undergoing transanal repair (33,34).

Transanal sutured repair

This is usually performed with the patient in the prone jack-knife position, and consists of reinforcing suture of the anterior rectal wall following mucosectomy overlying the rectocele (Fig. 11.3). It is well tolerated, with major morbidity rare. Minor perioperative complications include urinary tract infection, retention, secondary/reactionary haemorrhage and faecal impaction. Rectovaginal fistula is extremely rare with this approach.

In studies with 6–24 months median follow-up, subjective measures of symptomatic improvement report 'cure' or improvement in 75–93% per cent of patients (33,35). In studies with greater than 2 years follow-up, this figure falls to 50–62% (34,36,37), suggesting some diminution of efficacy with time. As discussed above, it has been suggested that coexistent animus predicts a poor subjective outcome (33,34). Other parameters that appear to benefit from repair include rectal distension sensation (35,36) and efficacy of evacuation (36). Whether the transanal approach adversely affects anal sphincter function is unclear. While some have shown a significant decrease in mean anal resting pressure (35) following transanal repair, others have shown no such effect (36). Moreover a beneficial effect of transanal rectocele repair on preoperative faecal incontinence symptoms has also been demonstrated (34,35,38). A selective operative approach has been advocated; whereby patients with significant preoperative

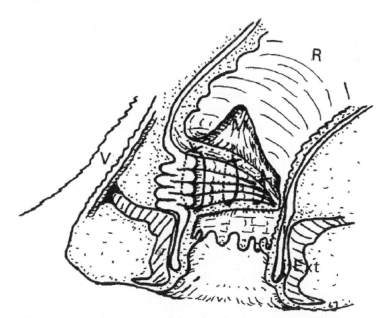

Fig. 11.3 Cross-section of the final phase of transanal anterior rectal wall repair before mucosal closure R. rectum V. vagina. Reproduced with permission from Janssen LW, Van Dijke CF. Selection criteria for anterior rectal wall repair in symptomatic rectocele and anterior rectal wall prolapse. *Dis Colon Rectum*. 1994 Nov;**37**(11):1100–7.

incontinence due to a sphincter defect undergo a transperineal or transvaginal repair, and those with incontinence thought due to mucosal prolapse undergo a transanal repair (38,39). While this approach has some logic, supportive data at the present time are lacking, and it may come at the expense of a greater rate of dyspareunia in the transvaginal group. Transanal repair has not been shown to adversely affect sexual function (36).

Transvaginal repair

Gynaecologists usually perform a transvaginal repair using one of three types of repair: non-selective plication of the deficient rectovaginal septum (posterior colporraphy); a defect-specific repair of identified tears in the rectovaginal septum; or a prosthetic reinforcement of the rectovaginal septum. A randomised trial of all three has shown similar anatomic and improved functional outcomes (40). For transvaginal prosthetic reinforcement of the rectovaginal septum, non-biological non-absorbable mesh (eg polypropylene), non-biological absorbable mesh (eg polyglactin), and biological mesh (eg porcine small intestine submucosa) have all been reported. While there are proponents of all of the above approaches, high quality comparative data in this area are lacking.

Enthusiasm for either a transanal or transvaginal approach is usually dictated by subspecialty interest. However a recent Cochrane review (41) found that posterior vaginal wall repair performed better than transanal repair in terms of a significantly lower recurrence rate. This was despite a higher perioperative blood loss and greater use of pain relief. The data were too few to comment on clinical outcomes such as flatus, faecal incontinence, or dyspareunia.

Transperineal repair

Repair via a transperineal incision has been reported using non-biological absorbable mesh (42), non-biological non-absorbable mesh (43) and biological mesh (44). This approach is attractive as it avoids anal sphincter stretch and facilitates concurrent anal sphincter repair where indicated. It may also minimise the risk of new-onset dyspareunia by avoiding a vaginal incision. Wound morbidity is a concern with this approach, with wound infection, haematoma, and mesh infection necessitating removal all described. While the results of these studies are generally encouraging, they are all small case series with short follow-up, and longer-term comparative data are necessary.

Transabdominal repair

This involves either open or laparoscopic dissection of the rectovaginal septum down to the pelvic floor, then reinforcement of the anterior rectal wall with prosthetic mesh. Results have been variable and seem to be related to technique. Anterolateral mesh placement has produced disappointing results (45), while solely anterior mesh placement (with perineal incision to bring the mesh right down to the perineal body) has been more encouraging (21). A retrospective matched cohort study favoured transanal repair over laparoscopic repair for alleviation of OD symptoms, although the authors noted a non-significant trend towards anal sphincter morbidity in the transanal group (46). The approach does appear to be safe and well tolerated. However more comparative data are required to establish whether these more invasive approaches with potentially greater morbidity offer any advantage over the local repairs described above.

On the other hand, transabdominal rectocele repair is more frequently reported in the situation of a more global pelvic floor dysfunction, such as uterovaginal prolapse eg sacrocolpopexy, or rectal prolapse/intussusception eg anterior mesh rectopexy (47–49). In these situations rectocele repair is a secondary outcome. This currently seems to be the main justification of the transabdominal approach to rectocele, where repair of the rectocele is a derivative of a more comprehensive pelvic floor repair.

Stapled transanal resection of the rectum (STARR procedure)

The STARR procedure consists of a transanal resection of rectal redundancy using either a circular or curved stapling device; the main indication is significant rectal intussusception causing OD (see chapter 19). As with transabdominal repair, the rectocele correction should be viewed as a by-product. There is no justification for performing the procedure just for rectocele in the absence of significant rectal intussusception or mucosal prolapse.

Key points

- Deficiency of or damage to the rectovaginal fascia is the pathological lesion predisposing to rectocele
- Female gender, vaginal childbirth, pregnancy and aging are the most important risk factors for rectocele formation
- Rectocele is a manifestation of pelvic organ prolapse
- Many symptoms are associated but the most specific to rectocele are awareness of a vaginal bulge, the need to self-digitate to achieve satisfactory evacuation, or a sense of incomplete evacuation
- Thorough physical examination and radiological assessment are important to demonstrate not only the rectocele but also any coexistent conditions
- Initial management must consist of conservative measures such as optimization of dietary factors and the use of biofeedback where indicated
- Rectocele can be repaired with low morbidity with several surgical approaches, the use of which is largely dictated by subspecialty expertise. There may be diminution of the initial surgical result with time. A lack of good-quality comparative studies means that, to date, the optimal repair method is not known.

Editor's summary

In our opinion isolated rectocele is uncommon, occurring in perhaps 10% of cases of obstructed defaecation. Therefore it is important to assess for and deal with coexistent patho-anatomical entities to achieve the optimum outcome. Rectocele repair in isolation, whether by transvaginal or transanal repair, is a relatively simple operation, but it is futile in the face of a more complex pelvic floor disorder. As a perineal procedure it suffers the same disadvantages as others, compared to an abdominal approach. Having said that, it is useful in elderly unfit patients; sometimes it provides enough relief on its own to justify its use in selected patients. However, as a general principle, rectocele is usually only one part in the pelvic floor jigsaw.

References

1. Milley PS, Nichols DH. A correlative investigation of the human rectovaginal septum. *Anat Rec.* 1969;**163**(3):443–51.
2. DeLancey JO. Anatomic aspects of vaginal eversion after hysterectomy. *Am J Obstet Gynecol.* 1992;**166**(6 Pt 1):1717–24; discussion 24–8.
3. Richardson AC. The rectovaginal septum revisited: its relationship to rectocele and its importance in rectocele repair. *Clin Obstet Gynecol.* 1993;**36**(4):976–83.
4. DeLancey JO. Structural anatomy of the posterior pelvic compartment as it relates to rectocele. *Am J Obstet Gynecol.* 1999;**180**(4):815–23.
5. Nagata I, Murakami G, Suzuki D, Furuya K, Koyama M, Ohtsuka A. Histological features of the rectovaginal septum in elderly women and a proposal for posterior vaginal defect repair. *Int Urogynecol J Pelvic Floor Dysfunct.* 2007;**18**(8):863–8.
6. Pescatori M, Spyrou M, Pulvirenti d'Urso A. A prospective evaluation of occult disorders in obstructed defecation using the 'iceberg diagram'. *Colorectal Dis.* 2006;**8**(9):785–9.
7. Thompson JR, Chen AH, Pettit PD, Bridges MD. Incidence of occult rectal prolapse in patients with clinical rectoceles and defecatory dysfunction. *Am J Obstet Gynecol.* 2002;**187**(6):1494–9; discussion 9–500.
8. Mant J, Painter R, Vessey M. Epidemiology of genital prolapse: observations from the Oxford Family Planning Association Study. *Br J Obstet Gynaecol.* 1997;**104**(5):579–85.
9. Schaffer JI, Wai CY, Boreham MK. Etiology of pelvic organ prolapse. *Clin Obstet Gynecol.* 2005;**48**(3):639–47.
10. MacLennan AH, Taylor AW, Wilson DH, Wilson D. The prevalence of pelvic floor disorders and their relationship to gender, age, parity and mode of delivery. *BJOG.* 2000;**107**(12):1460–70.
11. Kerkhof MH, Hendriks L, Brolmann HA. Changes in connective tissue in patients with pelvic organ prolapse—a review of the current literature. *Int Urogynecol J Pelvic Floor Dysfunct.* 2009;**20**(4):461–74.
12. Hendrix SL, Clark A, Nygaard I, Aragaki A, Barnabei V, McTiernan A. Pelvic organ prolapse in the Women's Health Initiative: gravity and gravidity. *Am J Obstet Gynecol.* 2002;**186**(6):1160–6.
13. Subak LL, Wing R, West DS, Franklin F, Vittinghoff E, Creasman JM, et al. Weight loss to treat urinary incontinence in overweight and obese women. *N Engl J Med.* 2009 29;**360**(5):481–90.

14. Kudish BI, Iglesia CB, Sokol RJ, Cochrane B, Richter HE, Larson J, et al. Effect of weight change on natural history of pelvic organ prolapse. *Obstet Gynecol.* 2009 Jan;113(1):81–8.

15. Shorvon PJ, McHugh S, Diamant NE, Somers S, Stevenson GW. Defecography in normal volunteers: results and implications. *Gut.* 1989;30(12):1737–49.

16. Samuelsson EC, Victor FT, Tibblin G, Svardsudd KF. Signs of genital prolapse in a Swedish population of women 20 to 59 years of age and possible related factors. *Am J Obstet Gynecol.* 1999;180(2 Pt 1):299–305.

17. Olsen AL, Smith VJ, Bergstrom JO, Colling JC, Clark AL. Epidemiology of surgically managed pelvic organ prolapse and urinary incontinence. *Obstet Gynecol.* 1997;89(4):501–6.

18. Subak LL, Waetjen LE, van den Eeden S, Thom DH, Vittinghoff E, Brown JS. Cost of pelvic organ prolapse surgery in the United States. *Obstet Gynecol.* 2001;98(4):646–51.

19. Luber KM, Boero S, Choe JY. The demographics of pelvic floor disorders: current observations and future projections. *Am J Obstet Gynecol.* 2001;184(7):1496–501; discussion 501–3.

20. Dietz HP, Korda A. Which bowel symptoms are most strongly associated with a true rectocele? *Aust N Z J Obstet Gynaecol.* 2005;45(6):505–8.

21. D'Hoore A, Vanbeckevoort D, Penninckx F. Clinical, physiological and radiological assessment of rectovaginal septum reinforcement with mesh for complex rectocele. *Br J Surg.* 2008;95(10):1264–72.

22. Altomare DF, Spazzafumo L, Rinaldi M, Dodi G, Ghiselli R, Piloni V. Set-up and statistical validation of a new scoring system for obstructed defaecation syndrome. *Colorectal Dis.* 2008;10(1):84–8.

23. Kelvin FM, Maglinte DD, Hornback JA, Benson JT. Pelvic prolapse: assessment with evacuation proctography (defecography). *Radiology.* 1992;184(2):547–51.

24. Mellgren A, Johansson C, Dolk A, Anzen B, Bremmer S, Nilsson BY, et al. Enterocele demonstrated by defaecography is associated with other pelvic floor disorders. *Int J Colorectal Dis.* 1994;9(3):121–4.

25. Bump RC, Mattiasson A, Bo K, Brubaker LP, DeLancey JO, Klarskov P, et al. The standardization of terminology of female pelvic organ prolapse and pelvic floor dysfunction. *Am J Obstet Gynecol.* 1996;175(1):10–7.

26. Greenberg T, Kelvin FM, Maglinte DD. Barium trapping in rectoceles: are we trapped by the wrong definition? *Abdom Imaging.* 2001;26(6):587–90.

27. Kelvin FM, Maglinte DD, Hale DS, Benson JT. Female pelvic organ prolapse: a comparison of triphasic dynamic MR imaging and triphasic fluoroscopic cystocolpoproctography. *AJR Am J Roentgenol.* 2000;174(1):81–8.

28. Perniola G, Shek C, Chong CC, Chew S, Cartmill J, Dietz HP. Defecation proctography and translabial ultrasound in the investigation of defecatory disorders. *Ultrasound Obstet Gynecol.* 2008;31(5):567–71.

29. Beer-Gabel M, Teshler M, Schechtman E, Zbar AP. Dynamic transperineal ultrasound vs. defecography in patients with evacuatory difficulty: a pilot study. *Int J Colorectal Dis.* 2004;19(1):60–7.

30. Mellgren A, Lopez A, Schultz I, Anzen B. Rectocele is associated with paradoxical anal sphincter reaction. *Int J Colorectal Dis.* 1998;13(1):13–6.

31. Rao SS, Seaton K, Miller M, Brown K, Nygaard I, Stumbo P, et al. Randomized controlled trial of biofeedback, sham feedback, and standard therapy for dyssynergic defecation. *Clin Gastroenterol Hepatol.* 2007;5(3):331–8.

32. Chiarioni G, Whitehead WE, Pezza V, Morelli A, Bassotti G. Biofeedback is superior to laxatives for normal transit constipation due to pelvic floor dyssynergia. *Gastroenterology*. 2006;**130**(3):657–64.

33. Tjandra JJ, Ooi BS, Tang CL, Dwyer P, Carey M. Transanal repair of rectocele corrects obstructed defecation if it is not associated with anismus. *Dis Colon Rectum*. 1999;**42**(12):1544–50.

34. Abbas SM, Bissett IP, Neill ME, Macmillan AK, Milne D, Parry BR. Long-term results of the anterior Delorme's operation in the management of symptomatic rectocele. *Dis Colon Rectum*. 2005;**48**(2):317–22.

35. Janssen LW, van Dijke CF. Selection criteria for anterior rectal wall repair in symptomatic rectocele and anterior rectal wall prolapse. *Dis Colon Rectum*. 1994;**37**(11):1100–7.

36. Heriot AG, Skull A, Kumar D. Functional and physiological outcome following transanal repair of rectocele. *Br J Surg*. 2004;**91**(10):1340–4.

37. Roman H, Michot F. Long-term outcomes of transanal rectocele repair. *Dis Colon Rectum*. 2005;**48**(3):510–7.

38. Ayabaca SM, Zbar AP, Pescatori M. Anal continence after rectocele repair. *Dis Colon Rectum*. 2002;**45**(1):63–9.

39. Tsujinaka S, Tsujinaka Y, Matsuo K, Akagi K, Hamahata Y. Changes in bowel function following transanal and transvaginal rectocele repair. *Dig Surg*. 2007;**24**(1):46–53.

40. Paraiso MF, Barber MD, Muir TW, Walters MD. Rectocele repair: a randomized trial of three surgical techniques including graft augmentation. *Am J Obstet Gynecol*. 2006;**195**(6):1762–71.

41. Maher C, Baessler K, Glazener CM, Adams EJ, Hagen S. Surgical management of pelvic organ prolapse in women. *Cochrane Database Syst Rev*. 2007(3):CD004014.

42. Leventoglu S, Mentes BB, Akin M, Karen M, Karamercan A, Oguz M. Transperineal rectocele repair with polyglycolic acid mesh: a case series. *Dis Colon Rectum*. 2007;**50**(12):2085–92; discussion 92–5.

43. Mercer-Jones MA, Sprowson A, Varma JS. Outcome after transperineal mesh repair of rectocele: a case series. *Dis Colon Rectum*. 2004;**47**(6):864–8.

44. Smart NJ, Mercer-Jones MA. Functional outcome after transperineal rectocele repair with porcine dermal collagen implant. *Dis Colon Rectum*. 2007;**50**(9):1422–7.

45. Oom DM, Gosselink MP, van Wijk JJ, van Dijl VR, Schouten WR. Rectocele repair by anterolateral rectopexy: long-term functional outcome. *Colorectal Dis*. 2008;**10**(9): 925–30.

46. Thornton MJ, Lam A, King DW. Laparoscopic or transanal repair of rectocele? A retrospective matched cohort study. *Dis Colon Rectum*. 2005;**48**(4):792–8.

47. D'Hoore A, Cadoni R, Penninckx F. Long-term outcome of laparoscopic ventral rectopexy for total rectal prolapse. *Br J Surg*. 2004;**91**(11):1500–5.

48. Slawik S, Soulsby R, Carter H, Payne H, Dixon AR. Laparoscopic ventral rectopexy, posterior colporrhaphy and vaginal sacrocolpopexy for the treatment of recto-genital prolapse and mechanical outlet obstruction. *Colorectal Dis*. 2008;**10**(2):138–43.

49. Collinson R, Wijffels N, Cunningham C, Lindsey I. Laparoscopic ventral rectopexy for internal rectal prolapse: short-term functional results. *Colorectal Dis*. 2010;**12**:97–104.

Chapter 12

Solitary rectal ulcer syndrome (SRUS)

Will Chambers and Tony Dixon

Introduction

Solitary rectal ulcer syndrome (SRUS) describes an enigmatic condition, which combines disturbances to bowel function and symptoms specific to the ulcer including the passage of blood and mucus per rectum. Macroscopic ulceration is not always present but the cardinal feature is erythema or ulceration of the anterior rectal wall (1). The syndrome covers a spectrum of anterior rectal wall lesions from induration and erythema to frank ulceration, including polypoid lesions.

Aetiology

A lack of consensus exists as to the cause of SRUS. Physiological and histological studies have illustrated a spectrum of findings suggesting a possible variety of causes (2–5). However, most agree that patients with SRUS have at least internal or external rectal prolapse and a simultaneous opposing force on the rectal mucosa, the downward force of defaecation countered by upward force from the pelvic floor that generates the trauma required for the formation of SRUS. The forces may lead to mucosal ischaemia and subsequent ulceration. In addition, the prolapsed mucosa may be traumatised against the closed anal canal.

While the presence of rectal prolapse, external or internal, is clearly understood, the nature of the opposing upward physiological force is unclear. Some believe this to be a paradoxical contraction of the pelvic floor, anismus or paradoxical puborectalis contraction. However the nature of anismus itself is poorly understood and some doubt its existence. Current radiological criteria for anismus have been shown to be over-diagnostic and frequently, for reasons unclear, mask an underlying diagnosis of internal rectal prolapse (so-called radiological pseudoanismus) (6). It is difficult to see how true anismus can commonly coexist with prolapse. One is an uncommon disorder of skeletal musculature, with a urological external urethral sphincter correlate (Fowler's syndrome). The other has a completely different pathophysiology.

It seems more likely that the upward force opposing the downward force of the prolapse is generated by the involuntary internal anal sphincter (IAS). Endoanal ultrasound reveals characteristically marked thickening of IAS in SRUS (7). This thickening response of the IAS is also seen in obstructed defaecation from internal rectal prolapse without SRUS, but less prominently. Patients with SRUS are known to have higher maximum resting pressures than those with prolapse without SRUS. It is possible that the response of the IAS to the prolapse leads to the development of the

SRUS. If prolapse and anismus coexisted in SRUS one would expect to see poor results in nerve-sparing ventral rectopexy, which treats only the prolapse, and a requirement for biofeedback or Botulinum toxin postoperatively.

Some authors, including the editors, feel that rectal prolapse and ulceration are different elements of the same pathological process (4). Others think the two conditions occur separately with different aetiologies. It is clear however that the two conditions coexist in many patients (5).

Pathological features

Though usually single, SRUS is occasionally multiple. Usually the ulcers are situated on the anterior rectal wall but they may extend circumferentially. The microscopic histological features include thickening of the mucosa and distortion of the underlying glands. The lamina propria is oedematous and may contain an abundance of fibroblasts. There is thickening of the muscularis mucosae and extension of its fibres upward through the glandular crypts. Often, there is erosion of surface epithelium. This is accompanied by a fibrinous exudate and engorged vessels in the superficial lamina propria but perhaps surprisingly, no significant inflammatory cell infiltrate (8).

Chiang et al (8) summarised the histological findings of 158 cases. 56% showed an ulcerated, 24% a polypoid pattern, and 20% a flat lesion (also called erythematous lesions). Glandular crypt abnormalities were seen in 91%, fibromuscular obliteration of the lamina propria 98%, hypertrophied and splayed muscularis mucosae upwards into lamina propria in 96%, inflammatory cells and granulation tissue infiltration in lamina propria 75%, mucosal capillary abnormalities 48%, haemosiderin deposition in lamina propria in 53%, surface erosion with fully mature and normal epithelium in 56% and misplaced glands in the submucosa in 7%.

Clinical features

SRUS is rare with an incidence estimated at 1 per 100,000 (1). There is a slight female predominance (1) and typically patients are young adults. A large series, however, recorded a mean age of 49 years with up to one quarter of patients presenting after 60 years of age (1). The commonest symptoms and signs of SRUS include rectal bleeding and passage of mucous, constipation and/or diarrhoea and prolonged straining at stool (1). There is often evidence of rectal prolapse, which may be internal or external and may be associated with abnormal perineal descent. Occasionally patients may be asymptomatic. Many have a delayed presentation, with an average of four years between symptom onset and diagnosis. Chiang et al (8) reported bleeding in 91%, mucous discharge in 77%, rectal pain in 61%, excessive straining in 63%, tenesmus in 64%, digitations in 29%, incontinence in 38%, constipation in 47%, and diarrhoea in 18%. Examination demonstrates combinations of perineal descent with straining; rectoanal incoordination with straining; palpable prolapse; and features of the SRU itself, induration/ulceration and fibrosis. In established fibrosis, it may not be possible to digitate the narrowed rectal lumen.

Investigations

SRUS is suggested by the combination of functional and ulcer symptoms, the macroscopic appearance of the rectal lesion on rigid sigmoidoscopy or colonoscopy, and confirmed histology of the biopsy specimen. Radiology and anorectal physiological testing are supportive but not definitive.

On rigid sigmoidoscopy different types of lesion (as described above) may be seen. The changes are usually anterior and at the apex of any high-grade (anal) internal rectal prolapse. Often the ulcer can be seen to correspond exactly with the top of the anal canal. Endoanal ultrasound reveals circumferentially thickened muscularis propria, a loss of the interface between mucosa and the muscularis propria and marked thickening of the internal anal sphincter (IAS) (7). This thickening response of the IAS is also seen in obstructed defaecation from internal rectal prolapse without SRUS, but less prominently. It is possible that the response of the IAS to the prolapse leads to the development of the SRUS.

Abnormalities may be demonstrated on defaecating proctography with two thirds of patients having evidence of internal or external rectal prolapse (9). This is often associated with delayed or incomplete evacuation. Halligan et al (9) demonstrated rectal prolapse in 68% of SRUS patients (internal 45%, external 23%). Proctography characteristically may also demonstrate prolonged and incomplete evacuation, often without prolapse, in patients with SRUS as compared with normal subjects. Overall, proctography disclosed delayed or incomplete emptying and/or rectal prolapse in 75% of patients. Only two patients in the control group showed low grade internal prolapse. This may be a form of pseudoanismus (see chapter 10). These functional rather than anatomical radiological appearances may result from the interaction between the prolapse and the thickening response of the IAS that potentially leads to the development of SRUS in the first place.

Anorectal physiology testing yields variable results in patients with SRUS. The tests neither make the diagnosis nor predict the patient's response to therapy. The most consistent finding with anorectal physiology is that of relatively high maximum resting pressures, excessive perineal descent and pudendal neuropathy (10).

Treatment

The main questions for the colorectal surgeon are:

- ◆ Can rectifying the abnormal anatomy (prolapse) cure or stop progression of the condition?
- ◆ Can it be assumed that if one treats high-grade internal rectal prolapse this will prevent the recto-anal interaction that leads to ulceration, and allow the SRU to heal?

Conservative management

It must be clear that an anatomical correction will not treat any supposed paradoxical puborectalis contraction. Should the potential complications of surgery be avoided; the anatomical abnormalities ignored; and SRUS be treated along functional lines with biofeedback or Botulinum toxin to re-educate patients in 'lifestyle change', to relax the pelvic floor appropriately, and learn to live with their condition? This strategy presupposes that in the face of marked anatomical abnormalities, pelvic floor re-education is possible.

Dietary fibre

The response rates vary from 19% to 70%, with rectal prolapse patients seeming to benefit the least from bulking agents alone (11). Most investigators have combined the use of additional dietary fibre with behavioural modification to reduce straining. The combination therapy was used successfully for symptom control in 14 of 21 patients. The literature suggests that fibre and straining avoidance only works with meticulous attention to therapy (1).

Topical agents

The first form of conservative treatment has been the application of local agents. All local agents may contribute to healing of the mucosa but they do not address the underlying defaecatory disorder and/or anatomy. Topical steroids and sulphasalazine enemas have not been shown to be effective. In contrast, a small study has demonstrated that sucral-fate enemas (2g twice daily for 3–6 weeks) have allowed symptomatic improvement and even sigmoidoscopic healing but the histological changes have persisted (12).

The application of human fibrin glue has also been shown to stimulate fibroblast and vascular proliferation leading to tissue regeneration and mucosal healing. In a small study, all six subjects treated with the topical fibrin, increased dietary fibre, and behavioural correction of straining had ulcer healing at 14 days. The healing had remained at 1-year follow-up. For the controls, treated with fibre and correction of straining alone, none had achieved ulcer healing by 14 days, yet half demonstrated healing at 1 year (13).

Biofeedback

Table 12.1 gives results of series using biofeedback to treat SRUS. The number of bio-feedback sessions varied between the studies, as did the exact nature of the treatment offered. Most of the patients included had failed more straight-forward conservative management.

Malouf et al (14) showed short-term benefit in 8 of 12 patients but longer-term benefit in only half this number. Jarrett et al (15) showed that biofeedback led to a significant rise in mucosal blood flow and postulated that this showed improved extrinsic autonomic nerve activity. Binnie et al (16) demonstrated a higher recurrence rate in 14 patients treated with surgery (posterior rectopexy) alone compared to a group of 17 who were treated with surgery and biofeedback either before or immedi-ately after surgery.

Surgery

The surgical options that have been tried for SRUS include perineal treatments (local excision, Delorme's procedure, STARR) and abdominal rectopexies of various kinds, almost always posterior, sometimes combined with resection. Anterior resection and stoma formation have also been used.

Table 12.1 Biofeedback for SRUS

Author	Year	Number	Success (%)	Follow-up (months)
Ho (10)	1995	7	54	n/s
Malouf (14)	2001	12	33	36
Jarrett (15)	2004	16	31	3–6
Rao (2)	2006	9	44	3

n/s not specified

Table 12.2 Stapled transanal rectal resection (STARR) for SRUS

Author	Year	Number	Success (%)	Follow-up (months)
Boccosanta (17)	2007	10	100	27
Dixon (unpublished)	2009	12	83	28

Stapled transanal rectal resection (STARR) (Table 12.2)

Boccosanta et al. (17) showed data on patients who had all received biofeedback and remained refractory to treatment. While ulcer healing was reported as occurring in 100% in this series, 20% of patients remained to some degree symptomatic, a finding repeated in our series where the number of symptomatic patients exceeded those with ulcer healing.

In our own unpublished series, two patients who did not have a successful outcome following STARR went on to have a laparoscopic ventral mesh rectopexy, both with successful outcome. Two patients with initial success post STARR developed recurrent symptoms at 18 months and 5 years. Both became asymptomatic after ventral mesh rectopexy.

Posterior rectopexy (Table 12.3)

Success with posterior rectopexy ranges from 50% to 100% (median of 70%). It should be noted that all published series are of posterior rectopexy, involving posterior rectal mobilization and rectal denervation. Posterior rectopexy leads to a high rate of postoperative constipation and is ill advised for internal prolapse. It also does not support the anterior rectal wall, the usual origin an internal prolapse. Tjandra et al (1) found

Table 12.3 Rectopexy for SRUS

Author	Year	Number	Success (%)	Follow-up (months)
Posterior rectopexy				
Schweiger (3)	1977	10	100	3–13
Stuart (18)	1984	15	73	n/r
Keighley (19)	1984	14	50	12
Nicholls (20)	1986	14	86	2–48
Tjandra (1)	1992	10	70	25
Binnie (16)	1992	19	74	n/r
Sitzler (21)	1998	49	59	21-177
Marchal (22)	2001	3	66	15–112
Tweedie (23)	2004	7	86	71–106
Meurette (24)	2008	19	74	36
Ventral rectopexy				
Dixon (unpublished)	2009	19	84	29
Lindsey (25)	2009	14	87	12

n/r not recorded

that the macroscopic appearance of the rectal lesion seemed to influence outcome, with polypoidal lesions doing better after surgery.

Sitzler et al (21) described a large experience of SRUS at St Mark's, 81 patients underwent surgical treatment over a 10-year period and 66 had at least 12 months follow-up. 49 underwent posterior rectopexy, nine a Delorme's procedure, two anterior resection and four patients a primary stoma. Rectopexy succeeded in 27/49 patients (55%). 19 of 22 failures underwent further surgery including rectal resection and colostomy formation. Eventually, 14 of these failures required permanent colostomy. For the nine patients treated initially with a Delorme's procedure there were four failures at a median follow up of 38 months (Table 12.4). Two of these patients ultimately required a stoma. Seven patients underwent an anterior resection as their initial treatment or as second line therapy for SRUS, four of these eventually required a colostomy. Anterior resection was not a successful salvage procedure. The overall stoma rate for the treatment of SRUS in this large series was 30 per cent. Posterior rectopexy resulted in a satisfactory long-term outcome in only 55–60% of patients. The poor outcome after surgery was related to two main factors: incontinence and incomplete evacuation, probably due to the rectal denervation associated with posterior rectal dissection.

Ventral rectopexy (Table 12.3)

While these figures do not make encouraging reading, it may be seen that when a ventral rectopexy is employed (Dixon and Lindsey (25)) the success is better. Ventral mesh rectopexy supports the anterior rectum where intussusception originates, without disturbing the autonomic innervation of the rectum as posterior rectopexy does. However, the number of series detailing the use of this novel treatment for SRUS is limited and further studies are needed to confirm the promising early results.

Summary

A reasonable proportion of patients with SRUS will respond to conservative measures such as advice to stop straining and stool modification with bulking agents and stool softeners. For those who do not respond, debate will continue as to the optimal course of treatment; the main choice being between biofeedback and surgery with rectopexy probably being the procedure of choice.

We would argue that structural abnormality should be corrected before defaecatory re-education commences. However, it is not unreasonable to try biofeedback before surgery if the clinician and patient want to take that course. Biofeedback seems to work in a proportion of patients although perhaps not for long. We believe rectopexy should be a laparoscopic ventral rectopexy rather than a posterior rectopexy.

Perineal procedures such as Delorme's procedure may result in ulcer healing but are also likely to lead to poor function and recurrence. The STARR procedure may be suitable

Table 12.4 Delorme's rectal mucosectomy for SRUS

Author	Year	Number	Success (%)	Follow-up (months)
Sitzler (21)	1998	9	55	19–107
Marchal (22)	2001	8	63	15–112

for those in whom the cervix and vaginal vault is well supported but in whom an abdominal approach is likely to be difficult (previous surgery, morbid obesity for instance), also in women who plan to have children and men. In our experience, men with SRU who show evidence of perineal descent invariably have a 'neo-rectocoele' at proctography and a gynaecoid pelvis at laparoscopy. In these cases we would consider ventral mesh rectopexy more appropriate. More studies are needed to assess the success of these two new techniques. Persistent post-operative urgency remains a problem of STARR.

Key points

♦ The hallmark feature of SRUS is chronic rectal ulceration with typical prolapse-associated changes, at about 6–7 cm from the anal verge

♦ SRUS is seen in internal and occasionally external prolapse; it is possible that the ulcer results from the interaction between the forces of the prolapse (downward) and the response of the internal anal sphincter (back upward), which is often very thickened

♦ SRUS has historically been regarded as a distinctly idiosyncratic and medically-managed condition, only appropriate to conservative approaches involving biofeedback/pelvic floor retraining

♦ Modern surgery is becoming the mainstay of treatment and while STARR is effective in patients with early change and good support, ventral rectopexy probably offers more long term control and an effective cure.

Editor's summary

Solitary rectal ulcer (SRU) has acquired almost mythical status in colorectal circles but one wonders whether the condition is a little more mundane. It probably just represents an unusual sequel of prolapse disease. It is seen in both internal and external prolapse, and there is some evidence that patients with SRU have higher resting pressures and thicker internal anal sphincters: it is possibly the result of the interaction between the prolapse and the response of the internal anal sphincter. Whilst STARR is effective in patients with early change and good support, ventral rectopexy offers greater long-term control and an effective cure.

References

1. Tjandra JJ, Fazio VW, Church JM, Lavery IC, Oakley JR, Milsom JW. Clinical conundrum of solitary rectal ulcer. *Dis Colon Rectum* 1992;**35**:227–34.

2. Rao S, Ozturk R, De Ocampo S, Stessman M. Pathophysiology and role of biofeedback therapy in solitary rectal ulcer syndrome. *Am J Gastroenterol* 2006;**101**:613–8.

3. Schweiger M, Alexander-Williams J. Solitary–ulcer syndrome of the rectum: its association with occult rectal prolapse. *Lancet* 1977;**i**:170–1.

4. Sun WM, Read NW, Donnelly TC, Bannister JJ, Shorthouse AJ. A common pathophysiology for full thickness rectal prolapse, anterior mucosal prolapse and solitary rectal ulcer. *Br J Surg* 1989;**76**:290–5.

5. Kang YS, Kamm MA, Nicholls RJ. Solitary rectal ulcer and complete rectal prolapse: one condition or two? *Int J Colorectal Dis* 1995;**10**:87–90.

6. Harmston C, Wijffels NA, Cunningham C, Lindsey I. Anismus, Botulinum toxin and 'Radiological Pseudo-anismus'. *Colorectal Dis.* 2009;**11**:(suppl 2) 27 [abst].

7. Halligan S, Sultan A, Rottenberg G, Bartram CI. Endoscopy of the anal sphincters in solitary rectal ulcer syndrome. *Int J Colorectal Dis* 1995;**10**:79–82.

8. Chiang JM, Changchien CR, Chen JR. Solitary rectal ulcer syndrome. *Int J Colorectal Dis* 2006;**21**:348–56.

9. Halligan S, Nicholls RJ, Bartram CI. Evacuation proctography in patients with solitary rectal ulcer syndrome. *AJR* 1995;**164**:91–5.

10. Ho YH, Ho JM, Parry BR. Solitary rectal ulcer syndrome: The clinical entity and anorectal physiology findings in Singapore. *Aust NZ J Surg* 1995;**65**:93–7.

11. van den Brandt Gradel V, Huibregtse K, Tytgat GN. Treatment of solitary rectal ulcer syndrome with high fibre diet and abstention of straining at defaecation. *Dig Dis Sci* 1984;**29**:1005–8.

12. Zagar SA, Khuroo MS, Mahajan R. Sucralfate retension enemas in solitary rectal ulcer. *Dis Colon Rectum* 1991;**34**:455–7.

13. Ederle A, Bulighin G, Orlandi PG, Pilati S. Endoscopic application of human fibrin sealant in the treatment of solitary rectal ulcer syndrome. *Endoscopy* 1992;**24**:736–7 (Letter).

14. Malouf AJ, Vaizey CJ, Kamm MA. Results of behavioural treatment (biofeedback) for solitary rectal ulcer syndrome *DCR* 2001;**44**:72–6.

15. Jarrett M, Vaizey CJ, Emmanuel AV et al. Behavioural therapy (biofeedback) for solitary rectal ulcer syndrome improves symptoms, mucosal blood flow. *Gut* 2004;**53**:368–70.

16. Binnie NR, Papachrysostomou M, Clare N, Smith AN. Solitary rectal ulcer: the place of biofeedback and surgery in the treatment of the syndrome. *World J Surg* 1992;**16**:836–40.

17. Boccasanta P, Venturi M, Calabro G, Maciocco M, Roviaro GC. Stapled transanal rectal resection in solitary rectal ulcer associated with prolapse of the rectum: a prospective study. *Dis Colon Rectum.* 2008;**51**:348–54.

18. Stuart M. Proctitis cystica profunda. Incidence, etiology, and treatment. *Dis Colon Rectum* 1984;**27**:153–6.

19. Keighley MR, Shouler P. Clinical and manometric features of the solitary rectal ulcer syndrome. *Dis Colon and Rectum* 1984;**27**:507–12.

20. Nicholls RJ, Simson JN. Anteroposterior rectopexy in the treatment of solitary rectal ulcer syndrome without overt rectal prolapse. *Br J Surg* 1986;**73**:222–4.

21. Sitzler PA, Kamm MA, Nicholls RJ. Surgery for solitary rectal ulcer syndrome. *Int J Colorectal Dis* 1996;**11**:136.

22. Marchal F, Bresler L, Brunaud L et al. Solitary rectal ulcer syndrome. a series of 13 patients operated with a mean follow-up of 4.5 years. *Int J Colorectal Dis* 2001;**16**:228–33.

23. Tweedie DJ, Varma JS. Long-term outcome of laparoscopic mesh rectopexy for solitary rectal ulcer syndrome. *Colorect Dis* 2005;**7**:151–5.

24. Meurette G, Siproudhis L, Regenet N, Frampas E, Proux M, Lehur PA. Poor symptomatic relief and quality of life in patients treated for 'solitary rectal ulcer syndrome without external rectal prolapse'. *Int J Colorectal Dis* 2008;**23**:521–6.

25. Evans C, Jones OM, Cunningham C, Lindsey I. Management of solitary rectal ulcer syndrome: Ignore the ulcer, treat the underlying posterior compartment prolapse. *Colorectal Dis* 2010;**12**:(suppl 1) 23 [abst].

Chapter 13

Slow transit constipation

Niels Wijffels

Introduction

Constipation and definitions

Slow transit constipation (STC) is a subgroup of constipation. A brief description of constipation is mandatory to understand its position in this broad group of patients. Constipation is a subjective symptom rather than a diagnosis. Symptoms may include incomplete, prolonged, difficult, rare, or painful defaecation; abdominal pain; and bloating (1). The original widely held definition of Drossman et al. described two or fewer bowel actions per week or straining at stool more than 25% of the time (2). At present the Rome II criteria are more frequently used to identify people with constipation. These require the presence in the last year (for at least 12 weeks and in more than 25% of defaecations) of two or more of the following: straining, lumpy or hard stools, sensation of incomplete evacuation, sensation of anorectal obstruction/blockade, manual manoeuvres to facilitate defaecation, and/or less than three defaecations per week. Loose stool are not present and there are insufficient criteria for irritable bowel syndrome (3). One must understand that whatever definition is used, it is used to identify patients with symptoms called 'constipation'. Constipation is not a disease or diagnosis by itself. (A diagnosis is the identification of a disease from a patient's symptoms (4)).

Indeed constipation might be induced by an organic cause (endocrine, metabolic, neurologic etc), an anatomic cause (neoplasm, prolapse, stricture etc), or by drugs, ie secondary constipation. When no such clear cause can be found it is referred to as 'functional' or 'idiopathic' constipation. In general there are three subgroups of functional constipation described:

1. Constipation-predominant IBS, constipation without prolongation of transit time, often associated with abdominal pain and bloating

2. Obstructed defaecation (OD), constipation characterized by the inability to initiate defaecation following the urge to do so

3. Slow transit constipation, constipation characterized by prolongation of transit time.

It is tempting to think of these subgroups as quite distinct but in practice there is overlap. OD caused by rectal prolapse might be referred to as 'functional constipation' but anatomical changes due to the prolapse are probably the cause of these symptoms. There is an overlap between the three different subtypes of functional constipation as well. It is known that some patients with OD might have STC as well and vice versa. One should bear in mind the grey area between these definitions. More research on functional constipation and a better understanding of underlying physiology (or pathology) in the future may change our view on constipation. In this chapter we have defined STC as 'symptoms of constipation with a prolongation of transit time, as measured by a transit study'. But it is possible to have a prolonged transit time without constipation symptoms (5) and that transit time may be prolongated secondary to anal stenosis, OD caused by anismus, etc (secondary STC).

Different points of perspective

For a good understanding of STC it is important to realise that there are different points of perspective. First of all one should exclude secondary causes of STC:

1. Secondary STC:
   - Neurogenic: neurological disorders are known to cause STC (eg spinal cord lesion, multiple sclerosis, Parkinson's disease, aganlionosis)
   - Organic/Systemic: different organic or systemic diseases may prolong colonic transit time (hypothroidism, hyper and hypocalcaemia, diabetes)
   - Anatomical: secondary STC can be due to an anatomical cause (eg polyp, stricture, aganlionosis)
   - Medical: numerous medicines are known to cause STC (eg anticholinergics, antipsychotics, antidepressants).

   Only a minority of patients will have secondary STC. If secondary causes are excluded a large group of patients with idiopathic STC will remain. In particular different points of perspective can be applied to this group:

2. Functional: In general, when organic and anatomical causes are excluded, STC is known to be a functional or idiopathic disorder. As in all functional disorders why some people develop this disorder and others do not is not clear. (A functional disorder is a disorder of physiological function which has no known organic basis)

3. Psychosocial: It is known that relatively more people who have been sexually abused or are depressive will develop STC. There is an association between eating disorders, anxiety disorders and STC as well.

4. Physiological (at organic level): Recent evidence shows that changes in the enteric nervous system are found in people with STC. The question remains is this cause or effect?

For optimal treatment shifting between these different perspectives might be very useful. More than one perspective can apply to one patient with STC which means that different treatment strategies can be used.

In this chapter we try to give an overview and description of what is known about the aetiology of STC. Different diagnostic tools and their relevance are discussed and an overview of different treatment strategies is given.

Normal colorectal motility

The aetiology of STC is not well understood and remains elusive. Research has been focused on colorectal motility. For a good understanding of the physiological changes seen in people with STC one should know the 'normal' physiology in people without STC. The function of the human colon is to mix, absorb and propel its contents, store it and finally expel the remnants (faeces). To fulfil this task the colon (and rectum) is equipped with unique motor activities. These motor activities can be measured with 24 hour manometry. Manometric investigations have shown that colonic motility may be grossly classified into two main types: Segmental activity (single contractions) and propagated activity (low-amplitude propagated contractions (LAPC); high-amplitude propagated contractions (HAPC)) (6).

Segmental contractile activity (amplitude 5–50 mmHg, 3 cycles/minute) is often measured in the distal colon (descending and sigmoid colon). The purpose of this activity is to propel the colonic contents distally. It creates an aborally directed pressure gradient which will move the contents towards the rectum.

LAPC (amplitude < 50 mmHg, > 100 events/day) are believed to distend viscus and pass flatus. HAPC (amplitude > 100 mmHg, about 6 events/day) are powerful contractions and able to propel large quantities of contents for some distance within the colon. HAPC are associated with defaecation itself and precede the expulsion of stool. Colonic motility is influenced by the daily cycle where awakening will provoke colonic motility and sleeping will inhibit motility. Ingestion of food will further stimulate colonic motor response.

Colorectal motility in STC

There is good evidence that colorectal motility is deranged in patients with STC. Almost all of the above described colonic activities are disturbed in patients with STC. Segmental contractile activity is impaired to cholinergic stimulation and its frequency is reduced to about half of that recorded in normal subjects. For propagated activity, data on LAPC activity is scarce and in fact might be preserved in patients with STC; but HAPC activity is deranged, and may be completely absent. The frequency of HAPC is decreased as well as the amplitude and duration. This results in a lack of propulsive forces which are mandatory for normal bowel action; and the early motor response following ingestion of a meal is decreased or absent. In severe cases HAPC are completely absent, combined with a complete disappearance of the segmental activity. These patients have true 'colonic inertia' and are unlikely to be helped with the use of laxatives.

Neuropathological changes in STC

Recently data has been published on the concept that colonic enteric autonomic innervation might be impaired. Selective sensory and autonomic neuropathy has been described in patients with STC and pathologic findings show a reduction in the total number of neurones and morphological neuronal and/or axonal abnormalities of the enteric nervous system (7). This could suggest a decrease of neurotransmission essential for the innervations of the colon. Excessive production of nitric oxide in the myenteric plexus of patients with STC could play a patho-physiological role, concurring in the persistent inhibition of contractions. The interstitial cells of Cajal, described as the intestinal pacemakers, are significantly decreased in patients with STC. Enteric Glial cells, originating from the neural crest and providing both mechanical and physiological support for neuronal elements, are also significantly decreased in patients with STC. Although incompletely understood, these neurological changes as seen on pathological examination in patients with STC, suggest an enteric neuropathy. The question remains whether these neurological changes are the cause of symptoms or if patients with STC will develop these in due time?

The aetiology of STC remains elusive and sometimes controversial. Changes in motility and pathological findings as described above are ample and suggest STC to be a real pathological entity. The concept of STC as a neuropathy is interesting and more research is needed to clarify this subject.

Diagnostic tests and their relevance

Most research on diagnostic tests for constipation has not differentiated between the different types of constipation. For STC the transit study has been best evaluated. The relevance of other tests is only briefly described and accounts for the broader group of patients with undifferentiated constipation.

Transit Study

Colonic transit time (CTT) of between 25 and 40 hours (8–11)is reported in healthy, normal subjects. Although there is no difference in age, there is a sex difference: females have significantly higher CTT compared to males. Two different techniques have been described to measure CTT. Radioisotopes scintigraphy can be used, although this technique has become less popular because of practical disadvantages and high costs. Although validated, reliable, and reproducible, this test is seldom used currently.

The 'marker study' with ingestion of radio-opaque markers followed by a plain abdominal X-ray (taken once or at variables times), is more commonly used to measure CTT. Different schedules have been described regarding when to take the markers and take the X-ray. For its practical advantages we advocate Arhan's method (12); 10 markers or pellets are ingested on six consecutive days (60 in total) and an abdominal X-ray is performed on the seventh day. Counting the number of markers and multiplying this number by 2.4 will give the CTT (in hours). More than 20 markers or 48 hours is defined as (total) delayed colonic transit. With this method it is also possible to analyse segmental delayed colonic transit time. The colon is subdivided in first (right colon), second (left colon) and third colonic segments (recto-sigmoid). Right colonic delayed transit time is strongly correlated with patients with low stool frequency (less than three bowel actions per week) which is suggestive of STC. Interestingly females have significantly higher right CTT compared to males. In patients with outlet obstruction left colonic or recto-sigmoidal delayed transit time will be observed.

Transit studies are found to be reliable and reproducible. Patients with symptoms of constipation and a delayed CTT on a transit study are believed to have STC (see introduction). With the introduction of segmental delayed CTT more subgroups can be identified. A new debate is arising about these subgroups. Could patients with left colonic or recto-sigmoidal delayed CTT have STC secondary to outlet obstruction for example? And if so, should all patients with a delayed CTT on transit study be further analysed for causes of outlet obstruction such as internal rectal prolapse or anismus? After a positive transit study, we suggest that patients with symptoms of constipation should have a complete analysis and not just be left in a separate 'slow transit constipation box'. Further research in this area might reveal an interesting new light on the complexity of patients with symptoms of constipation.

Laboratory blood tests

There is no evidence to support or reject routinely screening patients with symptoms of constipation with blood tests for endocrine or metabolic disorders. It must be recognized that these conditions are rare causes of constipation and judicious use of these tests rather than routine use is recommended (13).

Sigmoidoscopy, colonoscopy or barium enema

Rates of colon polyps or cancer found in patients with symptoms of constipation are similar to rates found in studies screening asymptomatic populations. Thus there is no evidence that patients with symptoms of constipation, without alarm symptoms, should routinely be screened by sigmoidoscopy, colonoscopy or barium enema (9). In children a barium enema appears to be a good screening test for identifying Hirschsprung's disease.

Plain abdominal X-ray

There is no evidence to support or reject routinely screening patients with symptoms of constipation with a plain abdominal X-ray. It might reveal an excessive amount of stool but is a poor indicator of colonic transit time (9).

Physiological tests and defaecography

For the relevance of physiologic tests and defaecography we refer to earlier chapters. Patients with symptoms of constipation (especially with symptoms of obstructed defaecation) should be analysed thoroughly and we believe that physiological tests and defaecography should be performed. In a cohort of patients diagnosed with high-grade internal rectal prolapse one-third of these patients were found to have been diagnosed with constipation-predominant IBS at an earlier stage. Two-thirds of patients with anismus may also exhibit delayed CTT. Anorectal manometry provides confirmatory evidence for anismus.

Treatment options

Diet and lifestyle changes

In general, as a first step approach, a physician should advise patients with symptoms of constipation to have a high fibre diet (20 grams daily) complemented with sufficient fluid intake (two litres daily); to avoid coffee, tea, and alcohol; and to have enough physical exercise. Although evidence for this advice is scarce it seems to significantly increase stool frequency and decrease laxative use. For patients with STC, following this advice will rarely be sufficient to improve symptoms and other treatment strategies will be necessary.

Pharmacological treatment: laxatives (Table 13.1) and lubricants

Bulking laxatives or hydrophilic agents (fibre supplements) interact with water to increase water content and volume in the stool, improving propulsion of the stool in the colon. Fibre supplement can be divided into insoluble and soluble fibre. Insoluble fibre resists bacterial degradation in the colon and can retain more water than soluble fibre can. Interestingly fibre may only have a beneficial effect on patients with normal transit constipation. In patients with STC 80% will not have an improvement of symptoms with the use of fibre (14). Side effects such as bloating, excessive gas production and abdominal cramping may limit the use of fibre.

Osmotic laxatives are molecules that are either not absorbed or only poorly absorbed and draw water into the bowel lumen to maintain isotonicity. Use of osmotic laxatives leads to a significantly higher number of bowel movements and better stool consistency compared with the use of fibre alone (15). This class of laxatives can cause bloating, diarrhoea, electrolyte disturbances, volume overload or dehydration. They should be used with caution; side effects limit their use. An exception is polyethylene glycol. It is not absorbed and does not contain electrolytes, which makes it an attractive option in patients with underlying renal or cardiac dysfunction.

Stimulant laxatives are used when bulking or osmotic laxatives fail. They influence intestinal motility and fluid secretion. Historically these laxatives have only been used for short periods although they can be used on a more regular basis when bulking or osmotic laxatives fail. Although they are believed to cause damage to the enteric nervous system and cause laxative dependency there is little evidence to support this. Excessive use can lead to diarrhoea and can cause electrolyte disturbances.

Table 13.1 Laxatives

Bulking or hydrophilic laxatives	
Insoluble fibre	Bran
Soluble fibre	Psyllium, Methylcellulose
Osmotic laxatives	
Poorly absorbed Ions	Magnesium sulphate, Magnesium hydroxide, Magnesium citrate, Sodium phosphate, Sodium sulphate, Potassium sodium tartrate
Poorly absorbed disaccharides, sugar alcohols	Lactulose, Sorbitol, Mannitol
Other	Glycerine, Polyethylene glycol
Stimulant laxatives	
Surface-active agents	Docusates, Bile acids
Diphenylmethane derivates	Phenolphthalien, Bisacodyl, Sodium picosulphate
Anthaquinones	Senna, Cascara sagrada
Other	Ricinoleic acid

Mineral oil is chemically inactive. It acts on the rectum lining as a lubricant. Long-term use can cause malabsorption of fat soluble vitamins. It can also cause foreign body reactions in the intestinal mucosa and regional lymph nodes. Anal seepage of oil is another side-effect.

Pharmacological treatment: Neuromuscular agents

5-HT4 or serotonin agonists stimulate acetylcholine release in the myenteric plexus and stimulate coordinated contraction. Tegaserod and cisapride (which is a 5-HT3 antagonist as well) have been widely used as prokinetic drugs. Because of adverse cardiovascular effects it has been suspended from the market. More specific and selective 5-HT4 agonists such as renzapride and prucalopride are under investigation.

Chloride channel (subtype 2) agonists such as lubiprostone increase chloride secretion into the bowel, enhancing fluid secretion. Although it has been reported to improve symptoms of constipation it has not yet been compared to conventional laxatives. High costs prohibit it becoming a first line drug at this moment.

Pharmacological treatment: pre- or probiotics

Prebiotics are nondigestable preparations that stimulate the growth or activity of beneficial bacteria. Probiotics are live beneficial bacteria preparations. Bacteria of the colon influence peristalsis. Because of their potential influence on improving symptoms of constipation they have been gaining interest as a potential therapy. Evidence however is lacking because of the paucity of data from randomised controlled clinical trials.

In summary, many patients with STC will, after diet and lifestyle changes, benefit from conventional laxatives. Because bulk laxatives may not work very well in patients with STC and may even worsen symptoms, polyethylene glycol seems to be a better alternative. Stimulant laxatives can be used on a long-term basis as well and should be offered more frequently to patients with STC. Neuromuscular agents are potent drugs which are still under investigation and may have an important role in future pharmacological therapy for STC patients.

Biofeedback

Biofeedback training is designed to teach patients to relax the pelvic floor while straining to defaecate. It may benefit constipated patients with anismus unresponsive to conventional treatments. Originally the St Mark's group reported that biofeedback was equally effective in patients with anismus and STC (16–18). Later publications disagreed with this finding and reported very poor short- and long-term effect in patients with STC (19–21). Chiarioni et al found that there is another subgroup of patients, those with anismus and STC. They acknowledged that in this subgroup the STC is likely to be secondary to the outlet obstruction caused by anismus. These patients responded better to biofeedback that the 'STC alone' group and this is reflected by the finding that the transit studies normalized in this subgroup in 65% against 22% in the 'STC alone' group. This supports our view on secondary STC as described earlier in this chapter. We conclude that there is no evidence that biofeedback is a reasonable treatment for STC with the exception for STC secondarily caused by outlet obstructive disorders such as anismus.

Colonic irrigation

Colonic irrigation can be either retrograde or antegrade and can be considered if other conservative measures fail. Most research has been done on children and patients with spina bifida. Although retrograde colonic irrigation (RCI) avoids surgery and has low morbidity, long-term efficacy can be disappointing. It requires a lot of patient motivation and consumes valuable time. In the long-term more than 50% of patients will discontinue its use (22). Antegrade colonic enema (ACE) can be instituted after the formation of a Malone appendicostomy. Success rates are satisfactory although lower in the adult population compared with children. The appendicostomy can be complicated by sepsis, stenosis and leakage of fluid stool. Formation of a caecal neoappendicostomy, an ileal neoappendicostomy, or a colonic conduit are more complex but have a lower occurrence of stenosis.

Sacral nerve stimulation (SNS)

SNS (or sacral nerve modulation) is a promising new technique for treating patients with STC when conservative measures have failed. A coincidental simultaneous positive effect on coexisting chronic constipation was observed in some patients with urinary incontinence (23). More reports seem to confirm this effect (24–26)and a recent study has confirmed this on a small selective group of patients with STC (27). It is an attractive alternative to a subtotal colectomy but the high cost of the implant and the lack of a well designed randomized controlled trial at the moment work against SNS as a widely accepted treatment for patients with STC not responding to conservative measures.

Subtotal colectomy

If all other treatments fail a subtotal colectomy may be indicated. Although a subtotal colectomy with the formation of an ileorectal anastomosis is the most widely accepted surgical procedure, this has a significant associated morbidity and one-third of patients develop diarrhoea, ten percent remained constipated and ten percent progress to a permanent ileostomy (28–30). If patients are well selected and in patients with whole gut slow transit (including stomach and small bowel) functional results after a subtotal colectomy are better.

Key Points

- Slow transit is suspected in patients with constipation complaining of infrequent stools, and is diagnosed on marker studies
- Slow transit constipation is largely a medical condition managed by combinations of laxatives and dietary manipulation
- Occasionally surgical intervention is warranted for severe symptoms resistant to medical therapy
- Subtotal colectomy has fallen out of favour due to high complication rates and persistent symptoms of pain and bloating

Editor's summary

The clinical significance of slow transit constipation (STC) is becoming less rather than more clear. There has been a shift in functional surgery away from colonic surgery (subtotal colectomy) towards outlet surgery (ventral rectopexy, STARR). Recent data from Oxford have shown that isolated STC is uncommon (5%), and is more often associated with outlet obstruction, where it is present in 35%. Moreover, the results of outlet obstruction surgery are equally good in the presence or absence of associated STC, further casting doubt over the clinical significance of STC. This would also explain the poor results and persistent symptoms after subtotal colectomy.

References

1. Lennard-Jones JE (1994). Clinical classification. In Kamm MA, Lennarde-Jones JE (eds). *Constipation*. Petersfield, Wrightson Biomedical Publishing;3–10.

2. Drossman DA, Sandler RS, McKee DC, Lovitz AJ. Bowel patterns among subjects not seeking health care. Use of a questionnaire to identify a population with bowel dysfunction. *Gastroenterology* 1982; **83**(3):529–34.

3. Thompson WG, Longstreth GF, Drossman DA, Heaton KW, Irvine EJ, Müller-Lissner SA. Functional bowel disorders and functional abdominal pain. *Gut* 1999;**45** Suppl 2:II43–7.

4. Shorter Oxford English Dictionary. Sixth Edition. Oxford: Oxford University Press; 2007.

5. Ducrotte P, Rodomanska B, Weber J, Guillard JF, Lerebours E, Hecketsweiler P, Galmiche JP, Colin R, Denis P. Colonic transit time of radiopaque markers and rectoanal manometry in patients complaining of constipation. *Dis Colon Rectum* 1986;**29**(10):630–4.

6. Bassotti G, de Roberto G, Castellani D, Sediari L, Morelli A. Normal aspects of colorectal motility and abnormalities in slow transit constipation. *World J Gastroenterol*, 2005;**14**;11(18):2691–6.

7. Bassotti G, Villanacci V. Slow transit constipation: a functional disorder becomes an enteric neuropathy. *World J Gastroenterol* 2006;**12**(29):4609–13.

8. Metcalf AM, Phillips SF, Zinsmeister AR, MacCarty RL, Beart RW, Wolff BG. Simplified assessment of segmental colonic transit. *Gastroenterology* 1987;**92**(1):40–7.

9. Ke MY, Li RQ, Pan GZ. Gastrointestinal transit time (GITT) in normal Chinese and patients. *Zhonghua Nei Ke Za Zhi* 1990;**29**(12):723–6, 65. Chinese.

10. Meir R, Beglinger C, Dederding JP, Meyer-Wyss B, Fumagalli M, Rowedder A, Turberg J, Brignoli R. Age- and sex-specific standard values of colonic transit time in healthy subjects. *Schweiz Med Wochenschr* 1992;**122**(24):940–3. German.

11. Escalante R, Sorgi M, Salas Z. Total and segmental colonic transit time. Clinical and prospective study using radiopaque markers in normal subjects. *G E N* 1993;**47**(2):88–92. Spanish.

12. Arhan P, Devroede G, Jehannin B, Lanza M, Faverdin C, Dornic C, Persoz B, Tétreault L, Perey B, Pellerin D. Segmental colonic transit time. *Dis Colon Rectum* 1981;**24**(8):625–9.

13. Rao SS, Ozturk R, Laine L. Clinical utility of diagnostic tests for constipation in adults: a systematic review. *Am J Gastroenterol* 2005;**100**(7):1605–15.

14. Voderholzer WA, Schatke W, Mühldorfer BE, Klauser AG, Birkner B, Müller-Lissner SA. Clinical response to dietary fiber treatment of chronic constipation. *Am J Gastroenterol* 1997;**92**(1):95–8.

15. Quah HM, Ooi BS, Seow-Choen F, Sng KK, Ho KS. Prospective randomized crossover trial comparing fibre with lactulose in the treatment of idiopathic chronic constipation. *Tech Coloproctol* 2006;**10**(2):111–4.

16. Koutsomanis D, Lennard-Jones JE, Roy AJ, Kamm MA. Controlled randomised trial of visual biofeedback versus muscle training without a visual display for intractable constipation. *Gut* 1995;**37**(1):95–9.

17. Chiotakakou-Faliakou E, Kamm MA, Roy AJ, Storrie JB, Turner IC. Biofeedback provides long-term benefit for patients with intractable, slow and normal transit constipation. *Gut* 1998;**42**(4):517–21.

18. Emmanuel AV, Kamm MA. Response to a behavioural treatment, biofeedback, in constipated patients is associated with improved gut transit and autonomic innervation. *Gut* 2001;**49**(2):214–9.

19. Battaglia E, Serra AM, Buonafede G, Dughera L, Chistolini F, Morelli A, Emanuelli G, Bassotti G. Long-term study on the effects of visual biofeedback and muscle training as a therapeutic modality in pelvic floor dyssynergia and slow-transit constipation. *Dis Colon Rectum* 2004;**47**(1):90–5.

20. Kairaluoma M, Raivio P, Kupila J, Aarnio M, Kellokumpu I. The role of biofeedback therapy in functional proctologic disorders. *Scand J Surg* 2004;**93**(3):184–90.

21. Chiarioni G, Salandini L, Whitehead WE. Biofeedback benefits only patients with outlet dysfunction, not patients with isolated slow transit constipation. *Gastroenterology* 2005;**129**(1):86–97.

22. Koch SM, Melenhorst J, van Gemert WG, Baeten CG.koch. Prospective study of colonic irrigation for the treatment of defaecation disorders. *Br J Surg* 2008;**95**(10):1273–9.

23. Caraballo R, Bologna RA, Lukban J, Whitmore KE. Sacral nerve stimulation as a treatment for urge incontinence and associated pelvic floor disorders at a pelvic floor center: a follow-up study. *Urology* 2001;**57**(Suppl 1):121.

24. Kenefick NJ, Nicholls RJ, Cohen RG, Kamm MA. Permanent sacral nerve stimulation for treatment of idiopathic constipation *Br J Surg* 2002;**89**(7):882–8.

25. Kenefick NJ, Vaizey CJ, Cohen CR, Nicholls RJ, Kamm MA. Double-blind placebo-controlled crossover study of sacral nerve stimulation for idiopathic constipation. *Br J Surg* 2002;**89**(12):1570–1.

26. Mowatt G, Glazener C, Jarrett M. Sacral nerve stimulation for fecal incontinence and constipation in adults: a short version Cochrane review. *Neurourol Urodyn* 2008; **27**(3):155–61. Review.

27. Naldini G, Martellucci J, Moraldi L, Balestri R, Rossi M. Treatment of Slow Transit Constipation with Sacral Nerve Modulation. *Colorectal Dis* 2009; (E-pub) Oct 19.

28. Kamm MA, Hawley PR, Lennard-Jones JE. Outcome of colectomy for severe idiopathic constipation. *Gut* 1998;**29**:969–73.

29. Lubowski DZ, Chen FC, Kennedy ML, King DW. Results of colectomy for severe slow transit constipation. *Dis Colon Rectum* 1996;**39**:23–9.

30. Knowles CH, Scott M, Lunniss PJ. Outcome of colectomy for slow transit constipation. *Ann Surg* 1999;**230**:627–38.

Chapter 14

Perineoproctology (fissures and haemorrhoids)

Oliver M. Jones

Perineoproctology is a neologism. It is a reference to the fact that pelvic floor disorders and proctological problems are not necessarily distinct entities. More specifically, there is an increasing belief that anal fissures and haemorrhoids in some patients may be a reflection of a global underlying pelvic floor problem.

Anal fissure

The conventional view

The traditional view from the early nineteenth century has been that spasm of the internal anal sphincter is central to chronicity in anal fissure (1). Spasm is said to render the anoderm ischaemic and prevent healing (2).

Overcoming spasm and improving blood supply to the anal canal is the basis of traditional surgical approaches to anal fissure in the form of manual dilatation of the anus or lateral internal sphincterotomy. Concerns over long-term incontinence rates following these procedures (3) and the permanence of such side effects were the driving force behind the development of alternative medical therapies for anal fissure that treat internal sphincter hypertonia in a reversible, 'sphincter-preserving' manner. However, healing rates in some studies with these agents have been disappointing. For example, between 20% (4) and 70% (5) of patients treated with glyceryl trinitrate (GTN) paste fail to heal on a single course of treatment.

In the non-healing fissure, one should consider other diagnoses including Crohn's disease. In others, the fissure appears to be 'idiopathic' but persistently fails to heal with conventional therapies. This might reflect the fact that the ischaemic theory of chronicity may be oversimplistic.

Are all chronic anal fissures ischaemic?

In recent years there has been increasing recognition that some patients with anal fissure may have normal or low resting anal pressures (6). These patients may have other abnormalities in anorectal physiology including a lack of recto-anal inhibitory reflex, a longer high pressure zone, and more frequent ultraslow pressure waves (7).

There has been a recent report from Jenkins et al. (8) suggesting that anterior and posterior fissures may have a differing aetiology and pathophysiology. They examined

70 consecutive patients with chronic anal fissure and compared them to 39 asymptomatic controls. They reported that anterior fissures were more commonly seen in young women. Patients with anterior fissures more commonly had a history of obstetric injury and an external sphincter injury demonstrable on endoanal ultrasound. Physiology showed that whilst posterior fissures were associated with a significantly increased maximum resting pressure, resting pressure in those with anterior fissures was not significantly higher. Squeeze pressure was lower in the anterior fissure group. These results are summarised in table 14.1.

Corby et al. performed a prospective study on women to investigate the effect of parturition on the pelvic floor (9). In this study, manometry was performed six weeks before and after 209 primigravid women without a history of anorectal disease. Postpartum studies only were performed on a further 104 primiparae. Overall, 29 (9%) of women developed postpartum anal fissure. Antepartum pressures were similar for women who did and those who did not develop anal fissure, though in both groups, postpartum resting and squeeze pressures were lower compared to antepartum values. This study concluded that patients with postpartum fissures tended to have low sphincter pressures. The aetiology of the fissures was unclear. Patients with anal fissure tended to have postpartum incontinence but whether this was the cause or a consequence of the fissure was unclear. The authors concluded that in view of the low sphincter pressures, surgery should be avoided in this patient group.

Is identification of the low pressure fissure important?

It is controversial whether an effort should be made to identify the patient with a low pressure fissure. A questionnaire study of consultant members of the Association of Coloproctology of Great Britain and Ireland revealed that 57% of those responding would perform lateral sphincterotomy for anal fissure without pre-operative anorectal physiology and endoanal ultrasound. Overall, 36% of surgeons selectively performed manual dilatation and of these, 65% would do so without pre-operative physiology and ultrasound. In part, this reflects differing views on the prevalence and significance of the low pressure fissure. Prohm and Bonner (10) performed anorectal manometry on 177 patients with anal fissure and found that whilst only one fifth of patients in their cohort had a normal or low pressure fissure, this was not predictive of either failure of sphincterorotomy or indeed development of postoperative incontinence.

Table 14.1 Comparison of characteristics of anterior and posterior fissures from study of Jenkins et al. [8]

	Anterior fissure N = 28	Posterior fissure N = 39	P value
Gender (M:F)	1:27	14:25	
Obstetric trauma (number)	15	3	P = 0.0005
IAS defect	5/28	1/39	p = 0.078
EAS defect	21/28	9/39	p = 0.0005

By contrast, Jenkins et al. (8) commented in their study on the high incidence of low pressure fissures and occult sphincter injuries in women with anterior fissures and suggested a potential danger of incontinence if sphincterotomy was performed in this group. Indeed, the recent Position Statement from the Association of Coloproctology of Great Britain and Ireland (11) suggested that an anal flap (12) (V–Y advancement or a rotational flap (13)) should be employed for the low pressure fissure rather than a sphincterotomy or anal dilatation.

Is there another aetiology to 'idiopathic' anal fissure?

The conventional view, as we have seen, is that anal fissures are caused by a tear to the anoderm and that chronicity is brought about by ischaemia of the anal canal secondary to internal anal sphincter spasm. It is clear, however, that in many patients there is no history of constipation and the persistence of fissures in the absence of a raised maximum resting pressure in the anal canal makes the ischaemic hypothesis for all fissures untenable.

Post partum fissures may be caused by a different mechanism to 'conventional' idiopathic fissures. They are generally anterior and they might be caused by the shearing forces applied to the anal canal during vaginal delivery. Anterior fissures in women, it has been suggested by Neal (14), often coexist with a rectocele. He hypothesized that trauma to the anoderm occurred during distension of the rectocele resulting in a chronic anal fissure. To test this theory, he performed a trial on 54 consecutive women with an anterior fissure and rectocele and randomized them between lateral sphincterotomy and levatorplasty. The groups were well matched and pre-operative manometry suggested that most of these were not high pressure fissures, though the data presented in the paper is not detailed. Post-operatively, fissure healing was reported in all 29 patients having a levatorplasty and in all but one of the 25 patients undergoing sphincterotomy. Resting pressures fell significantly in the sphincterotomy group, though this did not cause incontinence, whilst pressures were unchanged in the levatorplasty group.

It is our observation in Oxford that anal fissures resistant to treatment often have an underlying rectoanal intussusception (15). In this report, we described 11 patients with average symptom duration of five years, all of whom had failed GTN treatment and additionally either diltiazem, botulinum toxin or both. One patient had also had a sphincterotomy and another a manual dilatation of the anus at their referring hospital. Of these patients, nine complained of obstructed defaecation. On proctography, five patients had recto-anal intussusception. Furthermore, the mean internal sphincter thickness on endoanal ultrasound was 3.5mm, with seven of the patients having a thickened internal sphincter. A thickened internal anal sphincter is highly predictive for high-grade internal prolapse (16).

There is some support for a role of high-grade intussusception in resistant anal fissure from a small study of five patients with anal fissure all of whom had failed glyceryl trinitrate or diltiazem and botulinum toxin. They were all subjected to proctography and all five had high-grade (recto-anal) intussusception. Three patients also had a rectocele. All five patients healed their fissure after a stapled transanal rectal resection (STARR procedure) (17).

Haemorrhoids

The conventional view

The aetiology of haemorrhoids was investigated by Thomson in his landmark paper from 1975 (18). He considered the three main theories on the pathogenesis of haemorrhoids: the varicose vein theory, the vascular hyperplasia theory and the sliding anal lining theory. His study included anatomical work based on post-mortem specimens and a questionnaire assessment of patients with haemorrhoids. He concluded that the sliding anal lining theory was probably correct.

This theory supposes that the haemorrhoidal venous plexus is supported by a scaffold of smooth muscle and elastic tissue arising partially from the internal sphincter and partially from the conjoined longitudinal muscle. Indeed, Thomson describes in his paper how haemorrhoids are more likely to occur in patients who strain and/or pass hard stools. Such straining might be expected to push the haemorrhoids out of the anal canal, both engorging the haemorrhoids and impeding venous return.

Does constipation cause haemorrhoids?

There have been a number of studies of the aetiology of haemorrhoids and in particular their relationship to constipation. One of the problems is that many of these studies have not used a tight definition of constipation. However, many authors have commented that constipation does seem to be a risk factor for the development of haemorrhoids (19).

A recent study from Sweden looked at the bowel habits of 100 consecutive patients with haemorrhoids who had participated in a randomized study on haemorrhoidectomy and compared them to 200 age- and gender-matched control subjects and a further 100 gender-matched consecutive patients undergoing an orthopaedic procedure (20). This study, interestingly, concluded that bowel frequency was similar in the study and control groups and patients in the haemorrhoid group did not report hard stools. However, it did show that the patients in the haemorrhoid group had an increased tendency to 'disturbed defaecation' including an exaggerated desire to strain and a feeling of incomplete evacuation and urgency. The authors concluded that irritable bowel syndrome-type symptoms commonly coexisted with haemorrhoids. It seems possible, however, that many of these patients in fact had an underlying pelvic floor problem, though they were labelled as 'IBS' and not investigated further.

Haemorrhoids and prolapse

The conventional classification system for haemorrhoids grades haemorrhoids from I–IV on the basis of the degree of prolapse. The weakness of the classification system is that it simply considers prolapse and not symptom severity (21). It is useful, however, in that the degree of prolapse serves as a useful guide to treatment (22). It is perhaps intuitive that if the haemorrhoidal prolapse is not addressed, the diverse haemorrhoidal symptoms (bleeding, pruritis, incontinence) are unlikely to resolve. Indeed in most patients, Thomson suggests, prolapse precedes bleeding (18) and thus it seems sensible that prolapse must be dealt with before the other symptoms resolve.

The next issue is whether haemorrhoidal prolapse is part of a continuum of internal rectal prolapse. The literature is confusing on this subject as some authors talk of rectal internal mucosal prolapse and intussusception (full thickness internal prolapse) almost as if they are synonymous. Interestingly, although Longo believes that rectal mucosal prolapse is part of the pathophysiology of haemorrhoidal disease (23), colo-proctologists report considerable variation in their detection of rectal mucosal prolapse in patients with haemorrhoids (24). In this same study, almost half of respondents considered rectal mucosal prolapse and haemorrhoids to be distinct clinical entities. In an important study in the 1980s Sun et al. found similar patho-physiological characteristics in patients with mucosal prolapse (25).

Many colorectal surgeons, however, will be familiar with inserting a circular anal dilator (CAD) into the anal canal with a plan to perform a stapled anopexy, only to find a surprisingly large amount of prolapsing tissue within the CAD. The PPH-03™ gun is capable of resecting only a limited amount of tissue and there is a concern that these patients are at risk of persistent prolapse into the staple line or an early recurrence of symptoms (26). In a randomised controlled trial, 68 patients with haemorrhoids associated with rectal mucosal prolapse and/or intussusception were randomised to stapled anopexy or STARR (27). At mean follow-up of eight months, the incidence of residual disease in the anopexy group was 29% versus 6% in the STARR group (p = 0.007). The authors commented that if the prolapse extended over one half of the length of the CAD, then this was associated with a 100% incidence of residual tissue after anopexy. How this correlated with symptoms was unclear.

Fissures and haemorrhoids: a proposed algorithm for treatment

A proposed new classification in perineoproctology

The data presented in this chapter reflect a growing understanding that the aetiology of both anal fissures and haemorrhoids may be multifactorial. In particular, there is an increased recognition that many patients with these proctological conditions have abnormal defaecatory habits and clinical evidence of a pelvic floor disorder. There is a need for more studies in these patients looking at abnormalities in proctography, anorectal physiology, and endoanal ultrasound. Set against this, it is undoubtedly true that many patients have 'uncomplicated' fissures and haemorrhoids and should not have treatment delayed by inappropriate investigation. So which patients need pelvic floor investigations (anorectal manometry, endoanal ultrasound, proctogram, and transit studies)?

We propose that patients may be considered in four categories. Type A refers to patients with a pelvic floor disorder in whom the clinician detects incidental asymptomatic haemorrhoids or a fissure. This type of patient should be investigated and treated as a pelvic floor problem. Type B patients present with symptomatic haemorrhoids or a fissure but on further questioning are found to have pelvic floor symptoms, such as obstructed defaecation. In such patients, it is reasonable to instigate therapy for the proctological problem (eg banding or topical treatments) whilst undertaking pelvic floor investigations. Treatment of any detected pelvic floor problem may be necessary if proctological treatments fail.

Type C patients have a proctological problem with clinically detectable, asymptomatic pelvic floor dysfunction (eg ballooning of the perineum on straining). These patients

Table 14.2 A proposed new classification for perineoproctology. For patients with an anal fissure or haemorrhoids, it is reasonable to start simple treatments such as stool softeners, laxatives, glyceryl trinitrate or diltiazem paste. The classification gives a guide to the need to investigate a possible underlying pelvic floor problem which may require treatment before the fissures or haemorrhoids resolve. For types B and C, pelvic floor investigations can be reserved for those patients failing simple measure to treat their fissure or haemorrhoids

Patient Category	Proctology symptoms	Pelvic floor symptoms	Pelvic floor signs	Pelvic floor investigations
A	−	+	+	Yes
B	+	+	+/−	If persists
C	+	−	+	If persists
D	+	−	−	Rarely

can be treated as a proctological problem without pelvic floor investigations unless they develop recurrent or persistent proctological problems. Type D patients have haemorrhoids or a fissure without symptoms or signs of a pelvic floor problem and should be treated conventionally. Pelvic floor investigation is rarely needed in this group. This classification is outlined in table 14.2.

Key points

♦ Pelvic floor problems and fissures/haemorrhoids often coexist

♦ The pathophysiology of fissures and haemorrhoids may be multifactorial

♦ Selective investigation of 'proctology' patients with physiology, endoanal ultrasound and proctography/transit studies may be necessary

♦ Grading patients with proctological problems may help to guide investigation and management.

Editor's summary

It is emerging that more substantial pelvic floor disorders sometimes underlie apparently straightforward proctological problems. Some anal fissures, particularly the low pressure anterior variety, have always appeared to be different in some way to the standard chronic anal fissure; and recalcitrant anal fissures, resistant to standard medical management seem to be different too. Haemorrhoids and mucosal prolapse share many characteristics with rectal prolapse, so it is not entirely unexpected to find these conditions commonly associated.

References

1. Brodie BC. Lectures on diseases of the rectum; lecture III; preternatural contraction of the sphincter ani. *London Medical Gazette* 1835; **16**:26–31.

2. Gibbons CP, Read NW. Anal hypertonia in fissures: cause or effect? *Br J Surg* 1986; **73**:443–5.

3. Khubchandani IT, Reed JF. Sequelae of internal sphincterotomy for chronic fissure-*in-ano*. *Br J Surg* 1989; **76**:431–4.

4. Gorfine SR. Treatment of benign anal disease with topical nitroglycerin. *Dis Colon Rectum* 1995; **38**:453–7.

5. Richard CS, Gregoire R, Plewes EA et al. Internal sphincterotomy is superior to topical nitroglycerin in the treatment of chronic anal fissure. *Dis Colon Rectum* 2000; **43**: 1048–58.

6. Jones OM, Ramalingam T, Lindsey I, Cunningham C, George BD, Mortensen NJ. Digital rectal examination of sphincter pressures in chronic anal fissure is unreliable. *Dis Colon Rectum* 2005; **48**:349–52.

7. Lund JN, Scholefield JH. Aetiology and treatment of anal fissure. *Br J Surg* 1996; **83**:1335–44.

8. Jenkins JT, Urie A, Molloy RG. Anterior anal fissures are associated with occult sphincter injury and abnormal sphincter function. *Colorectal Dis* 2007; **10**:280–5.

9. Corby H, Donnelly VS, O'Herlihy C, O'Connell PR. Anal pressures are low in women with post-partum anal fissure. *Br J Surg* 1997; **84**:86–8.

10. Prohm P, Bonner C. Is manometry essential for surgery of chronic fissure-in-ano? *Dis Colon Rectum* 1995; **38**:735–8.

11. Cross KLR, Massey EJD, Fowler AL, Monson JRT. The management of anal fissure: ACPGBI Position Statement. *Colorectal Dis* 2008; **10** (Suppl. 3):1 7.

12. Leong AF, Seow-Choen F. Lateral sphincterotomy compared with anal advancement flap for chronic anal fissure. *Dis Colon Rectum* 1995; **38**:69–71.

13. Singh M, Sharma A, Gardiner A, Duthie GS. Early results of a rotational flap to treat chronic anal fissures. *Int J Colorectal Dis* 2005; **20**:339–42.

14. Ellis CN. Anterior levatorplasty for the treatment of chronic anal fissures in females with a rectocele: a randomized, controlled trial. *Dis Colon Rectum* 2004; **47**:1170–3.

15. Wijffels N, Collinson R, Cunningham C, Lindsey I. Rectoanal intussusception frequently underlies recalcitrant chronic anal fissures. *Colorectal Dis* 2008; **10** (suppl 2):15.

16. Marshall M, Halligan S, Fotheringham T, Bartram C, Nicholls RJ. Predictive value of internal anal sphincter thickness for diagnosis of rectal intussusception in patients with solitary rectal ulcer syndrome. *Br J Surg* 2002; **89**:1281–5.

17. Clarke AD, Chand M, Tarver D, Nash GF, Lamparelli M. Stapled transanal rectal resection in the management of resistant anal fissures. *Colorectal Dis* 2008; **10** (suppl 1): 6.

18. Thomson WHF. The nature of haemorrhoids. *Br J Surg* 1975; **62**:542–52.

19. Delco F, Sonnenberg A. Associations between hemorrhoids and other diagnoses. *Dis Colon Rectum* 1998; **41**:1534–41.

20. Johannsson HO, Graf W, Pahlman L. Bowel habits in hemorrhoid patients and normal subjects. *Am J Gastroenterol* 2005; **100**:401–6.

21. Thomson JPS, Leicester RJ, Smith LE. Haemorrhoids. In: Henny MM, Swash M (eds). *Coloproctology and the Pelvic Floor*. 2nd Ed. Oxford: Butterworth-Heinemann; 1992. pp. 272–93.

22. Acheson AG, Scholefield JH. Management of haemorrhoids. *BMJ* 2008; **336**:380–3.

23. Longo A. Stapled anopexy and stapled haemorrhoidectomy: two opposite concepts and procedures. *Dis Colon rectum* 2002; **45**:571–2.

24. Gaj F, Trecca A. Hemorrhoids and rectal internal mucosal prolapse; one or two conditions? A national survey. *Tech Coloproctol* 2005; **9**:163–5.

25. Sun WM, Read NW, Donnely TC, Bannister JJ, Shorthouse AJ. A common pathophysiology for full thickness rectal prolapse, anterior mucosal prolapse and solitary rectal ulcer. *Br J Surg* 1989; **76**:290–5.

26. Ortiz H, Marzo J, Armendariz P. Randomized clinical trial of stapled haemorrhoidectomy versus conventional diathermy haemorrhoidectomy. *Br J Surg* 2002; **89**:1376–81.

27. Boccasanta P, Venturi M, Roviaro G. Stapled transanal rectal resection versus stapled anopexy in the cure of hemorrhoids associated with rectal prolapse. A randomized controlled trial. *Int J Colorectal Dis* 2007; **22**:245–51.

Chapter 15

Pudendal pain syndrome

Andrew Paul Baranowski

Introduction

The classification of conditions associated with pain perceived within the pelvis and its adjacent areas is complex and controversial. Pain associated with peripheral nerve injury is well described and many of the mechanisms are clearly understood. When an obvious injury involves the pudendal nerve and is associated with pain then the diagnosis of pudendal neuralgia may be made. Following nerve injury, secondary changes within the central nervous system may occur and as a result areas beyond the classical areas associated with the pudendal nerve may be symptomatic and this may confuse the diagnosis. The term 'pudendal pain syndrome' is used when there is no obvious injury/disease process to account for the pain.

Pudendal anatomy

Understanding the anatomy of the pudendal nerve is essential for an understanding of the aetiology, diagnosis, and treatment of pudendal neuralgia (1).

Branches of the pudendal nerve (Fig. 15.1)

The pudendal nerve has its origins at the S2, S3, and S4 levels. S2 and 3 also contribute to the sciatic nerve and S4 to the coccygeal plexus and the anococcygeal nerves. The pudendal nerve has three main branches: the inferior anorectal nerve, the superficial perineal nerve (which terminates as cutaneous branches in the perineum and posterior aspect of the scrotum), and the deep perineal nerve, which is distributed to the pelvic structures (innervating parts of the bladder, prostate, and urethra). This branch terminates as the dorsal nerve of the penis/clitoris, innervating the glans. As well as sensory branches the pudendal nerve provides motor innervation to anal and urethral sphincters as well as to the bulbospongiosus and ischiocavernous muscles (involved in the bulbo cavernosal response and ejaculation). Autonomic fibres also pass with the pudendal nerve and are derived from the presacral parasympathetics as well as sympathetic fibres via the hypogastric plexus.

Anatomical relations of the pudendal nerve (Fig. 15.2)

The course of the nerve may be variable but the three roots that form the pudendal nerve usually merge anterior to the sacrum and ventral to the piriformis muscle.

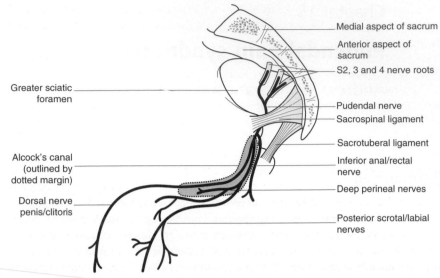

Fig. 15.1 Divisions of the right pudendal nerve, looking from inside the pelvis at the pelvic wall. Adapted from diagram courtesy of Natasha Marie Baranowski.

The pudendal nerve leaves the pelvis via the greater sciatic notch to enter the sub-gluteal region. In the sub-gluteal triangle (the area bordered by the inferior edge of the piriformis superiorly, the sacro-tuberous ligament medially and the upper border of quadratus femoris inferiorly) the nerve emerges from under the inferior border of the piriformis muscle with its associated pudendal artery and veins. The nerve lies medial to

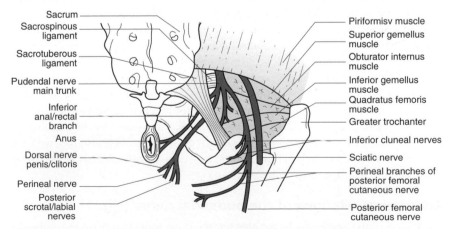

Fig. 15.2 Relations of the pudendal nerve to other structures, posterior view. Adapted from diagram courtesy of Natasha Marie Baranowski.

the nerve to the obturator internus muscle, which is medial to the posterior femoral cutaneous nerve (that divides into its cutaneous branch but also the inferior cluneal nerves and perineal nerves), which in turn is medial to the sciatic nerve. These anatomical relations are important for neurotracing techniques used for nerve blocks and because symptoms in those nerve territories will also help in the diagnosis.

The pudendal nerve leaves the sub-gluteal region as it wraps around the superficial surface of the ischial spine/sacro-spinous ligament to re-enter the pelvis via the lesser sciatic notch (between the more ventral sacro-spinous ligament and the more dorsal sacro-tuberous ligaments) (Fig. 15.3). This occurs 15% of the time at the enthesis of the spine and the ligament, 75% of the time it is more medial and 10% of the time it wraps around the spine. The sacro-tuberous ligament may have a sharp superior border, be wide and as a result close to the sacro-spinous ligament, or be divided with the pudendal nerve passing through it. All of these features may predispose to nerve injury.

As the pudendal nerve re-enters the pelvis below the levator muscles, it runs within a fascial canal medial to the internal obturator muscle (Alcock's canal) (Fig. 15.3).

The inferior anorectal branch may never be a true branch of the pudendal nerve, and may have its origins directly from the roots. As a consequence pain associated with pudendal nerve injury may not involve the anorectal area. Similarly pain may only be perceived in the anorectal area if the main pudendal nerve is not involved. In 11% the inferior anorectal nerve pierces the sacro-spinous ligament possibly increasing the risk of entrapment. Other variations of the anorectal branch exist with the nerve branching off from the main pudendal nerve at any point in the gluteal region or within the pelvis. In 56% of cases the pudendal nerve is a single trunk as it re-enters the pelvis. Some people will have 2 or 3 pudendal nerve trunks.

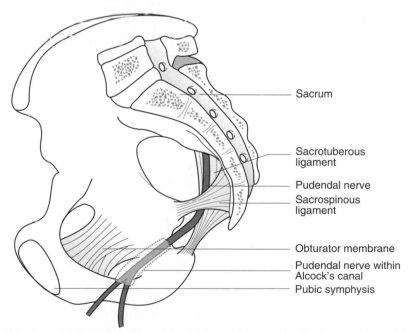

Sacrum

Sacrotuberous ligament

Pudendal nerve
Sacrospinous ligament

Obturator membrane
Pudendal nerve within Alcock's canal
Pubic symphysis

Fig. 15.3 Right hemipelvis, looking from inside. Adapted from diagram courtesy of Natasha Marie Baranowski.

Aetiology of pudendal neuralgia

Anatomical variations

Anatomical variations may predispose the patient to developing pudendal neuralgia over time or with repeated low-grade trauma (such as sitting for prolonged periods of time or cycling) (2).

The pudendal nerve may be damaged due to local anatomical variation at the level of:

1. The piriformis muscle (for instance as a part of a piriformis syndrome where in certain cases the nerve may pass through the muscle and hence be trapped or in other cases muscle hypertrophy or spasm has been implicated)

2. The sacro-spinous/sacro-tuberous ligaments (see above) possibly accounting for 42% of cases

3. Within Alcock's canal (medial to the obturator internus muscle, within the fascia of the muscle), possibly accounting for 26% of cases.

4. Multiple levels in 17% of cases.

The site of injury will determine the site of perceived pain (Fig. 15.4) and the nature of associated symptoms (eg the more distal the damage, the less likely the anal region will be involved).

Surgery

In orthopaedic hip surgery pressure from the positioning of the patient, where the perineum is placed up hard against the brace, has been reported to produce pudendal nerve damage (3). The surgery itself may also directly damage the nerve. Pelvic surgery such as sacro-spinous colpopexy is clearly associated with pudendal nerve damage in some cases (4). In many types of surgery pudendal injury is implicated even if less clear cut and this would include colorectal, urological and gynaecological surgery. Even minimally invasive procedures such as trans vaginal tape and trans obturator tape procedures for incontinence may be implicated. Trauma to the pudendal nerve during gender reassignment surgery has also been seen in our centre.

Trauma

Fractures of both the sacrum and/or pelvis may result in pudendal nerve/root damage and pain. Falls and trauma to the gluteal region may also produce symptoms if associated with significant tissue injury.

Cancer

Tumours in the pre-sacral space must be considered. Tumours invading the pudendal nerve are not uncommon.

Birth trauma

This is more difficult to be certain about. The pudendal neuralgia of birth trauma is thought to resolve in most cases over a period of months. However, rarely, it appears to continue as a painful neuropathy. Multiple pregnancies and births may predispose to stretch neuropathies in later life.

Elderly women

Childbirth (5) and repeated abdominal straining associated with chronic constipation (6) are thought to predispose elderly women to post menopausal pelvic floor descent and stretching of the pudendal nerve with associated pain. Changes in the hormone status may also be a factor.

In our Urogenital Pain Management Centre the commonest associations with pudendal neuralgia appear to be: history of pelvic surgery, prolonged sitting (especially young men working with computer type technology) and post menopausal older women. Trauma and cancer related pain is less frequent and we rarely see patients where cycling appears to have been the cause.

Differential diagnosis

Other forms of neuropathic pain

As well as the pudendal nerve there are several other nerves that if they are damaged may mimic the symptoms of pudendal neuralgia.

Inferior cluneal nerve. This is a branch of the posterior femoral cutaneous nerve (Fig. 15.2). This nerve is prone to injury in the region of the ischium. The neuropathy affects the skin more lateral in the perineum than that innervated by the pudendal nerve (Fig. 15.4).

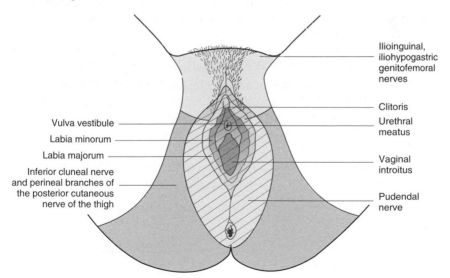

Fig. 15.4 Perineal dermatomes. Adapted from diagram courtesy of Natasha Marie Baranowski.

Sacral nerve roots. The S2, 3 or 4 nerve roots may be involved. This is an important differential diagnosis as tumours must be excluded.

Cauda equina syndrome. Lumbar spinal pathology involving the cauda equina may result in an intractable neuropathic pain.

Ilioinguinal, iliohypogastric and genitofemoral nerves. Injury to these nerves or their roots may occur from thoracolumbar pathology, abdominal posterior wall conditions, surgery and entrapment in the groin. The pain may extend into the groin, anterior perineum and scrotum/labia majorum. If the femoral branch of the genitofemoral nerve is involved, pain may extend into the inner thigh.

Referred spinal pain (7)

Pain from thoracolumbar pathology may refer to the groin. Spinal pain may become associated with muscle hyperalgesia and trigger points. The muscle associated pain may spread to involve a range of muscles, including the pelvic floor muscles with resultant pelvic pain.

Musculoskeletal disorders

Trigger points associated with localized tenderness and pain may be detected in the piriformis muscle, obturator internus muscle, levator ani muscles, bulbocavernosal and ischiocavernosal muscles, as well as the gluteal, adductors, rectus abdominus, and spinal muscles. All of these may refer the pain into or close to the pelvis.

Pathology of the joints (sacroiliac, pubic symphysis, hip, and spinal) may also refer into the pelvis.

Coccydynia, a painful coccyx may occur for a number of reasons. There may be local mechanical, inflammatory, infective, or infiltrative reasons. A neuropathic coccydynia has also been described.

Other conditions that may mimic pudendal neuralgia

Many disease processes involving the pelvis and its organs may be associated with pain and need to be excluded. Those involving inflammation, infection and infiltration are obvious candidates. Actual pudendal neuralgia also needs to be separated out from the pain syndromes that affect the pelvis. The pelvic pain syndromes have no obvious local cause and are considered to be mediated by the central nervous system. These syndromes are described in several texts (8) and include:

Prostate pain syndrome (also referred to as prostatitis)

Bladder pain syndrome (also referred to as interstitial cystitis, painful bladder syndrome)

Both of the above are not associated with infection; whereas inflammatory cells may be present in certain subgroups.

Neuropathic pain

Much has been written on the subject of neuropathic pain (9). There are some fundamental principles that are worth considering.

Nerve injury is associated with a number of changes both within the peripheral nervous system and the whole of the central neural axis right up to the higher centres. These changes serve to produce an increasing mismatch between stimulus and response. Windup is a progressive increase in elicited action potentials per unit stimulus and is mediated by N-methyl-D-aspartic acid (NMDA) glutamate receptors. An acute insult to the nervous system or repeated stimulation may result in transient windup phenomena becoming permanent, through immediate gene activation resulting in regulatory chemical changes as well as structural changes within the central nervous system. These long-term changes will be associated with both afferent sensory dysfunction as well as efferent motor dysfunction within the pathways of the injured nerve. However, the changes will also be associated with wider reaching abnormalities within the central nervous system and indeed the body as a whole. These abnormalities may include a spread of the abnormal afferent processing to nerves outside of the originally damaged nerve so that increased perception (pain and allodynia) from an area greater than the expected dermatomal pattern may occur. In the case of those organs with a nervous innervation that overlaps with the injured nerve, visceral hypersensitivity (sensory urge and as a result increased frequency of voiding/evacuation) and pain may result. Efferent dysfunction of striated and smooth muscle function may also be seen and the role of changes in the sympathetic and parasympathetic nervous system is still not fully understood.

Essentially, what may be considered a simple nerve injury may be magnified by the central nervous system so that a whole region may be involved and a nonspecific regional pain syndrome may occur. There is also a suggestion that involvement of the nervous system in the control of the endocrine and immunological systems may also become abnormal. Certainly, there is a complex interaction between nerve injury, emotional well being, disability and widespread pain. A proportion of patients will go on to develop Chronic Fatigue Syndrome and fibromyalgia.

Clinical presentation of pudendal neuralgia

There is a wide age range as one would expect with a condition that has so many potential causes. There is a suggestion that the younger the patient the better the prognosis. Essentially the sooner the diagnosis is made, as with any compression nerve injury, the better the prognosis and the older patient may represent a more protracted problem. 60% of the cases will present in women.

History

A proportion of patients will be able to relate the onset of pain to an acute event such as surgery, sepsis or trauma and occasionally cycling for a prolonged period. Chronic injury is more frequent, such as associated with sitting for prolonged periods over time. Many will be idiopathic.

The pain is classically perceived in the perineum from anus to clitoris/penis. However, a less specific pain distribution may occur and this may be due to anatomical variation (10); involvement of branches of the nerve rather than the main nerve; central nervous system central sensitization; and as a consequence the involvement of other organs and systems in a regional pain syndrome. Other nerves in the vicinity may also be involved eg inferior cluneal nerve and perineal branches of the posterior femoral cutaneous nerve (Fig 15.2 and 15.4). The musculoskeletal system may become involved confusing the pain picture as aches and pains develop in the muscles due to immobility and disability, possibly magnified by the central nervous system changes.

Burning is the most predominant adjective. Crushing and electric may also be used, indicating the two components—a constant pain often associated with acute sharp episodes. Many patients may have the feeling of a swelling or foreign body in the rectum or perineum, often described as a golf ball or tennis ball. The term pain has different meanings to patients and some would rather use the terms discomfort or numbness.

Aggravating factors include any cause of pressure being applied either directly to the nerve or indirectly by pressure to other tissue resulting in pudendal traction. Allodynia, pain on light touch due to the central nervous system involvement, may make sexual contact and the wearing of clothes difficult. These patients often remain standing and as a consequence develop a wide range of other aches and pains. Soft seats are often less well tolerated, while sitting on a toilet seat is said to be much better tolerated. If unilateral, sitting on one buttock is common. The pain may be exacerbated by bowel or bladder evacuation.

Associated features

Pudendal nerve damage may be associated with a range of sensory phenomena. In the distribution of the nerve itself, as well as unprovoked pain, the patient may have paraesthesia (pins and needles); dysaesthesia (unpleasant sensory perceptions usually secondary to provocation, but not necessarily so, the sensation of running cold water would be one such sensation); allodynia (pain on light touch); and hyperalgesia (increased pain perception following a painful stimulus but also hot and cold stimuli). Similar sensory abnormalities may be found outside of the territory of the damaged nerve and in particular visceral and muscle hyperalgesia may occur.

The cutaneous sensory dysfunction may be associated with superficial dyspareunia, but also irritation and pain associated with clothes brushing the skin at one extreme. At the other extreme there may be a lack of sensation and pain may occur in the presence of numbness. Visceral hypersensitivity may result in an urge to defaecate or urinate. This is usually associated with voiding frequency with small amounts being passed. Pain on visceral filling may occur. Anal pain and loss of motor control may result in poor bowel activity with constipation and/or incontinence. Ejaculation and orgasm may also be painful or reduced.

Many of those suffering with pudendal neuralgia will complain of fatigue and generalized muscle cramps, weakness and pain. Being unable to sit is a major disability, over time patients struggle to stand and they often become bedbound. The immobility produces generalized muscle wasting and minimal activity hurts. As a consequence of the widespread pain and disability, patients will often have emotional problems, in particular depression. Patients with chronic pelvic pain are also often anxious and have the tendency to catastrophize. Depression, catastrophizing and disability are all poor prognostic markers (11).

Skin colour may change due to changes in innervation but also possibly due to neurogenic oedema. The patient may describe the area as swollen because there is oedema but also when there is a lack of afferent perception.

Clinical examination

A full clinical examination of the spinal, muscular and nervous system as well as the urogenital and colorectal systems are necessary to aid in the diagnosis and especially to detect signs indicating another pathology. Often there is little to find in pudendal neuralgia and frequently findings are nonspecific. The main pathognomonic features would be the signs of nerve injury in the appropriate distribution, eg allodynia or numbness. Tenderness by pressure over the pudendal nerve may aid the clinical diagnosis. This may be elicited by per rectal or per vaginal examination and palpation in the region of the ischial spine and or Alcock's canal. Muscle tenderness and the presence of trigger points in the muscles may confuse the picture. Trigger points may be present in a range of muscles both within the pelvis (levator ani muscles, obturator internus) or externally (eg the piriformis, adductors, rectus abdominus or paraspinal muscles).

Investigations

Magnetic resonance imaging (MRI) scans of the pelvis are usually normal. However, MRI scans of the pelvis and spine (mid thoracic to coccyx) are considered essential to help with the differential diagnosis. Electrophysiological studies may reveal signs of perineal denervation, increased pudendal nerve latency, or an impaired bulbocavernosal reflex. However, for an abnormality to be detected significant nerve damage is probably necessary. As pain may be associated with limited nerve damage these investigations are often normal in patients thought to have pudendal neuralgia.

Treatment

The approach to treating pudendal neuralgia is essentially the same as for the treatment of any neuropathic pain. There is a suggestion that early treatment has a better prognosis.

Injections

The role of injections may be divided into two. Firstly, an injection of local anaesthetic and steroid at the sight of nerve injury may produce a therapeutic action (12). The possible reasons for this are related to the fact that steroid may reduce any inflammation and swelling at the sight of nerve irritation; but also, the steroid may have a sodium channel blocking activity and reduce irritable firing from the nerve. The second possible benefit of local infiltration is diagnostic. Above, we have already indicated that when the pudendal nerve is injured there are several sites where this may occur. Differential nerve blocks of the pudendal nerve will help to provide information in relation to the site where the nerve may be trapped.

Infiltration at the ischial spine requires the use of a nerve stimulator/locator. Both motor (anal contraction) and sensory endpoints may be noted. The anatomical endpoint may be localized by fluoroscopy (the most frequently used technique); computerized tomography (CT) guidance (involves a significant amount of radiation); or ultrasound. Currently, infiltration of the pudendal nerve within Alcock's canal is primarily undertaken with the use of CT.

As well as injecting around the pudendal nerve, specific nerve blocks of other nerves arising from the pelvis may be undertaken. Similarly, trigger point injections into tender areas within muscles may also be considered.

Surgery

Decompression of an entrapped or injured nerve is a routine approach and probably should apply to the pudendal nerve as it applies to all other nerves (13). There are several approaches and the approach of choice probably depends upon the nature of the pathology. The most traditional approach is the transgluteal approach; however, a transperineal approach may be an alternative, particularly if the nerve damage is thought to be related to previous pelvic surgery.

Currently there is only one prospective randomized study (13). This suggests that if the patient has had the pain for less than six years, 66% of patients will see some improvement with surgery (compared to 40% if the pain has been present for more than six years). Surgery is by no means the answer for all patients. On talking to patients that have undergone surgery, providing the diagnosis was clear-cut, most patients are grateful to have undergone surgery but many will still have symptoms that need management.

Drug therapy

There are numerous texts on the use of neuropathic analgesics to reduce the pain associated with nerve injury. Most of the literature uses diabetic neuropathy or post-herpetic neuralgia as the model. There is little published on the use of neuropathic analgesics specifically in pudendal neuralgia. A review of the drugs that may be used can be found in a chapter on pharmacotherapy for neuropathic pain with special reference to urogenital pain written by Sam Chong and Joan Hester (14).

Antidepressants

The gold standard antidepressant is amitriptyline; with a mean analgesic dose of around 70 mg and a number needed to treat (NNT) of about 2–3 depending upon the study. Essentially a NNT of 3 suggests that if we had three patients with the same neuropathic pain and an effective dose, one out of three patients would see a 50% (in some studies 30%) reduction in pain. An NNT of 2–3 is considered as representing a very effective drug. Other antidepressants are also used and are often chosen depending upon other symptoms that are present. For instance imipramine and duloxetine may be helpful if there are significant irritable bladder symptoms. Mertazapine and fluoxetine may have a particular role if depression is a significant feature. Studies looking at the NNT for these other drugs have usually only used small numbers of patients and as such the results are unreliable.

Antiepileptic drugs

Most of the research on antiepileptic drugs and neuropathic pain has been done with gabapentin with NNTs of about 3.8. Pregabalin is thought to be equally as effective. The starting dose for gabapentin is 300 mg a day; doses up to 3.6 g have been used. The maximum dose of pregabalin is 600 mg per day. Other antiepileptic drugs may be considered and prescribed by specialist pain clinics or neurologists.

Opioids

The use of opioids in neuropathic pain is controversial. However, there is evidence that opioids can reduce neuropathic pain and, providing appropriate guidelines are instigated and followed, (such as the guidelines of the British Pain Society (15)) opioids can be considered.

Other medications

There are a range of specialist neuropathic analgesics that are prescribed from the pain clinic. The availability of these will depend upon local formulary regulations. The drugs may include the cannabinoids, sodium channel blockers and NMDA (N-methyl-D-aspartate) antagonists.

Management of associated symptoms

Patients with persistent pelvic pain are best managed within a centre that can provide multidisciplinary and multi-speciality care. In view of the effect of pudendal nerve damage on multiple systems it is important to have access to multiple speciality clinics. In an ideal world, joint clinics between pain specialists, urologists, urogynae-cologists, and bowel specialists would occur. In the absence of this form of close collaboration, then detailed communication between specialists is important. Within any speciality there will be numerous disciplines such as medical, physiotherapy, psychology, and nursing, all of which have an important role.

Psychology and physiotherapy

Is well established that low mood, catastrophizing, and inappropriate resting are all associated with a poor prognosis in a chronic pain patient (16,17). The best way to manage these features is through an appropriate programme, usually organized and run by chronic pain psychologists and physiotherapists. These programmes are usually organized on a one-to-one basis for patients with chronic pelvic pain. More recently group pain management programmes have also started. The use of pain management programmes in the management of chronic pain is well established and in patients where the pain is likely to be persistent and unresolving there is significant evidence that these programmes can provide a major improvement in quality of life (18–20).

Neuromodulation

There is good scientific evidence that spinal cord stimulation is helpful in reducing the pain associated with nerve injury (21). For pain relief with spinal cord stimulation it is necessary to have paraesthesia perceived in the same area as the pain. To achieve this for pelvic pain, some specialists have turned the spinal cord stimulator electrode around so that it passes in a caudal direction to stimulate the sacral nerve roots. Others have used a S3 transforaminal approach. The beauty of the latter approach is that a trial is relatively easy to undertake. However, it must be noted that the action of a spinal cord stimulator upon the nervous system is different to the action of stimulating the sacral nerve roots, which is different to stimulating the dorsal root ganglia and peripheral nerve with sacral transforaminal stimulation.

Future

Prevention

Currently education appears to be the most important way forward in terms of preventing the condition. It is important to educate the medical profession about the risks of surgery and in particular the consequence of nerve damage. As far as educating the general population is concerned the importance of appropriate posture, chairs and pacing sitting needs to be emphasized. Cyclists need to be educated on appropriate saddles, cycling posture and appropriate attire.

Pudendal neuralgia is a problem that both family doctors and hospital specialists need to be aware of so the patient may be identified early on.

Investigation

Currently there are no specific investigations for pudendal neuralgia. In many patients treated as suffering with pudendal neuralgia the diagnosis is vague to say the least. Tests that can confirm nerve injury would significantly help in the management of this group of patients.

Treatment

Currently the only specific treatments for pudendal neuralgia are injections and surgery. The results of these are poor but may be improved by early diagnosis. The main impetus in nerve injury research is to look at treatments that may reduce nerve injury damage or possibly reverse it.

Key points

- Understanding chronic pelvic pain requires detailed appreciation of normal and disordered pelvic anatomy as well as physiology, psychology, behaviour silence, and peripheral and central chronic pain mechanisms. Involvement of a specialized multispeciality, multidisciplinary pain management centre is therefore an important consideration

- A cause for pudendal neuralgia should be considered. Pain will be perceived in the distribution of the nerve and may be associated with sensory changes, other symptoms of nerve injury should be looked for and other nerve injuries and non-neurological conditions may mimic the diagnosis

- Pudendal neuralgia is a nerve injury involving the classical pathological processes, and therefore its basic treatment is as for any other nerve injury (ie injections, surgical decompression, neuropathic analgesics, neuromodulation, cognitive behavioural therapy)

- Pudendal neuralgia patients often have significant secondary distress and disablement, and treatment must be multidisciplinary (surgeons, physicians, and pain medicine doctors, psychologists, physiotherapists and specialist nurses).

Editor's summary

Pudenal pain syndrome is uncommon in pelvic floor practice but is vital to recognise because it is highly debilitating and treatment is so specific. Only about 5% of pelvic floor patients present with a pain syndrome and pudendal pain will contribute a fraction of these cases. The pain is characteristically worse on sitting and relieved by standing: this is the key distinguishing feature. In our experience it is associated with gross pelvic floor descent (> 6 cm) and often is associated in parallel with obstructed defaecation. A challenge is the sequencing of treatment if there is associated prolapse disease. In general, evaluation and treatment of the pudendal pain syndrome is the priority because of the severity of the pain and risk of aggravation with antiprolapse surgery.

References

1. Mahakkanukrauh P, Surin P, Vaidhayakarn P. Anatomical study of the pudendal nerve adjacent to the sacrospinous ligament. *Clin Anat* 2005; **18**(3):200–5.

2. Antolak SJJ, Hough DM, Pawlina W, et al. Anatomical basis of chronic pelvic pain syndrome: the ischial spine and pudendal nerve entrapment. *Med Hypotheses* 2002; **59**:349–53.

3. Amarenco G, Ismael SS, Bayle B, Denys P, Kerdraon J. Electrophysiological analysis of pudendal neuropathy following traction. *Muscle Nerve* 2001; **24**:116–9.

4. Alevizon SJ, Finan MA. Sacrospinous colpopexy: management of postoperative pudendal nerve entrapment. *Obstet Gynecol* 1996; **88**:713–5.

5. Sultan AH, Kamm MA, Hudson CN. Pudendal nerve damage during labour: prospective study before and after childbirth. *Br J Obstet Gynaecol* 1994; **101**:22–8.

6. Amarenco G, Le Cocquen-Amarenco A, Kerdraon J, Lacroix P, Adba MA, Lanoe Y. Les névralgies périnéales. *Presse Med* 1991; **20**:71–4.

7. Maigne R. Le syndrome de la jonction dorso-lombaire. *Douleur lombaire basse, douleur pseudoviscérale, pseudo douleur de hanche et pseudo douleur pubienne. Sem Hop (Paris)* 1981; **57**:545–54.

8. EAU CPP guidelines. Fall M, Baranowski AP, Elneil S, Engeler D, Hughes J,. Messelink E.J, Oberpenning F, Williams AC de C; members of the European Association of Urology (EAU) Guidelines Office. *Guidelines on Chronic Pelvic Pain*. In: *EAU Guidelines, edition presented at the 23rd EAU Annual Congress, Milan*, 2008. http://www.uroweb.org/nc/professional-resources/guidelines/online

9. Apkarian AV, Baliki MN, Geha PY. Towards a theory of chronic pain. *Prog Neurobiol* **87** (2009) 81–97.

10. Robert R, Prat-Pradal D, Labat JJ, et al. Anatomic basis of chronic perineal pain: role of the pudendal nerve. *Surg Radiol Anat* 1998; **20**:93–8.

11. Sullivan MJL, Bishop S, Pivik J. The pain catastrophizing scale: development and validation. *Psychol Assess* 1995; **7**:524–32.

12. Amarenco G, Kerdraon J, Bouju P, et al. Treatments of perineal neuralgia caused by involvement of the pudendal nerve. *Rev Neurol (Paris)* 1997; **153**(5):331–4.

13. Robert R, Labat JJ, Bensignor M, et al. Decompression and transposition of the pudendal nerve in pudendal neuralgia: a randomized controlled trial and long-term evaluation. *Eur Urol* 2005; **47**:403–8.

14. Chong MS, Hester J. Pharmacotherapy for neuropathic pain with special reference to urogenital pain. In: Baranowski AP, Abrams P, Fall M (eds). *Urogenital pain in clinical practice.* New York: Informa Health Care; 2007. pp.427–440.

15 . The British Pain Society, *Recommendations for the appropriate use of opioids for persistent non-cancer pain* http://www.britishpainsociety.org/book_opioid_main.pdf (accessed 28.09.2009)

16. Sullivan MJL, Martel M, Tripp DA, Savard A, Crombez G. The relation between catastrophizing and the communication of pain experience. *Pain* 2006; **122**:282-288.

17. Nickel JC, Tripp DA, Chuai S, Litwin MS, McNaughton-Collins M, Landis JR, Alexander, RB, Schaeffer AJ, O'Leary MP, Pontari MA, White P, Nyberg L, Kusek J, Mullins C and the NIH-CPCRN Study Group. Psychosocial Parameters Impact Quality of Life in Men Diagnosed with Chronic Prostatitis/Chronic Pelvic Pain Syndrome (CP/CPPS). *Brit J Urol* 2007; **101**:59–64.

18. Klaber Moffett J, Torgerson D, Bell-Syer S, et al. A randomised trial for exercise for primary care back pain patients: clinical outcomes, costs and preferences. *Br Med J* 1999; **319**:279–83.

19. Vlaeyen JWS, Linton S. Fear-avoidance and its consequences in chronic musculoskeletal pain: a state of the art. *Pain* 2000; **85**:317–32.

20. Fishbain DA, Cutler R, Rosomoff HL, et al. Chronic pain-associated depression: antecedent or consequence of chronic pain? A review. *Clin J Pain* 1997; **13**(2):116–37.

21. National Institute for Health and Clinical Excellence. *Spinal cord stimulation for chronic pain of neuropathic or ischaemic origin.* Issue date: October 2008 http://www.nice.org.uk/nicemedia/pdf/TA159Guidance.pdf

Chapter 16

Obstetric sphincter injury

Oliver M. Jones

Introduction

Whilst vaginal delivery is the physiological method of childbirth, it is also the most common cause of anal sphincter injury. Overt injury to the perineum and sphincter is usually recognized at the time of childbirth and repaired. Functional problems after repair may persist or recur. There may also be occult structural damage to the muscles of the sphincter not recognized at the time of delivery. Furthermore, childbirth may cause neurological (motor and sensory) injury to the anorectum without obvious morphological abnormality.

This chapter examines the classification, prevalence, and risk factors for obstetric sphincter injury. It also examines the longer term prognosis of obstetric sphincter injury and examines the evidence for advising patients about subsequent mode of delivery.

Classification of obstetric sphincter injury

The traditional classification of obstetric tears describes four degrees of injury. A first degree tear involves only skin or vaginal epithelium, whilst a second degree tear extends into the perineum to include the perineal muscles. Third degree tears involve the external anal sphincter and are subdivided into three further categories: (a) involving less than 50% of the external sphincter, (b) more than 50% of the external sphincter, (c) involving the internal anal sphincter. Fourth degree tears involve either the anal or rectal mucosa.

This is a clinical classification for obstetric injury and as such might be thought to have some limitations. Andrews et al. (1) studied 254 women having their first vaginal delivery over a twelve month period. The midwife or doctor delivering the baby made an assessment of the presence or absence of a sphincter injury and this assessment was then repeated by the research fellow who was first author of the study. Initial assessment showed that a sphincter injury was found in 11% of patients though this increased to 24.5% when they were re-examined. The gold standard was taken to be endoanal ultrasound and this was performed immediately post-partum (before perineal repair) and seven weeks post delivery. Ultrasound detected all 59 patients picked up clinically and a further three patients not detected clinically. Two of these three had isolated internal sphincter injuries, whilst one had both internal and external sphincter disruption. Midwives missed 87% of injuries whilst doctors missed 28%. These findings are consistent with another study in which sphincter injury rates were found to 'double' when the patients were re-examined.

Apart from poor recognition of the acute injury as noted in the Andrews study, there are widely held misunderstandings about the classification itself. Whether, therefore, rates of third and fourth degree sphincter injury are a valid tool for assessing quality in obstetric units is open to debate and it also raises some concerns about its use in other areas too. It is also a classification system which takes account only of physical injury to the sphincter and does not include, for example, any measure of pudendal neuropathy.

Prevalence of obstetric sphincter injury

The prevalence of obstetric sphincter injury can be considered on three levels: patients with symptoms of faecal incontinence, patients with overt signs of acute sphincter injury during delivery and patients with occult sphincter injury evident either at delivery or in the post-partum phase. Each of these is considered below.

Prevalence of faecal incontinence symptoms after childbirth

The prevalence of faecal incontinence after childbirth is dependent on a number of factors. The principle issue is whether the baby is delivered vaginally or by Caesarean section. Fynes et al. (2) undertook a prospective observational study of 278 nulliparous women. Patients were assessed antenatally and postnatally by questionnaire and by physiological methods. None of the 15 patients delivered by Caesarean section reported any symptoms of faecal incontinence, whilst 19% of the 200 women who delivered vaginally without instrumentation had some symptoms of faecal incontinence at six weeks. Many such symptoms might recover with time, but set against this is the fact that minor incontinence symptoms in younger life can be unmasked later in life by ageing and the menopause (3).

When one considers patients undergoing instrumental delivery, the rate of incontinence is higher still. In a study of 949 women, Eason et al. (4) reported that forceps delivery was associated with a relative risk of 12.3 for development of anal incontinence. By contrast, the relative risk for vacuum-assisted delivery was 7.4. The finding that forceps usage produces a higher rate of incontinence symptoms has been supported by a number of randomized trials.

Prevalence of overt sphincter injury after childbirth

Third or fourth degree sphincter injury is detected clinically in 1.5–9% of vaginal deliveries (5). Many studies report an incidence lower than this (6), though whilst this may reflect good practice, it might also be a manifestation of poor recognition (1). Recognition may be difficult at the time of delivery due to bleeding, oedema and lack of training. Injury to the transverse perineal muscles may, for example, be falsely labelled as a third degree tear.

Prevalence of occult abnormalities after childbirth

The development of endoanal ultrasound superceded older methods of assessing sphincter integrity such as electromyography. When studying 62 consecutive patients with flatus or faecal incontinence, Burnett et al. reported that 90% of patients had ultrasound evidence of an external sphincter defect, 65% of damage to the internal sphincter and 44% evidence of perineal body damage. By contrast, none of 18 asymptomatic parous controls had ultrasound evidence of a sphincter defect.

Sultan et al. studied 202 consecutive pregnant women six weeks before delivery, 150 of them six weeks after delivery and 32 with abnormal findings six months after delivery. Of the 150 patients studied both before and after birth, 23 had delivery by Caesarean section. The incidence of clinically evident sphincter injury (ie grade 3 or 4) was 3% in the primiparous group but 0% in the multiparous patients. Of the 79 primiparous women, 35% had an endosonographic sphincter defect at six weeks postpartum, which persisted in all 22 patients studied at six months. By contrast, of the 48 multiparous women, 40% had a sphincter defect before delivery and 44% had a defect after delivery. This work has been supported by eight further studies suggesting that between 20 and 41% of women sustain occult sphincter injuries from childbirth.

The relevance of these asymptomatic endosonographic sphincter injuries is disputed, however. Halligan and co-workers recently reported 5- and 10-year questionnaire follow-up of 156 patients recruited prenatally to a pre- and post-partum assessment of bowel function and study by anal endosonography. Their long-term questionnaire study suggested that patients with a sphincter defect on ultrasound associated with post partum incontinence suffered a further significant deterioration in symptoms over the ten years of the study. However, in the patient group with sphincter defects but no post partum incontinence, there was no deterioration in continence over the subsequent decade.

Risk factors for obstetric sphincter injury

Maternal and foetal risk factors for obstetric sphincter injury

Race seems to be a significant predictive factor for sphincter injury with Afro-Caribbean women having a low risk for injury as compared to Caucasians (7). Asian, Indian and Hispanic subjects have a higher risk of injury (8).

Overweight mothers are at greater risk of obstetric injury though the reasons for this are not clear (9,10). Higher foetal birth weight is also associated with an increased risk of tear (11,12). Perhaps the most significant risk factor for sphincter tear, however, is history of previous tear. This is considered in more detail below.

Mode of delivery as a risk factor for obstetric injury

Occipito-posterior foetal head position is significantly associated with third and fourth degree tears (13). A long second stage of delivery increases the risk of sphincter laceration (14). Women who are encouraged to push at full cervical dilatation also seem to increase their risk of injury (15).

Episiotomy is used for a number of indications; the control of perineal tearing, the facilitation of instrumental delivery and for shortening the second stage of labour. There are two main techniques: midline and mediolateral. A Cochrane review comparing restrictive versus routine use of episiotomy suggested that there is insufficient evidence to favour one technique over the other, though there are few high quality studies in this area (16).

A recent systematic review on episiotomies suggested that there was no evidence to suggest that episiotomy was either protective against or a risk factor for sphincter laceration (17). However, it did point out that there was a lack of long-term data for functional sequelae of episiotomy.

Non-muscular injuries to the anal sphincter

Pudendal neuropathy

The pudendal nerve is a mixed nerve derived from the anterior rami for S2–4. As well as being a motor nerve for the external anal sphincter, it also carries afferent fibres for the anal canal and perineum. The contribution of the pudendal nerves to puborectalis is debated with conflicting anatomical (18) and physiological (19) studies.

The measurement of pudendal terminal motor latency (PNTML) has surpassed electromyography for assessment of pudendal neuropathy. PNTML measures the conduction time from stimulation of the pudendal nerve in the region of the ischial spine to external sphincter contraction. Prolonged latencies are surrogate markers for neuropathy and measure axonal injury and demyelination, though normal latencies (as they reflect the fastest conducting fibres only) may mask underlying damage to many or most of the nerve fibres.

Vaginal delivery is associated with significant stretching of the pelvic floor and pudendal neuropathy. In a study from St Mark's Hospital, Sultan et al. (20) measured PNTML in 128 unselected pregnant ladies beyond 34 weeks gestation and repeated the measurements six to eight weeks after delivery. They found that vaginal delivery resulted in significant prolongation of the PNTML in both primiparous and multiparous women. By contrast, women who underwent elective Caesarean section did not experience alteration of PNTML, though PNTML was prolonged if Caesarean section was performed during labour. Risk factors for prolongation of PNTML were a heavier baby and a longer second stage of labour. The finding that prolonged PNTML are not prevented by Caesarean section performed during or late in labour suggests that it is the labour itself that causes neuropathy. A similar finding has been reported in other studies (3,21).

Pudendal neuropathy has been shown to be associated with a decreased resting and squeeze pressure of the anal canal (22). This is not simply a reflection of global sphincter damage. In a review of 1,404 patients evaluated for faecal incontinence from a single centre, Ricciardi et al. (23) reported that 83 patients had intact sphincters on endoanal ultrasound and no evidence of internal or external prolapse on proctography. When the PNTML was measured in these patients (using a 2.4 ms threshold), 18% had unilateral prolongation whilst a further 8% had bilateral prolongation. Bilateral (but not unilateral) neuropathy was associated with poor function. Resting pressure was reduced whilst squeeze pressure was unchanged in the patients with neuropathy in this study.

One of the important factors surrounding pudendal neuropathy is that its presence has been suggested in a number of studies to be predictive of poor outcome after sphincter repair. Gilliland et al. (24) reported that in their series of 100 patients undergoing sphincter repair, 62% of those patients with bilateral normal PNTMLs had a successful outcome. By contrast, only 17% of those with unilateral or bilateral neuropathy had a good result.

Rectal sensory dysfunction and prolapse

Anal and rectal sensory function may be disrupted after obstetric injury. Sensory dysfunction is dealt with in more detail in chapter 17. Both external and internal rectal prolapse are important 'non-muscular' injuries to the pelvic floor but are dealt with separately in chapter 9.

Immediate versus delayed sphincter repair

Immediate sphincter repair

Primary sphincter repair is performed at the time of delivery and in the UK is usually performed by obstetricians. The most commonly employed technique is an end to end approximation of the sphincter muscles, though sometimes an overlapping repair is used. Short term outcomes after sphincter repair are good in the overwhelming majority of patients (25). Endoanal ultrasound, however, shows that a residual sphincter defect is common, with one study of ultrasound within seven days after sphincter repair suggesting that defects were present in 37% of cases (26). Furthermore, whilst initial functional results may be good, these deteriorate, perhaps unsurprisingly, with time (27).

Delayed sphincter repair

Delayed repair may be performed if the initial injury is missed, the initial repair fails or the patient develops symptoms many years later. The surgical technique of sphincter repair is addressed in more detail in chapter 23.

Delayed repairs are usually undertaken by colorectal surgeons using an overlapping technique. Whilst delayed sphincter repair improves continence in the majority of women, those who do not demonstrate early improvement in squeeze pressure are likely to derive least benefit in the medium term (28). Certainly, results of sphinctero-plasty deteriorate with time. In the largest reported follow-up study of sphincter repair, Bravo-Gutierrez et al. (29) looked at 191 patients who were a median of 10 years post-surgery, of whom 130 returned questionnaires. Of these patients, only 6% reported full continence and 58% were incontinent to solid stool.

A summary of all series of sphincter repair with greater than 12 months of follow-up, more than 30 patients, and predominantly containing obstetric injuries are shown in table 16.1.

Alternatives to delayed sphincter repair

Conservative measures

These are considered in chapter 8.

Sacral nerve stimulation

Initial trials of sacral nerve stimulation for faecal incontinence focussed on patients with intact or minimally disrupted sphincters (30). However, more recent studies

Table 16.1 Summary of sphincter repair results from several series. Outcome is defined by Park's classification. Parks I/II is full continence or incontinence to flatus only. Parks II/IV is incontinence to liquid or solid stool. Only studies with over 30 patients and at least 12 months of follow-up have been included. Data from Dudding et al. (51)

Reference	No patients	Follow-up (months)	Parks I/II (%)	Parks III/IV (%)
Fleshman	55	12	72	28
Rothbarth	39	12	62	38
Engel	55	15	76	24
Pinta	39	22	59	41
Karoui	86	40	51	49
Buie	158	43	62	38
Halverson	49	69	46	54
Malouf	38	77	11	89
Barisic	65	80	48	52
Bravo Gutierrez	130	120	22	78

have reported good outcomes for patients with significant external sphincter injuries. A study from Chan and Tjandra (31), though non-randomized, looked at 53 successive patients undergoing sacral nerve stimulation. Of these, 21 had external sphincter defects whilst 32 had intact sphincters. Weekly incontinent episodes decreased from 13.8 to 5 (p < 0.0001) for patients with external sphincter defects. These findings have been replicated in other studies (32,33).

This data suggests that sacral nerve stimulation is a real alternative to sphincter repair. A possible algorithm for the patient with a sphincter defect, therefore, is a test of sacral nerve stimulation (Fig 16.1). This can be done under local anaesthetic, is associated with little cost (if unsuccessful and a permanent implant is not used) and runs

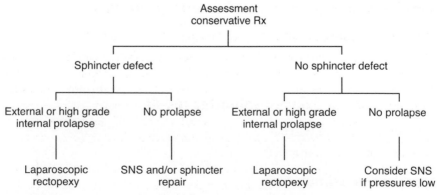

Fig. 16.1 An algorithm for the treatment of obstetric sphincter injury related incontinence.

no risk of making the patient's incontinence worse. Such an approach makes a number of assumptions, however. It assumes that sacral nerve stimulation is similar in efficacy (both in the short and long term) to sphincter repair for patients with a sphincter defect. This has not been proven and it may be that only certain subgroups, such as those with pudendal neuropathy (34), should be pushed to sacral nerve stimulation rather than sphincter repair. It is as yet unproven whether correction of a sphincter defect (ie repair) and then sacral nerve stimulation is better than one or other treatment on its own.

Laparoscopic ventral rectopexy

Rectal intussusception is underdiagnosed. It is commonly found in fully investigated patients with 'unexplained' faecal incontinence. In a study of 40 patients from Oxford (35), two thirds of patients with unexplained incontinence had evidence of recto-anal intussusceptions on their proctogram. Indeed only one in six patients had a normal proctogram.

Laparoscopic ventral rectopexy has been shown to improve symptoms in incontinent patients with both internal and external rectal prolapse (36). Furthermore, it can be undertaken safely with minimal morbidity and very few patients are worse afterwards. It seems reasonable, therefore, for patients with high-grade internal prolapse (and external prolapse) to undergo anti-prolapse surgery before sphincter repair, though again this has not been subjected to a randomized trial.

Follow up after sphincter injury

There is no high quality data on the subject of how women with third and fourth degree tears should be followed up. Follow-up with a colorectal surgeon for these women has certainly been suggested in some publications (37). A consensus conference recommended that all women with persistent bowel symptoms should be assessed in a multidisciplinary clinic (38). Despite this, fewer than 10% of obstetricians in the UK offer women with a sphincter laceration follow-up beyond six months (39).

Prediction and prevention of sphincter injuries

Risks of Caesarean section to mother and neonate

Maternal mortality in the United Kingdom is a rare event, with recent data suggesting it occurs at a rate of 11.4/100,000, the relative risk of Caesarean section being 2.0 (42). Much of this risk lies in relation to an increased risk of thromboembolism with Caesarean section (41). Caesarean section also has a higher rate of puerperal infection compared with vaginal delivery, though the rates of postpartum haemorrhage and transfusion requirements are lower compared to those undergoing vaginal delivery (44).

Caesarean section also has implications for subsequent childbirth. One potential problem for future childbirth is the risk of uterine rupture which was a high as 0.7% in one study of women having a trial of vaginal delivery for their second baby. The same trial also showed an increased rate of foetal hypoxaemia in the trial labour group (45).

Placenta previa is also increased in patients who have a history of Caesarean section (44). The morbidity increases with repeated Caesarean sections.

The risks of Caesarean section to the neonate are clearly important too. The relative risk of Caesarean section is difficult to quantify in patients failing vaginal delivery as there are many variables that introduce potential bias. However, in an analysis of neonatal mortality for primary Caesarean section and vaginal delivery in low-risk women, MacDorman et al. (45) concluded that the relative risk of neonatal mortality with Caesarean section was 1.69. More specifically, the relative risk of hypoxic, ischaemic encephalopathy may be 20 times higher after vaginal delivery compared with elective Caesarean section (46).

A blanket recommendation to patients with a history of obstetric sphincter injury to undergo Caesarean section is therefore impractical and inappropriate.

Risk of vaginal delivery in women with a history of obstetric sphincter injury

Women with a history of transient faecal incontinence with their first delivery are at increased risk of developing incontinence with a subsequent delivery (48). There have been a number of studies looking at the risk of recurrent anal sphincter lacerations in women who sustained a tear in their delivery. Elfaghi et al. (48), in their Swedish Birth Registry study, estimated that women having a third or fourth degree tear are at a five to seven fold risk of tear with subsequent delivery, even after stratification for birthweight, year of birth, parity and maternal age. In a similar study from Norway, the odds ratio was 4.3 for sphincter laceration at second delivery in those patients with prior laceration (49). Given that sphincter laceration is a rare event, however, the authors made the point that only 10% of women with a sphincter laceration at second delivery had had one after their delivery.

Advising women with faecal incontinence or a history of sphincter injury about the best mode of subsequent delivery is difficult. Women should be counselled and informed of the risk of both vaginal delivery to continence and Caesarean section. Assessment of symptoms, clinical examination and investigation with endoanal ultrasound and physiology may be a helpful adjunct. Many women will have few symptoms and no demonstrable abnormalities on testing. They are unlikely to suffer significant deterioration in symptoms from further vaginal delivery.

Key points

♦ Obstetric sphincter injury is common and often not recognized

♦ Investigation reveals that the rate of occult injury is even higher

♦ Treatment of incontinence after obstetric sphincter injury is moving away from a 'sphincter-centred' approach

♦ Careful examination, investigation and counselling is needed when advising women about the mode of subsequent delivery after a sphincter injury.

Editor's summary

In some patients, pregnancy and vaginal delivery has an adverse affect on the pelvic floor in many ways. Historically, surgeons have concentrated on what they could surgically correct, and this usually meant obstetric defects in the external and sometimes also the internal anal sphincter. While the results of surgical repair are good in selected patients, the modest longer-term outcomes indicate the complexity of obstetric pelvic floor damage (pudendal neuropathy, direct pelvic floor musculo-aponeurotic injury, sphincter disruption, or a combination of these). This complexity is reflected in the broadening of the range of therapeutic options in faecal incontinence to include such newer approaches as sacral neuromodulation, anal sphincter bulking, and anti-prolapse surgery including ventral rectopexy.

References

1. Andrews V, Sultan AH, Thakar R, Jones PW. Occult sphincter injuries-myth or reality. *BJOG* 2006;**113**:195–200.

2. Fynes M, Donnelly VS, O'Connell PR, O'Herlihy C. Caesarean delivery and anal sphincter injury. *Obstet Gynecol* 1998;**92**:496–500.

3. Donnelly VS, O'Connell PR, O'Herlihy C. The influence of oestrogen replacement on fecal incontinence in post-menopausal women. *Br J Obstet Gynaecol* 1997;**104**:311–5.

4. Eason E, Labrecque M, Marcoux S, Mondor M. Anal incontinence after childbirth. *Can Med Assoc J* 2002;**166**:326–30.

5. Adams EJ, Fernando RJ. *Management of Third- and Fourth degree Perineal Tears Following Vaginal Delivery*. Guideline No. 29 London, UK. Royal College of Obstetricians and Gynaecologists; 2001.

6. Sultan AH, Kamm MA, Hudson CN, Bartram CL. Third degree obstetric sphincter tears: risk factors and outcome of primary repair. *BMJ* 1994;**308**:887–91.

7. Howard D, Davies PS, DeLancey JO et al. Differences in perineal lacerations in black and white primiparas. *Obstet Gynecol* 2000;**96**:622–4.

8. Handa VL, Danielsen BH, Gilbert WM. Obstetric anal sphincter lacerations. *Obstet Gynecol* 2001;**98**:225–30.

9. Kabira W, Raynor BD. Obstetric outcomes associated with increase in BMI category during pregnancy. *Am J Obstet Gynecol* 2004;**191**:928–32.

10. Castro LC, Avina RL. Maternal obesity and pregnancy outcomes. *Curr Opin Obstet Gynecol* 2002;**14**:601–6.

11. Sultan AH, Kamm MA, Hudson CN et al. Third degree obstetric anal sphincter tears: risk factors and outcome of primary repair. *BMJ* 1994;**308**:887–91.

12. Dupuis O, Madelenat P, Rudigoz RC. Faecal and urinary incontinence after delivery: risk factors and prevention. *Gynecol Obstet Fertil* 2004;**32**:540–8.

13. Fitzpatrick M, McQuillan K, O'Herlihy C. Influence of persistent occiput posterior position on delivery outcome. *Obstet Gynecol* 2001;**98**:1027–31.

14. Cheng YW, Hopkins LM, Laros RK Jr, Caughey AB. Duration of the second stage of labor in multiparous women: maternal and neonatal outcomes. *Am J Obstet Gynecol* 2007;**196**:585.e1–6.

15. Fraser WD, Marcoux S, Krauss I et al. Multicenter, randomized controlled trial of delayed pushing for nulliparous women in the second stage of labor with continuous epidural analgesia. The PEOPLE (Pushing Early or Pushing Late with Epidural) Study Group. *Am J Obstet Gynecol* 2000;**182**:1165–72.

16. Carroli G, Mignini L. Episiotomy for vaginal birth. *Cochrane Database Syst Rev* 2009;**1**:CD000081.

17. Hartmann K, Viswanathan M, Palmieri R, Gartlehner G, Thorp J Jr, Lohr KN. Outcomes of routine episiotomy: a systematic review. *JAMA* 2005;**293**:2141–8.

18. Schraffordt SE, Tjandra JJ, Eizenberg N, Dwyer PL. Anatomy of the pudendal nerve and its terminal branches: a cadaver study. *ANZ J Surg* 2004;**74**:23–6.

19. Percy JP, Neill ME, Swash M, Parks AG. Electrophysiologic study of motor nerve supply of pelvic floor. *Lancet* 1980;**1**:16–7.

20. Sultan AH, Kamm MA, Hudson CN. Pudendal nerve damage during labour: prospective study before and after childbirth. *Br J Obstet Gynaecol* 1994;**101**: 22–8.

21. Allen R, Hosker G, Smith A, Warrell D. Pelvic floor damage and childbirth: a neurophysiological study. *Br J Obstet Gynaecol* 1990;**97**:770–9.

22. Gooneratne ML, Scott SM, Lunniss PJ. Unilateral pudendal neuropathy is common in patients with fecal incontinence. *Dis Colon Rectum* 2007;**50**:449–58.

23. Ricciardi R, Mellgren AF, Madoff RD, Baxter NN, Karulf RE, Parker SC. The utility of pudendal nerve terminal motor latencies in idiopathic incontinence. *Dis Colon Rectum* 2006;**49**:852–7.

24. Gilliland R, Altomare DF, Moreira H Jr, Oliveira L, Gilliland JE, Wexner SD. Pudendal neuropathy is predictive of failure following anterior overlapping sphincteroplasty. *Dis Colon Rectum* 1998;**41**:1516–22.

25. Faltin DL, Boulvain M, Floris LA, Irion O. Diagnosis of anal sphincter tears to prevent fecal incontinence: a randomized controlled trial. *Obstet Gynecol* 2005;**106**:6–13.

26. Starck M, Bohe M, Valentin L. Results of endosonographic imaging of the anal sphincter 2-7 days after primary repair of third or fourth degree obstetric sphincter tears. *Ultrasound Obstet Gynecol* 2003;**22**:609–15.

27. Nazir M, Stien R, Carlsen E, Jacobsen AF, Nesheim BI. Early evaluation of bowel symptoms after primary repair of obstetric perineal rupture is misleading: an observational cohort study. *Dis Colon Rectum* 2003;**46**:1245–50.

28. Oliveira L, Pfeifer J, Wexner SD. Physiological and clinical outcome of anterior sphincteroplasty. *Br J Surg* 1996;**83**:502–5.

29. Bravo Gutierrez A, Madoff RD, Lowry AC, Parker SC, Buie WD, baxter NN. Long-term results of anterior sphincteroplasty. *Dis Colon Rectum* 2004;**47**:727–31.

30. Leroi AM, Parc Y, Lehur PA, Mion F, Barth X, Rullier E, Bresler L, Portier G, Michot F; Study Group. Efficacy of sacral nerve stimulation for fecal incontinence: results of a multicenter double-blind crossover study. *Ann Surg* 2005;**242**:662–9.

31. Chan MK, Tjandra JJ. Sacral nerve stimulation for fecal incontinence: external anal sphincter defect vs. intact anal sphincter. *Dis Colon Rectum* 2008;**51**:1015–24.

32. Boyle DJ, Knowles CH, Lunniss PJ, Scott SM, Williams NS, Gill KA. Efficacy of sacral nerve stimulation for fecal incontinence in patients with anal sphincter defects. *Dis Colon Rectum* 2009;**52**:1234–9.

33. Jarrett ME, Dudding TC, Nicholls RJ, Vaizey CJ, Cohen CR, Kamm MA. Sacral nerve stimulation for fecal incontinence related to obstetric anal sphincter damage. *Dis Colon Rectum.* 2008;**51**:531–7.

34. Tjandra JJ, Chan MK, Yeh CH, Murray-Green C. Sacral nerve stimulation is more effective than optimal medical therapy for severe fecal incontinence: a randomized, controlled study. *Dis Colon Rectum* 2008;**51**:494–502.

35. Collinson R, Cunningham C, D'Costa H, Lindsey I. Rectal intussusceptions and unexplained faecal incontinence: findings of a proctographic study. *Colorectal Dis* 2009;**11**:77–83.

36. Slawik S, Soulsby R, Carter H, Payne H, Dixon AR. Laparoscopic ventral rectopexy, posterior colporraphy and vaginal sacrocolpopexy for the treatment of recto-genital prolapse and mechanical outlet obstruction. *Colorectal Dis* 2008;**10**:138–43.

37. Walsh CJ, Mooney EF, Upton GJ, Motson RW. Incidence of third degree perineal tears in labour and outcome after primary repair. *Br J Surg* 1996;**83**:218–21.

38. Keighley MRB, Radley S, Johanson R. Consensus on prevention and management of post-obstetric bowel incontinence and third degree tear. Clinical Risk 2000;**6**:231–7.

39. Fernando RJ, Sultan AH, Radley S, Jones PW, Johanson RB. Management of obstetric anal sphincter injury: a systematic review and national practice survey. *BMC Health Serv Res* 2002;**2**:9.

40. National Institute of Clinical Excellence Scottish Executive Health Department of Helath Social Service and Public Safety. Why Women Die, report on Confidential Enquiries into Maternal Deaths in the United Kingdom 1997-9. London: RCOG Press, 2001.

41. Jacobsen AF, Skjeldestad FE, Sandset PM. Incidence and risk patterns of venous thromboembolism in pregnancy and puerperium-a register-based case-control study. *Am J Obstet Gynecol* 2008;**198**:233.e1–7.

42. Simoes E, Kunz S, Bosing-Schwenkglenks M, Schmahl FW. Association between method of delivery and puerperal infectious complications in the perinatal database of Baden-Wurttemberg 1998-2001. *Gynecol Obstet Invest* 2005;**60**:213–7.

43. Landon MB, Hauth JC, Leveno KJ et al. Maternal and perinatal outcomes associated with a trial of labor after prior Caesarean delivery. *N Engl J Med* 2004;**351**:2581–9.

44. Oyelese Y, Smulian J. Placenta previa, placenta accreta and vasa previa. *Obstet Gynecol* 2006;**107**:771–8.

45. Macdorman M, Declercq E, Menacker F, Malloy MH. Neonatal mortality for primary Caesarean section and vaginal births to low risk women: application of an 'intention-to-treat' model. *Birth* 2008;**35**:3–8.

46. Badawi N, Kurinczuk J, Alessandri L et al. Intrapartum risk factors for newborn encephalopathy: the Western Australian case-control study. *BMJ* 1998;**317**:1554–8.

47. Fynes M, Donnelly V, Behan M, O'Connell PR, O'Herlihy. Effect of second vaginal delivery on anorectal physiology and faecal incontinence: a prospective study. *Lancet* 1999;**354**:983–6.

48. Elfaghi I, Johansson-Ernste B, Rydhstroem H. Rupture of the sphincter ani: the recurrence rate in second delivery. *BJOG* 2004;**111**:1361–4.

49. Spydslaug A, Trogstad LI, Skrondal A, Askild A. Recurrent risk of anal sphincter laceration among women with vaginal deliveries. *Obstet Gynecol* 2005;**105**:307–13.

50. Dudding TC, Vaizey CJ, Kamm MA. Obstetric anal sphincter injury. Incidence, risk factors and management. *Ann Surg* 2008;**247**:224–37.

Chapter 17

Rectal sensory dysfunction

Martijn P. Gosselink

Introduction

There is growing evidence of the role of rectal sensory perception in the pathogenesis of defaecatory disorders. The sensation of urgency is mediated by extrinsic afferent neurons activated by superficial mucosal mechanoreceptors in the rectal wall, and deeper muscular and serosal receptors in the rectum and surrounding pelvic floor musculature (1). Superficial receptors are connected with sympathetic afferent nerves whilst the deeper receptors are under parasympathetic control. Under normal circumstances, when the rectum is empty and the internal anal sphincter is closed, there is no urge to defaecate. Entry of stool into the rectum and the distention of the rectal wall cause a sudden drop in the internal anal sphincter (IAS) tone ie the rectoanal inhibitory reflex (involuntary phase). Relaxation of the IAS allows stool to descend further and come into contact with the anal canal. During this phase, anal sensory receptors discriminate the consistency of the rectal content and create awareness that defaecation is imminent. Further distention leads to a series of rectal contractions; evacuation is then completed by a voluntary increase in intra-abdominal pressure and relaxation of the puborectalis and levator ani muscles of the external sphincter (voluntary phase). If it is not socially acceptable to evacuate, defaecation can be inhibited by voluntary contraction of the pelvic muscles and relaxation of the rectal wall to increase compliance. The rectum is considerably more elastic than the sigmoid because the longitudinal muscle is substantially thinner compared to the rest of the colon.

Rectal physiological investigation

The viscoelastic properties of the rectal wall allow it to maintain a low intraluminal pressure whilst being filled and so preserve continence. Although the rectum is sensitive to electrical and thermal stimulation, mechanical distention is the most reliable and physiologic stimulus for assessment of its compliance and sensory perception. A balloon is placed in the rectum and inflated with increasing volumes of air. The volume at which the first sensation is appreciated can be recorded. With increasing volumes the first urge to defaecate and finally the maximum tolerable volume, characterized by an irresistible and painful urgency, can be reached. Latex balloons on a catheter connected with a syringe were initially used to perform volume-controlled distention. However, compliance and sensory perception are more accurately assessed using an 'infinitely' compliant polyethylene bag mounted on a catheter connected to a computer

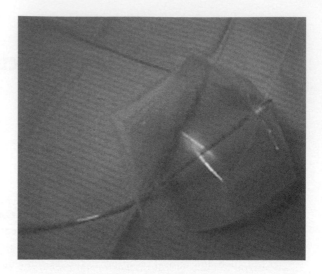

Fig. 17.1 'Infinitely' compliant polyethylene bag.

controlled distention pump (Fig. 17.1). The pressure within this bag represents the pressure exerted upon the rectal wall. Inflation can follow two protocols: (i) slow ramp distention (cumulative) where the bag is continuously inflated at a rate of approximately 40 ml of air per minute (Fig. 17.2) and (ii) fast phasic (intermittent) distention – the bag is inflated to a baseline pressure of 5 mmHg and then increased in steps of 5 mmHg for 20 seconds (Fig. 17.3). Basal pressures within the rectum range from 5 to 25 cm H_2O, corresponding with the intra-abdominal pressure. Taking into account this large range, and inter- and intra-individual variations, care must be taken to describe the examination method properly and to establish laboratory specific normal values.

Rectal compliance

The measurement of rectal volume in response to cumulative pressure steps reveals a characteristic triphasic compliance curve representative of rectal storage function (Fig. 17.4). During the first phase, the increasing pressure only gives rise to a small

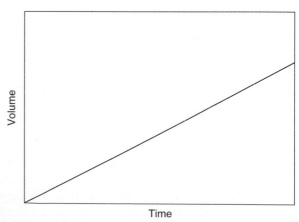

Fig. 17.2 Representation of slow ramp distension protocol.

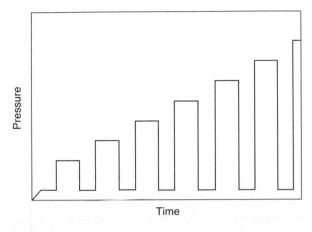

Fig. 17.3 Representation of fast phasic distention protocol.

increase of volume, ie the initial resistance of the rectal wall. The second phase is situated around the point of inflection and is characterized by a larger increase of volume, presumably reflecting an adaptive relaxation of the rectal wall. The last phase of the curve is more flattened and is probably representative of increasing resistance of the rectal wall to further distention. At this point, the distensibility of the rectal wall is starting to reach its limits and the patient perceives pain and discomfort. There is little data concerning the triphasic shape of the curve and the morphology of the rectal wall; passive mechanical properties and active muscular components may be involved. Passive mechanical properties are represented by connective tissue and non-contractile muscle fibres. Collagen fibres are coiled at low pressures. This aspect probably accounts for the plateau of the first phase. When the load is increased collagen fibres gradually un-crimp, which might in turn explain the steep increase of the second phase or the point of inflection. In the final third phase the collagen fibres are actually overstretched.

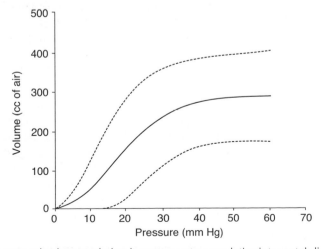

Fig. 17.4 Intrarectal volume variation in response to cumulative intrarectal distention. Mean values are represented by the solid line. The dotted lines indicate normal range.

The tone of the smooth muscle fibres within the rectal wall might also contribute to the curve's shape. Active muscular resistance may account for the first and third phase and adaptive relaxation of the smooth muscle fibres for the second phase. This is supported by the observation that the rectal compliance curve is almost linear in patients with complete spinal cord lesions (2), and after implantation of sacral spinal stimulators the pressure-volume curve regains its characteristic triphasic shape.

Sensory perception

Parasympathetic and sympathetic afferent nerves both transport rectal sensory signals. Parasympathetic nerves are thought to mediate rectal filling sensations (1) and are stimulated by both slow ramp (cumulative) and fast phasic (intermittent) distention of the rectum and run from the rectum through branches situated on each side of the rectum and around the cervix uteri. They also run on both lateral vaginal surfaces and the lateral surfaces and base of the bladder. All these parasympathetic afferents join in the inferior hypogastric plexus and then run to the second and third sacral segments of the spinal cord.

Goligher and Hughes investigated rectal sensory perception in six patients before and after induction of low spinal anaesthesia (3) where all parasympathetic afferent nerves were blocked. None of the patients experienced any sensation during continuous (ramp) distention of the rectum with a balloon. Gunterberg et al. examined anorectal function in patients with both unilateral and bilateral loss of sacral nerves after radical tumour excision (4). In patients with unilateral loss, no significant impairment of anorectal function was noted. However, in patients with bilateral loss, there was a serious impairment of rectal filling sensation. In patients with a complete thoracic spinal cord lesion below T7, the parasympathetic pathway is blocked completely, whereas the sympathetic pathway through the splanchnic thoracolumbar nerves remains partially intact. These patients experience no awareness of rectal filling sensations during either slow ramp or fast phasic distention. However, during fast phasic distention, the majority of subjects report a nonspecific sensation within their pelvis or lower abdomen characterized by 'fullness', 'stool', or 'discomfort' (5). The sympathetic afferent nerves supposedly mediate this sensation. Therefore, it has been suggested that the sympathetic afferent nerves are only stimulated by fast phasic (intermittent) distention. The sympathetic afferent nerves run from the rectum together with the parasympathetic afferent branches. They cross the inferior hypogastric plexus and run through the superior hypogastric plexus to the spinal cord between the third thoracic and third lumbar segments. Some sympathetic branches run directly to the sacral portion of the sympathetic trunk and run upward via the thoracolumbar sympathetic trunk to the third thoracic and third lumbar segments. Although the exact role of the sympathetic afferent nerves is still not clear, there is growing evidence that these nerves mediate feelings of abdominal pain in patients with IBS. Patients with a high cervical lesion, in whom the parasympathetic and sympathetic pathways are both blocked totally, perceive no sensation during balloon distention (6). On the basis of the assumption that different distention protocols stimulate distinct afferent nerve pathways, it might be possible to use slow ramp and fast phasic distention protocols to differentiate between a parasympathetic or sympathetic afferent deficit.

Rectal hyposensitivity and obstructed defaecation

There is growing evidence that attention needs to be paid to the contribution of rectal wall properties in the development of symptomatic obstructed defaecation. Akervall et al. found that patients with severe slow transit constipation, but with normal rectal sensory function had satisfactory functional results after subtotal colectomy and ile-orectal anastomosis, whereas patients with blunted sensation did not improve (7). These authors suggested that determination of the distention pressures required to elicit rectal sensation is an important step in selecting patients suitable for surgery. Straining in patients with obstructed defaecation forces the mucosa of the rectal wall into the anal canal, where the anal sphincter may repeatedly damage it leading to rupture of overstretched submucosal vessels and extramural damage to the afferent and efferent nerves. Furthermore, repeatedly ignoring the call to stool results in development of insensitivity to the reflex initiated by faeces moving into the rectum. This then results in adaptation of the sensory mechanism such that the arrival of further propulsive waves fails to produce an adequate call to stool and ultimately, all natural periodic urges disappear. Gosselink and Schouten reported that in women with obstructed defaecation, the threshold for rectal sensory perception is significantly increased indicating rectal hyposensitivity (8). They also found that the tonic response of the rectum to an evoked urge to defaecate is absent or significantly blunted (9).

Others have also described hyposensitivity in obstructed defaecation. Gladman and colleagues observed rectal hyposensitivity in 29% of patients with ODS (10). Comparing patients with and without rectocele or rectal prolapse, the incidence of rectal hyposensitivity was found to be equal. The cause of this alteration in rectal sensory perception is not clear although increased rectal compliance might be a contributing factor; larger volumes would be required to reach an adequate stimulating pressure on the rectal wall. Sensory threshold volumes are significantly elevated in patients with megarectum. However, De Medici et al. and Gosselink et al. (11,12) reported that rectal compliance was normal in most patients with constipation in whom rectal sensory perception was impaired. There is limited evidence that rectal hyposensitivity is caused by impairment of afferent pathways caused by pelvic nerve injury. It is well known that in some females, obstructed defaecation starts, or deteriorates, after pelvic surgery. Patients who have undergone open posterior rectopexy frequently experience diminished rectal sensory perception. This has been attributed to the division of the lateral ligaments, which contain branches of both the parasympathetic and sympathetic afferent nerves. After hysterectomy, changes in bowel function have been reported by 43% (13). This is perhaps not surprising given that the parasympathetic afferent nerves run from the rectum through branches situated on each side of the rectum, around the cervix uteri, and on both lateral vaginal surfaces. This extensive network of nerve fibres is difficult if not impossible to spare during hysterectomy and dissection of the rectovaginal septum; most surgeons will have little knowledge of their existence. Gumari et al. showed that constipation occurred more frequently the more radical the hysterectomy (14). It has also been suggested that a central neurogenic deficit contributes to rectal hyposensitivity in patients with ODS. It is thought most likely that this central deficit is situated in the anterior side of the pons cerebri, where the coordinating centre of micturition is also located. Neurons in the reticular area of the pons respond to stimulation of parasympathetic afferent nerves that run from the rectum. Moreover, patients with a vascular lesion of their pons loose any rectal sensation during balloon distention.

Biofeedback therapy, especially sensory retraining improves rectal sensitivity as assessed during physiological evaluation; improved rectal hyposensitivity is associated with symptom improvement. There is little evidence to suggest that patients with more severely impaired rectal sensitivity are less likely to improve their sensory function (15). Chang et al. (16) reported that electrical stimulation therapy using an anal plug with pulse generator resulted in clinical improvement and enhancement of rectal sensitivity on physiological testing. It has been suggested that improvement in rectal sensitivity may be one of the mechanisms by which symptoms of obstructed defecation improve following sacral nerve modulation (17), although direct evidence for this is currently lacking.

Two recently introduced surgical procedures are also based on the assumption that impaired rectal sensitivity contributes to obstructed defaecation. Vertical reduction rectoplasty was developed on the premise that reducing rectal capacity and compliance would restore the perception of rectal fullness in patients with idiopathic megarectum (18). The second procedure is stapled trans-anal rectal resection (STARR) whose main goal is to remove the distal part of the insensitive and dysfunctional rectum; preliminary results are promising. The results from the European STARR registry of 2224 patients (19) indicate the procedure to be safe and effective; a significant reduction of the 'obstructed defaecation score' was observed in 85% of patients at one year. Reboa et al. showed that this clinical improvement after surgical correction was associated with increased rectal sensitivity (20).

Rectal hypersensitivity and faecal incontinence

Whilst the bulk of published work on faecal incontinence has concentrated on anal sphincter disorders, it is now recognized that rectal hypersensitivity can be an independent risk factor. Rectal hypersensitivity is observed in about 45% of patients with urge faecal incontinence (21) and is associated with increased stool frequency and urgency, reduced ability to defer, increased pad usage, and negative lifestyle effects when compared to patients with faecal incontinence and normal rectal sensation. The mechanisms mediating rectal hypersensitivity remain unclear. Patients with inflammatory bowel disease or radiation-damage may be incontinent because of rigid noncompliant rectums generating high pressures that overcome normal sphincters. Rasmussen et al. (22) studied rectal compliance in 31 patients with faecal incontinence. All experienced a constant defaecation urge at a lower rectal volume. They also had a lower maximal tolerable volume and a lower rectal compliance compared to controls.

The role of compliance is controversial. Chan et al. (23) studied 27 patients with urge faecal incontinence and rectal hypersensitivity. Only 11 patients had a reduced rectal compliance. The fact that most patients had a normal compliance suggests that the hypersensitivity is caused by abnormal afferent pathway mechanisms. Read et al. (24) have demonstrated that serial distention of the rectum in patients with faecal incontinence shows that the anus relaxes more profoundly at lower volumes than in normal subjects. These data suggest that these patients have a degree of rectal irritability and intolerance to lower rectal volumes, and resemble the published results from patients with irritable bowel syndrome. It follows that high rectal pressures and precipitous anal relaxation in response to rectal distention are particularly likely to cause incontinence if either rectal sensation or external sphincter contraction is impaired.

The treatment of urge faecal incontinence is largely empirical. Biofeedback might work by enhancing the ability of the patient to perceive and respond to rectal distention, known as sensory training. Chiarioni et al. (15) reported that sensory retraining is indeed the key to biofeedback treatment of faecal incontinence. Although they observed an increase of maximum anal squeeze pressure and squeeze duration after biofeedback, the sphincter strength did not separate responders from non-responders. However, responders had a lower threshold for first sensation at the end of the treatment. A better coordination between rectal sensory perception and sphincter activity might also contribute to the effectiveness of biofeedback. Critics of this treatment modality argue that the improvement may well be a result of the supportive interaction between the therapist and the patient, resulting in decreased anxiety and increased confidence. This opinion underlines the importance of psycho-behavioural issues in urge faecal incontinence. Amitriptyline, a tricyclic antidepressant that inhibits parasympathetic nerve impulses seems to have a beneficial effect on the symptoms of faecal incontinence but with variable outcomes (25). Two operative techniques have been designed to attenuate the contribution of rectal hypersensitivity to faecal incontinence. Sacral neuromodulation (SNS) has rapidly evolved as an attractive method for treating faecal incontinence with excellent medium-term results. Until now, it is still not clear why and how SNS works. Convincing evidence that SNS has an affect on anal resting pressure and squeeze pressure is lacking. It has also been suggested that an increased rectal sensitivity is one of the mechanisms of action (26). If sacral neuromodulation is not effective, ileal rectal augmentation can be considered (27). Rectal augmentation is developed upon the primary hypothesis that normalizing rectal capacity and compliance would in turn normalize rectal sensibility. The procedure comprises longitudinal division of the anterior rectal wall; followed by augmentation of the defect with an ileal patch which increases rectal sensory thresholds with corresponding improvements in faecal incontinence.

Sensory perception after sphincter saving operations

Resection of the rectum necessitates substitution of the rectal storage function and continuity of the normal route of defaecation. Developments in surgical techniques have focused on increasing the capacity of the neo-rectum (colonic J-pouch or ileal pouch-anal anastomosis). Several studies have evaluated compliance and sensory perception threshold volumes in patients with and without a pouch. A recent meta-analysis conducted by Heriot et al. revealed that pouch sensory perception threshold-volumes are larger in patients with a colonic J-pouch, than in those with a straight anastomosis and that this results in better function (28). It has been suggested that this better function might be due to the design of the pouch with the anti-isoperistaltic limb resulting in reversal of propulsive movements. Gosselink et al. investigated the influence of neo-rectal wall properties on the functional outcome amongst patients with a uniform pouch design (29). In this study they observed a significant correlation between an increasing faecal incontinence score and a decrease in sensory perception thresholdvolumes. Furthermore, the results indicated, the higher the compliance, the better the outcome. The configuration of the pouch should not be too large as long-term evacuatory problems can and do occur. Data reported by Van Duijvendijk et al. also illustrate the impact of compliance and sensory perception (30). They examined the influence of pre-operative radiotherapy on the functional outcome after transanal double-stapled low colo-rectal anastomosis, by comparing patients with and without radiotherapy. They found that in the patients who had received radiotherapy, compliance was significantly lower and that this was associated with a higher defaecation frequency as well as faecal incontinence. Rectal sensory testing with phasic distention showed impairment at six months and recovery at two years, suggesting that postoperative recovery of residual afferent sympathetic nerves may play a role in functional long-term improvement.

Defaecation disturbances post proctectomy are managed conservatively using combinations of loperamide and retrograde bowel irrigation. Some authors have shown a beneficial effect of SNS in patients with faecal incontinence post resection (31). Whilst functional outcome after pouch surgery is good in most, a pouch is not functionally identical to the original rectum. The development of potential alternatives has focused on rectal preservation ie an ileo-neorectal anastomosis. This operation aims to restore bowel continuity by replacing rectal mucosa with a vascularised ileal mucosal graft without pelvic dissection. Despite its elegant concept, the functional outcome is less favourable than expected and probably reflects low compliance of the neo-rectum. After sphincter-saving surgery, rectum-saving surgery might be the next challenge for colorectal surgeons.

Key points

- Inclusion of rectal wall properties in the pre-operative work-up of patients with faecal incontinence or constipation is advocated
- Rectal sensory dysfunction predicts the outcome after biofeedback therapy and surgery in individual patients with urge faecal incontinence and obstructed defaecation
- The pathophysiological mechanisms of rectal sensory dysfunction in patients with obstructed defaecation or urge faecal incontinence may be the result of abnormal rectal wall properties and/or abnormal afferent pathway function
- Sacral root modulation seems to be a promising avenue to improve rectal sensory dysfunction
- Better understanding of neo-rectal wall properties after restorative colorectal resection may reveal new treatment options for patient suffering from postoperative defaecation disturbances
- There is growing evidence of the role of rectal sensory perception in the pathogenesis of defaecatory disorders, particularly obstructed defaecation
- The cause of this alteration in rectal sensory perception is not clear although increased rectal compliance or impairment of afferent pathways might be contributing factors
- Data from the use of STARR to excise internal rectal prolapse to treat obstructed defaecation showed that clinical improvement after surgery was associated with increased rectal sensitivity
- It has also been suggested that an increased rectal sensitivity is one of the mechanisms of action of sacral neuromodulation.

Editor's summary

The issue of whether ODS is primarily a disorder of sensory function or an anatomical/mechanical disorder, with secondary rectal sensory changes in some patients, remains debatable: more research data are needed. According to our data, only a modest subset of patients (about 30%) with a high-grade mechanical disorder (internal rectal prolapse) exhibit hyposensitivity, and in about 15% hypersensitivity can be demonstrated. What happens to the putative secondary rectal sensory disorder after anatomical/mechanical correction remains unclear.

References

1. Sabate JM, Coffin B, Jian R, Le Bars D, Bouhassira D. Rectal sensitivity assessed by a reflexologic technique: further evidence for two types of mechanoreceptors. *Am J Physiol Gastrointest Liver Physiol* 2000;**279**:G692–9.

2. Sun WM, McDonagh R, Forster D, Thomas DG, Smallwood R, Read NW. Anorectal function in patients with complete spinal transection before and after sacral posterior rhizotomy. *Gastroenterology* 1995;**108**:990–8.

3. Goligher JC, Hughes ES. Sensibility of the rectum and colon. *Lancet* 1951;**10**:543–8.

4. Gunterberg B, Kewenter J, Petersén I, Stener B. Anorectal function after major resections of the sacrum with bilateral or unilateral sacrifice of sacral nerves. *Br J Surg* 1976; **63**:546–54.

5. Lembo T, Munakata J, Mertz H, Niazi N, Kodner A, Nikas V, Mayer EA. Evidence for the hypersensitivity of lumbar splanchnic afferents in irritable bowel syndrome. *Gastroenterology* 1994;**107**:1686–96.

6. MacDonagh R, Sun WM, Thomas DG, Smallwood R, Read NW. Anorectal function in patients with complete supraconal spinal cord lesions. *Gut* 1992;**33**:1532–8.

7. Akervall S, Fasth S, Nordgren S, Oresland T, Hultén L. The functional results after colectomy and ileorectal anastomosis for severe constipation (Arbuthnot Lane's disease) as related to rectal sensory function. *Int J Colorectal Dis* 1988;**3**(2):96–101.

8. Gosselink MJ, Schouten WR. Rectal sensory perception in females with obstructed defecation. *Dis Colon Rectum* 2001;**44**:1337–44.

9. Schouten WR, Gosselink MJ, Boerma MO, Ginai AZ. Rectal wall contractility in response to an evoked urge to defecate in patients with obstructed defecation. *Dis Colon Rectum* 1998;**41**:473–9.

10. Gladman MA, Scott SM, Chan CL, Williams NS, Lunniss PJ. Rectal hyposensitivity: prevalence and clinical impact in patients with intractable constipation and fecal incontinence. *Dis Colon Rectum* 2003;**46**:238–46.

11. De Medici A, Badiali D, Corazziari E, Bausano G, Anzini F. Rectal sensitivity in chronic constipation. *Dig Dis Sci* 1989;**34**:747–53.

12. Gosselink MJ, Hop WC, Schouten WR. Rectal compliance in females with obstructed defecation. *Dis Colon Rectum* 2001;**44**:971–7.

13. Van Dam JH, Gosselink MJ, Drogendijk AC, Hop WC, Schouten WR. Changes in bowel function after hysterectomy. *Dis Colon Rectum* 1997;**40**:1342–7.

14. Gurnari M, Mazziotti F, Corazziari E, et al. Chronic constipation after gynaecological surgery: a retrospective study. *Br J Gastroenterot* 1988;**20**:183–6.

15. Chiarioni G, Bassotti G, Stanganini S, Vantini I, Whitehead WE. Sensory retraining is key to biofeedback therapy for formed stool fecal incontinence. *Am J Gastroenterol* 2002; **97**:109–17.

16. Chang HS, Myung SJ, Yang SK, Jung HY, Kim TH, Yoon IJ et al. Effect of electrical stimulation in constipated patients with impaired rectal sensation. *Int J Colorectal Dis* 2003;**18**:433–8.

17. Kenefick NJ, Nicholls RJ, Cohen RG, Kamm MA. Permanent sacral nerve stimulation for treatment of idiopathic constipation. *Br J Surg* 2002;**89**:882–8.

18. Williams NS, Fajobi OA, Lunniss PJ, Scott SM, Eccersley AJ, Ogunbiyi OA. Vertical reduction rectoplasty: a new treatment for idiopathic megarectum. *Br J Surg* 2000;**87**:1203–8

19. Jayne DG, Schwandner O, Stuto A. Stapled transanal rectal resection for obstructed defecation syndrome: one-year results of the European STARR Registry. *Dis Colon Rectum* 2009;**52**:1205–12.

20. Reboa G, Gipponi M, Logorio M, Marino P, Lantieri F. The impact of stapled transanal rectal resection on anorectal function in patients with obstructed defecation syndrome. *Dis Colon Rectum* 2009;**52**:1598–604.

21. Chan CL, Scott SM, Williams NS, Lunniss PJ. Rectal hypersensitivity worsens stool frequency, urgency, and lifestyle in patients with urge fecal incontinence. *Dis Colon Rectum* 2005;**48**:134–40.

22. Rasmussen O, Christensen B, Sorenson M, et al. Rectal compliance in the assessment of patients with fecal incontinence. *Dis Colon Rectum* 1990;**33**:650–53.

23. Chan CL, Lunniss PJ, Wang D, Williams NS, Scott SM Rectal sensorimotor dysfunction in patients with urge faecal incontinence: evidence from prolonged manometric studies. *Gut* 2005;**54**:1263–72.

24. Read NW, Haynes WG, Bartolo DC, et al. Use of anorectal manometry during rectal infusion of saline to investigate sphincter function in incontinent patients. *Gastroenterology* 1983;**85**:105–113.

25. Santoro GA, Eitan BZ, Pryde A, Bartolo DC. Open study of low-dose amitriptyline in the treatment of patients with idiopathic fecal incontinence. *Dis Colon Rectum* 2000;**43**: 1676–82.

26. Uludag O, Morren GL, Dejong CH, Baeten CG. Effect of sacral neuromodulation on the rectum. *Br J Surg* 2005;**92**:1017–23.

27. Murphy J, Chan CL, Scott SM, Vasudevan SP, Lunniss PJ, Williams NS. Rectal augmentation: short- and mid-term evaluation of a novel procedure for severe fecal urgency with associated incontinence. *Ann Surg* 2008;**247**:421–7.

28. Heriot AG, Tekkis PP, Constantinides V, Paraskevas P, Nicholls RJ, Darzi A et al. Meta-analysis of colonic reservoirs versus straight coloanal anastomosis after anterior resection. *Br J Surg* 2006;**93**:19–32

29. Gosselink MP, Zimmerman DD, West RL, Hop WC, Kuipers EJ, Schouten WR. The effect of neo-rectal wall properties on functional outcome after colonic J-pouch-anal anastomosis. *Int J Colorectal Dis* 2007;**22**:1353–60.

30. van Duijvendijk P, Slors JF, Taat CW, van Tets WF, van Tienhoven G, Obertop H et al. Prospective evaluation of anorectal function after total mesorectal excision for rectal carcinoma with or without preoperative radiotherapy. *Am J Gastroenterol* 2002;**97**:2282–9.

31. Holzer B, Rosen HR, Zaglmaier W, Klug R, Beer B, Novi G, Schiessel R. Sacral nerve stimulation in patients after rectal resection—preliminary report. *J Gastrointest Surg* 2008;**12**:921–5.

Part C

Techniques

Chapter 18

Laparoscopic ventral rectopexy (with posterior colporraphy and vaginal sacrocolpopexy)

Tony Dixon

Introduction

It was D'Hoore (1) and Dixon (2) who independently first proposed laparoscopic ventral rectopexy (LVR) as a new surgical approach to the management of both full thickness rectal prolapse and obstructed defaecation syndrome (ODS) associated with internal rectal prolapse and rectocele. The technique is particularly effective in patients with faecal incontinence, urgency (see chapter 4: faecal incontinence; a pathophysiological approach) and/or evidence of synchronous uro-genital prolapse. The approach uses either a polyester or polypropylene mesh anchored between the sacral promontory and perineal body to achieve level I, II and III reinforcement of the rectovaginal septum, rectum, and uterus ie it restores the vaginal suspensory axis and stabilises the pericervical ring and restores the rectovaginal septum (see chapter 5: OD; a pathophysiological approach). The technique of anterior dissection avoids any potential for postoperative constipation secondary to autonomic nerve damage, which is inherent to traditional posterior approaches (3). The Leuven, Bristol, and Oxford groups (1,2,4–7) have data to support the safety, reproducibility, and efficacy of this technique. The aim of this chapter is to present the technical aspects involved in LVR accompanied by a brief overview of the evidence relating to the safety and efficacy and discussion relating to the relative merits and indications. It is worth emphasizing that this surgery is technically demanding, and very difficult to carry out via an open approach.

Indications for laparoscopic LVR

Before describing the technical aspects of the operation, it is important to consider the indications and contraindications for LVR; like any other operation, inappropriate patient selection is likely to result in a poor outcome. All patients should be assessed with a careful history to evaluate symptoms of obstructed defaecation, rectal intussusception, and pelvic organ prolapse; and clinical examination to document anatomical abnormalities. This is followed by appropriate radiological investigation to classify the type and severity of pelvic floor dysfunction. It is the author's usual practice to perform the following work up:

- Anorectal manometry is useful where there is a story of faecal incontinence and/or a clinical or proctographic suspicion of anismus
- Endoanal ultrasound when there is clinical suspicion of a significant sphincter defect
- Dynamic colpocysto-defaecating proctography with opacification of the small bowel looking for multi-compartmental prolapse
- Marker studies to document the presence or otherwise of slow transit constipation.

LVR itself is indicated in patients with external full thickness rectal prolapse and in those patients with intrusive ODS symptoms (includes faecal incontinence) in which there is sigmoidoscopy and radiological evidence of internal rectal prolapse (intussusception), a rectocele and/or enterocele or sigmoidocele. It should be appreciated that some 40–50% of patients presenting with ODS symptoms also have anterior and middle compartment prolapse (Fig. 18.1). A further 5% will have urinary stress incontinence sufficient to warrant placement of a synchronous tension vaginal tape (TVT).

Technical aspects

Preoperative preparation

Patients are informed about possible complications and side effects: voiding and continued evacuatory problems, stress incontinence (< 3%), mesh infection (0.3%), mesh erosion (1.2%), dyspareunia (0.6%) (Bristol data). A phosphate enema is administered to empty the rectum. A single dose of broad-spectrum antibiotics and DVT prophylaxis is given peri-operatively. The anaesthetised patient is placed in a modified Lloyd-Davis position with 20° Trendelenburg. An initial examination under anaesthetic (EUA) is performed to confirm the radiological findings of prolapse/intussusception and to

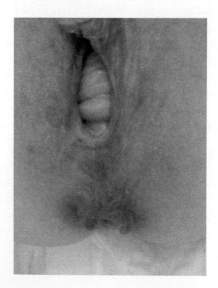

Fig. 18.1 Cystocele, grade III uterine prolapse, rectocele and posterior facing everted anal canal (patient in lithotomy).

exclude other anatomical deficiencies. This should include bimanual vaginal, speculum and rectal examination to assess for the presence of enterocele or sigmoidocele. The patient is then catheterised for the operative period. A Spakman retractor can be used to elevate the uterus when present (8), or a narrow Deaver used as a vaginal retractor. The surgeon and camera operator stand on the patient's left whilst the second assistant sits between the patients abducted legs. The video-monitor is positioned to the right of the patient.

Instrumentation

+ two 10mm, and one or two 5mm trocars
+ Johan fenestrated grasping forceps
+ diathermy hook or 5mm harmonic scalpel
+ two 5mm needle holders
+ 30° endoscope
+ Sims speculum, D&C set, Spakman retractor or vaginal trainer
+ Protacker (Covidien Healthcare)
+ Knot pusher (Karl Stortz)

Operative technique

The laparoscope is centred at the umbilicus with additional operating 5 and 10mm trocars placed lateral to the rectus muscle in the right iliac fossa (RIF) (superior 5mm port at level of umbilicus). The enterocele and sigmoidocele are then reduced from the pelvis using fenestrated grasping forceps (the latter may require sharp dissection, particularly if there has been any previous diverticulitis or hysterectomy). The rectosigmoid junction is retracted to the left and with the laparoscope facing downwards, a peritoneal incision made (using either hook diathermy or laparoscopic Ultracision) over the right side of the sacral promontory to expose the vertebral ligament but avoiding the median sacral vessels and right hypogastric nerve. The incision is then extended in an inverted J form along the rectum and over the deepest (back) part of the pouch of Douglas, with the right-hand side uterosacral ligament at the upper limit of the peritoneal incision (Fig. 18.2). A vaginal trainer is useful in defining the vagina in post hysterectomy patients; alternatively a vaginal retractor can be placed in the posterior vaginal pouch. Counter traction is applied to the rectum by the left-hand Johan grasper lying within the 5mm port. Denonvillier's fascia is then incised and the rectovaginal septum opened widely. No rectal mobilization or lateral dissection is carried out. Dissection is then continued on the ventral side of the rectum (with the laparoscope looking forwards ie 180° turn) as deep down as possible ie down to the perineal body (transverse white fibres), the residual fibres of the rectovaginal septum, and the external anal sphincter. Anteversion of the uterus (via the Spakman) helps with this dissection as well as defining the midline.

In the rare event of perforating the vagina or rectum (0.2%), provided it is small and there is no contamination, we repair with an absorbable suture and continue (a repaired rectum would be temporarily defunctioned). In patients with truncal obesity where their pouch of Douglas contains lots of fibrotic fat, it is important to carry out

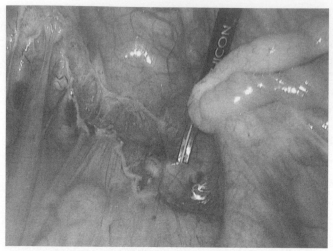

Fig. 18.2 Peritoneum incised from sacral promontory along the line of the right uterosacral ligament to the pouch of Douglas.

a Douglasectomy (Fig. 18.3) to ensure that the mesh is sutured to the seromuscular layer of the ventral rectum. The futility of repairing the 'bulge' of a rectocele by other methods is obvious from the above dissection.

A long mesh (polyester or mersilene) with a midline marking 3.5 x 17 cm (strip for hysterectomy patients and two taped for non-hysterectomy patients) (Fig. 18.4) is introduced through the 10mm RIF port and sutured to the anterior aspect of the perineal body/external anal sphincter and the distal rectum (Fig. 18.5) The mesh is then sutured to the anterior seromuscular layer of the rectum (Fig. 18.6) using approximately six non-absorbable 0 sutures placed with a taper-cut 26-mm needle (Ethibond Excel, Ethicon, Edinburgh, UK). A 'final' stitch is applied to the endocervical fascia

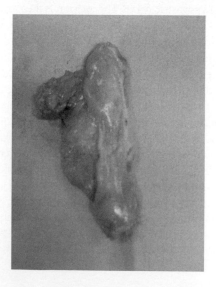

Fig. 18.3 Pouch of Douglasectomy.

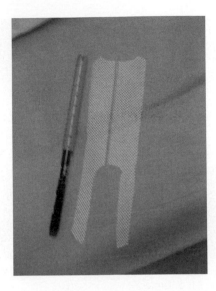

Fig. 18.4 'Bristol' polyester mesh (17 x 3.5 cm) for patients with a uterus in-situ.

with similar stitches placed between rectum, mesh and vagina/uterosacral ligament on either side (Fig. 18.7). This allows correction of any vaginal vault or uterine descent. It is important that the superior rectal sutures are placed above what was previously peritonealised rectum. If necessary, knots can be applied extra-corporally using a 5mm knot pusher.

In patients with a large rectocele and associated vaginal wall prolapse we also suture the anterior aspect of the mesh to the back of the vagina using a series of interrupted 2/0 vicryl sutures. (Non-absorbable suture material may increase the risk of mesh erosions (probably starting from a stitch sinus). D'Hoore (9) includes an additional perineal dissection in patients with a large rectocele. We believe this to be unnecessary

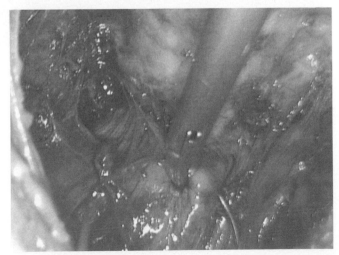

Fig. 18.5 Distal seromuscular suture placed in rectum at level of perineal body to anchor distal mesh (levator plate seen either side of rectal tube).

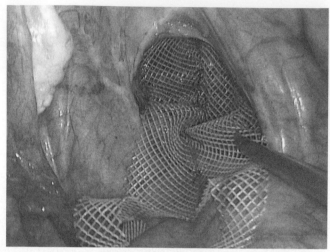

Fig. 18.6 Mesh sutured to ventral rectum with series of non-absorbable sutures placed in midline.

and accept that in the small group who have continued symptoms an anterior STARR or procedure for prolapse and haemorrhoids (PPH) may be required.)

The mesh is then applied at the right tension (checked by vaginal examination) to the vertebral ligaments (after first ensuring that the prolapse has been fully reduced), avoiding the median sacral vessels, fixed with four tacks (Fig. 18.8). The mesh is then covered with the free edge of the incised peritoneum, which in turn is sutured to the left uterosacral ligament. This manoeuvre elevates the new pouch of Douglas over the colpopexy. In patients with a large uterus or enterocele, in Bristol we employ a mesh with two 6cm tails which are passed either side of the rectum before been fixed in turn to the

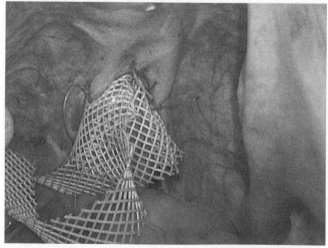

Fig. 18.7 Superior part of newly reinforced rectovaginal septum sutured to endo-cervical fascia and both uterosacral ligaments.

promontory; the pelvic peritoneum is used to cover each tape whose peritonealised medial edge is then sutured to the seromuscular edge of the adjoining rectum (Fig. 18.9). This closes off the pelvis and prevents both a high intussusception developing and a future enterocele. The final appearance is seen in figure 18.10. No drain is required.

In some patients an anterior colpopexy (which requires a second piece of mesh to be passed through the broad ligament when a uterus is in-situ) can be combined with a LVR. Here the bladder is mobilised from the vagina for 4–5cm, sometimes more in case of a large cystocele (Fig. 18.1). Absorbable sutures are used to fix the mesh to the vagina. The end anatomical result can be seen in figure 18.11. An additional, carefully executed PPH03 anopexy can be useful as it inverts an everted anal canal.

Postoperative care

Postoperatively the patient is provided with adequate analgesia: intravenous paracetamol/diclofenac in association with transversus abdominalis plane (TAP) local anaesthetic (0.375% bupivicane) blocks (10). Following this, oral, non-constipating agents are preferred. The patient is allowed to eat normally and encouraged to mobilize. Movicol (prn) is prescribed for the first week. Some 5% of patients will experience postoperative urinary retention necessitating insertion of a temporary catheter, which can usually be removed the following day. Most patients, including octogenarians (7) will be fit for discharge within 24 hours. Patients are warned that it takes about four weeks for them to start to see a benefit. It is our practice in Bristol to recommend courses of topical vaginal oestrogen to maintain vaginal 'plumpness' which might reduce the risk of mesh erosion. Patients are warned to consider any vaginal discharge as a potential warning of developing erosion and return to the clinic.

Complications and their management

Mesh erosions into the vagina are rare but do occasionally occur and are heralded by a vaginal discharge, usually blood stained. Erosions are readily dealt with by

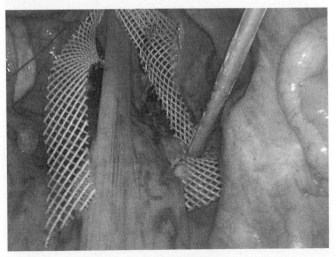

Fig. 18.8 Right limb of mesh fixed to sacral promontory.

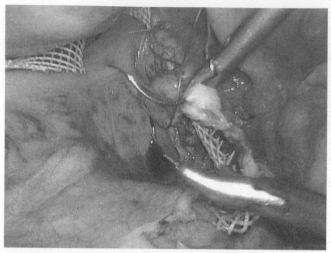

Fig. 18.9 Peritoneum closed over limbs of mesh with additional seromuscular suture to anchor rectum to tail of mesh.

transvaginal excision (including removal of the underlying suture/knot and a small area of mesh) and primary repair. Infected mesh can usually be removed transvaginally (utilising the erosion–usually at the apex). As with erosion repair, mesh removal is not associated with any loss of function (fibrous skeleton of repair remains). We have laparoscopically removed the mesh (with good effect) in one patient with dyspareunia. LVR has not precluded laparoscopic resection of a rectal cancer in one patient.

In patients with continued symptoms our approach is to re-visit biofeedback, repeat the proctograms and carry out a further EUA. About 2–3% of cases will have a

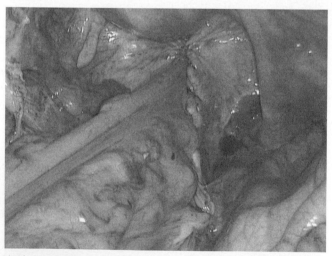

Fig. 18.10 Final appearance of peritonealised mesh (right-hand side limb) with elevated uterus and 'pouch of Douglas'.

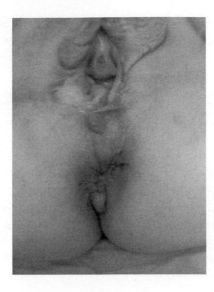

Fig. 18.11 Postoperative appearance after VMR and anterior laparoscopic colpopexy (note changes from pre op figure 18.1, particularly the now normal anal canal).

posterior or lateral prolapse component that will respond to STARR (single PPH (03) firing). Having corrected the prolapse and restored evacuation, a further group with severe global slow transit may benefit from subsequent laparoscopic subtotal colectomy and ileorectal anastomosis.

Outcomes following LVR

D'Hoore in 2004 (1) described the potential benefits of LVR in 42 external rectal prolapse patients with a median follow-up of 61 months. Outcomes were good, and have proved to be reassuringly reproducible (2), with no major postoperative complications and only two late recurrences (early in the series ascribed to the learning curve). There was a significant improvement in continence in 28 of 31 patients with incontinence and symptoms of obstructed defaecation resolved in 16 of 19 patients. New onset mild obstructed defaecation was seen in two patients. The Leuven group reported no problems with mesh erosion. Slawick's paper (2) detailed 80 patients (external prolapse 55%, internal prolapse 45%). Faecal incontinence improved in 39 of 43 patients (91%) and obstructed defaecation resolved in 20 of 25 patients (80%). Pelvic pain resolved in all but one.

The Oxford group (4) using D'Hoore's approach compared patients undergoing LVR for external rectal prolapse or high-grade internal rectal prolapse (the latter group after no response to biofeedback). Constipation improved similarly in external (71%) and internal prolapse (80%), and only worsened in one patient. In their larger series of 75 patients (6) with internal rectal prolapse and OD, at median follow-up of 12 months, preoperative constipation (median Wexner score 12) and faecal incontinence (median FISI score 28) had improved significantly at 3 months (Wexner 4, FISI 8, both $p < 0.0001$) and 12 months (Wexner 5, FISI 8, both $p < 0.0001$). No patient had experienced deterioration in function.

The same two UK groups confirmed the safety of LVR in the super-elderly (80 years and over). In a consecutive series of 80 patients with external prolapse (age median

84 (range 80–97), 3 ASA I, 42 II, 35 III, and 1 IV); the median length of stay was 3 days (range 1–37). There was no mortality, and morbidity in 10 patients (13%), most of which was minor (90%). At a median follow up of 23 (2–82) months, two (3%) developed recurrent full thickness prolapse.

Key points

- Laparoscopic ventral rectopexy is a new nerve-sparing technique for external rectal prolapse (including recurrence after perineal and posterior surgery) and high-grade internal rectal prolapse (including recurrence after perineal surgery, or associated solitary rectal ulcer)

- It is especially suited to co-treating pathoanatomical entities associated with these posterior compartment conditions, including enterocele, sigmoidocele, rectocele and middle compartment prolapse. It may be performed with additional gynaecological or colorectal surgery (anterior colpopexy for a large cystocele, TVT for stress urinary incontinence or stapled anopexy for mucosal prolapse/haemorrhoids).

References

1. D'Hoore A, Cadoni R, Penninckx F. Long-term outcome of laparoscopic ventral rectopexy for total rectal prolapse. *Br J Surg* 2004;**91**:1500–05.

2. Slawik S, Soulsby R, Carter H, Payne H, Dixon AR. Laparoscopic ventral rectopexy, posterior colporrhaphy and vaginal sacrocolpopexy for the treatment of recto-genital prolapse and mechanical outlet obstruction. *Colorectal Dis* 2008;**10**:138–43.

3. Solomon MJ, Young CJ, Eyers AA, Roberts RA. Randomized clinical trial of laparoscopic versus open abdominal rectopexy for rectal prolapse. *Br J Surg* 2002;**89**:35–9.

4. Collinson R, Vandjuivendiuk P, Cunningham C, Lindsay I. Laparoscopic anterior rectopexy improves obstructed defecation in patients with rectal intussusception. *Colorectal Dis* 2007;**9**(Suppl 1):31–104.

5. D'Hoore A, Pennincks F. Laparoscopic ventral recto(colpo)pexy for rectal prolapse: surgical technique and outcome for 109 patients. *Surg Endosc* 2007;**20**:1919–23.

6. Collinson R, Wijffels N, Cunningham C and Lindsey I. Laparoscopic ventral rectopexy for internal rectal prolapse: short-term functional results. *Colorectal Dis* 2010;**12**:97–104.

7. Wijffels N, Cunningham C, Dixon A, Greenslade GL, Lindsey I. Laparoscopic anterior rectopexy for external rectal prolapse is safe and effective in the elderly. Does this make perineal procedures obsolete? *Colorectal Dis* 2010;(E-pub) Feb 20.

8. Varey AH, Darweish A, Pandey S, Dixon AR. Laparoscopic anterior resection and uterine manipulation: why make things difficult? *Colorectal Dis* 2005;**7**:104–5.

9. D'Hoore A, Vanbeckevoort D, Penninckx F. Clinical, physiological and radiological assessment of rectovaginal septum reinforcement with mesh for complex rectocele. *Br J Surg* 2008;**95**:1264–72.

10. Zafar N, Davies R, Greenslade GL, Dixon AR. The evolution of analgesia in an 'Accelerated' recovery programme for resectional laparoscopic colorectal surgery with anastomosis. *Colorectal Dis* 2010;**12**(2):119–24.

Chapter 19

STARR and Transtar

David Jayne

Introduction

Stapled transanal rectal resection (STARR) was first proposed by Antonio Longo in 2002 as a novel surgical treatment for obstructed defaecation syndrome (ODS) associated with internal rectal prolapse and rectocele. The technique used a circular stapling device to achieve a full thickness, circumferential resection of the distal rectal prolapse and rectocele, resulting in a neorectum devoid of any mechanical obstruction to evacuation. The procedure attracted the attention of coloproctologists across Europe, enthused by a lack of other effective treatments, and was soon incorporated into clinical practice. Despite concerns expressed by some authors (1,2), the implementation of STARR has continued with accumulation of data to support its safety and efficacy. Despite its early success, the practicalities of performing STARR suffered from inherent limitations, which stemmed from the fact that the circular stapling device, the PPH-01 (Procedure for Prolapse and Haemorrhoids) stapler was not specifically designed for the procedure. In response, Ethicon Endosurgery designed and produced a further stapling device, the Contour30 Transtar™, which was dedicated to STARR. Currently, therefore, there are two stapling devices and two different methods for performing STARR. As yet, there has not been any prospective comparison of the two stapling techniques to assess their relative merits.

For the purpose of this chapter, the term STARR will be used as a generic term for stapled transanal rectal resection, performed with either of the two stapling devices. STARR performed with the original PPH-01 stapler will be referred to as PPH-01 STARR, whilst that performed with the Contour30 Transtar™ will be referred to as Transtar.

The aim of this chapter is to present the technical aspects involved in STARR as performed with both the PPH-01 and Contour30 Transtar™ staplers. This will be accompanied by a brief overview of the evidence relating to the safety and efficacy of STARR and discussion relating to the relative merits and indications for PPH-01 STARR and Transtar.

Indications for STARR

Before describing the technical aspects of the operation, it is important to consider the indications and contraindications for STARR. This is vitally important as, like any other operation, inappropriate patient selection is likely to result in a poor outcome (3).

Prior to considering STARR, patients should be assessed with a careful clinical history to evaluate obstructed defaecation symptoms; by clinical examination to document anatomical abnormalities and to exclude coexistent disease; and by appropriate radiological investigation to classify the type and severity of pelvic floor dysfunction.

It is the author's usual practice to perform the following preoperative work up:

- anorectal manometry and endoanal ultrasound to assess functional and structural integrity of the sphincter mechanism.
- either defaecating proctography or dynamic magnetic resonance imaging (MRI scanning). Defaecating proctography is preferred if the patient has isolated posterior compartment prolapse, whilst dynamic MRI is often more informative in the presence of multi-compartmental prolapse.
- Radio-opaque marker studies to document the presence or otherwise of slow transit constipation.
- Imaging of the colon, with flexible sigmoidoscopy as a minimum.

Based on the above, it is possible to exclude coexistent disease and to correlate patient's symptoms with any observed radiological abnormalities. STARR is indicated in patients who describe good ODS symptoms and in whom there is a radiological evidence of internal rectal prolapse (intussusception) with or without a rectocele. The severity of ODS symptoms is probably best assessed by the use an ODS scoring system (4,5). The presence of an enterocele or sigmoidocele, which forms on straining but is not present at rest, is not a contraindication to STARR. It should be appreciated that some 30–40% of patients presenting with ODS symptoms also have anterior and middle compartment prolapse; in these further evaluation by a urogynaecologist is desirable.

For a more detailed account of the pathophysiology underlying ODS, its investigation, and patient selection the reader is referred to 'Transanal Stapling Techniques for Anorectal Prolapse' (6).

The PPH-01 STARR procedure

Preoperative preparation

A phosphate enema is administered to prepare the bowel. The operation may be performed either under regional or general anaesthesia. A single dose of broad spectrum antibiotics is given perioperatively. The patient is placed in the lithotomy position with the legs in Allen stirrups or similar to facilitate wide exposure of the perineum. The use of the prone jack-knife position is not recommended as it precludes ease of access to the vagina.

An initial examination under anaesthetic (EUA) is performed to confirm the radiological findings of prolapse and to exclude other colorectal abnormalities. This should include bimanual vaginal and rectal examination to assess for enterocele or sigmoidocele.

Operative technique

Once it has been determined that the patient is suitable for STARR, the PPH-01 kit can be opened. The kit consists of a circular anal dilator (CAD), an obturator, an anoscope, the circular stapling device (PPH-01), and a 'hockey stick' for guiding sutures through the side holes of the stapler.

Four strong retaining sutures (1/0 silk) are place at the anal verge in the 12, 9, 6, and 3 o'clock positions. Traction is applied to these sutures whilst gently inserting the well lubricated CAD plus internal obturator into the anal canal. Once the CAD is fully inserted, the obturator is removed and the CAD secured with the retaining sutures.

Using a dry swab in a sponge holder, the extent of the internal rectal prolapse and its apex is determined. The operation proceeds in two parts: firstly, an anterior full-thickness distal rectal resection is performed with one PPH-01 stapler, followed by a second posterior resection with a further PPH-01 stapler.

For the anterior resection, 3 traction sutures are placed at the apex of the prolapse in the 10, 12, and 2 o'clock positions. It is usual to take a double, full thickness bit of the rectal wall with each suture. Each suture is loosely tied. The two strands of the middle (12 o'clock) suture are separated and individual strands are tied to the 10 and 2 o'clock sutures. In this way, there is in effect one traction suture on either side of the midline (Fig. 19.1A). Simultaneous traction on these sutures pulls the prolapse into

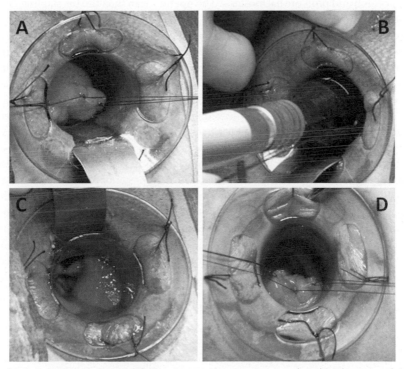

Fig. 19.1 A–D PPH-01 STARR (A) Anterior traction sutures are placed in the apex of the prolapse at the 10, 12, and 2 o'clock positions. The two strands of the 12 o'clock suture are separated and tied to either of the lateral sutures, such that there is in effect one traction suture on either side of the midline. (B) The PPH-01 stapler is inserted fully into the anorectum and closed tightly, checking the vagina to ensure that the mucosa has not been inadvertently incorporated into the stapler. (C) Following resection of the anterior prolapse, a mucosal bridge is frequently observed between the lateral ends of the stapled anastomosis; this should be divided with scissors. (D) The posterior resection proceeds in the same manner as the anterior resection, with one traction suture placed at each of the lateral 'dog-ears' and a third in the midline.

the CAD. A lubricated malleable retractor is inserted into the posterior gap in the outer flange of the CAD, and advanced between the CAD and the posterior anorectum for a distance of 7–8 cm. This serves to protect the posterior rectal wall during the course of the first anterior rectal resection. The PPH-01 stapler is opened fully and lubricated. It is passed into the distal rectum, with the anvil beyond the area of prolapse. The 2 traction sutures are passed through the side holes in the stapler with the aid of the 'hockey stick' and traction applied to bring the prolapse within the stapler housing. The stapler is then closed taking care to position the device such that the external reference marking on the stapler housing shows that the device is fully inserted into the anal canal. Once the stapler has been closed a digital vaginal examination is performed to ensure that the vaginal mucosa has not been inadvertently incorporated into the stapler; the vaginal wall should move freely over the stapler head (Fig. 19.1B). The stapler is held closed for approximately 30 seconds to aid tissue compression and promote haemostasis. The operator can then fire the stapling device to perform the anterior resection. Removal of the stapler is best accomplished by performing one-half turn of the release mechanism, which is sufficient to disengage the device without it becoming caught on the anastomotic line. Once removed, the stapler is fully opened to allow retrieval and inspection of the resection specimen, which should take the form of a rectangular segment of full thickness (mucosa, muscle, and fat) distal rectal wall. It is usual to send the specimen for histological analysis.

A mucosal bridge is frequently observed joining the two lateral ends of the anterior staple line. This should be divided with scissors prior to removal of the malleable retractor (Fig. 19.1C).

The posterior rectal resection proceeds in much the same manner as the anterior resection. Three traction sutures are placed at the apex of the posterior prolapse, such that two sutures each incorporate one of the 'dog-ears' left by the anterior resection, with a third suture placed midway between in the 6 o'clock position. Again, the individual strands of the middle (6 o'clock) suture are separated and tied separately with the lateral sutures, producing two traction sutures one either side of the midline (Fig. 19.1D). The malleable retractor is placed between the CAD and the anterior anorectum to protect the anterior rectal wall, with care being taken not the inadvertently damage the anterior staple line. A second PPH01 stapler is advanced into the distal rectum and the posterior prolapse drawn into the stapler housing using the 'hockey stick' to pull the traction sutures through the side holes of the stapler. The stapler is closed, again checking that the device is properly inserted into the anorectum as evidenced by the external reference markings on the stapler head. Following approximately 30 seconds for tissue compression, the stapler is fired to complete the posterior resection. The stapler is removed in a similar fashion and the resection specimen examined for full thickness resection. A mucosal bridge may again be encountered joining the two lateral ends of the posterior staple line. If so, this is divided with scissors prior to the malleable retractor being removed.

The final part of the procedure involves dealing with any lateral 'dog-ears', which are best inverted with a 'figure of 8' suture. Haemostasis is checked, and if necessary any bleeding points are under-run with a dissolvable suture (3/0 vicryl). A haemostatic sponge may be inserted into the anal canal if desired. The operation is completed by cutting the CAD retaining sutures, withdrawing the CAD, and infiltrating the anoderm with an appropriate anaesthetic solution.

Postoperative care

Postoperatively the patient is provided with adequate analgesia, which may involve the use of opioids in the first 24 hours. Following this, oral, non-constipating agents are preferred. The patient is allowed to eat normally and encouraged to mobilise early. Stool bulking agent (Ispaghula husk) and an osmotic laxative (Lactulose) are prescribed for the first week. If desired, a sphincter relaxing agent (Diltiazem 2% topical ointment) may be added. Some 5–10% of patients will experience postoperative urinary retention necessitating the insertion of a temporary bladder catheter, which can usually be removed the following day. Although some patients will be fit for discharge within 24 hours, the majority will go home on the second postoperative day.

Outcomes following STARR

The first publication to describe the potential benefits of PPH-01 STARR was that of Boccasanta in 2004 (7). This multicentre Italian study included 90 patients all of whom had previously tried and failed a course of biofeedback therapy. It did not include a control group for comparison. The outcomes demonstrated a significant improvement in obstructed defaecation score. Complications included faecal urgency in 17.8%, and incontinence to flatus in 8.9% of patients; no serious morbidity or mortality occurred. The mean follow-up was 16.3 months, at which point patient satisfaction was reported as either good or excellent in 90% of cases.

There shortly followed a number of case series, which generally included small numbers of patients with limited duration of follow-up (8–10). However, all reported good outcomes in approximately 90% of patients.

In 2006, the National Institute for Clinical Health and Excellence in the United Kingdom published its guidance on PPH-01 STARR and concluded, 'Current evidence on the safety and efficacy of stapled transanal rectal resection (STARR) for obstructed defaecation syndrome (ODS) does not appear adequate for this procedure to be used without special arrangements for consent and for audit or research' (11). Partly in response to this guidance, a European STARR Registry was established as a mechanism for rapidly accumulating data on the short-term safety and efficacy of the procedure. The registry was opened in 2006 and closed 2 years later in 2008, with the recruitment of just under 3000 PPH-01 STARR cases. Although the majority of patients (77%) were provided by Italy, the results showed the same trends across the 3 countries involved (Italy, Germany, and United Kingdom). A significant reduction in ODS score, symptom severity score, and quality of life (PAQ-QoL and EQ-5D) was observed. In addition, incontinence for the cohort as a whole was improved with this effect being most marked in the Italian subgroup. Complications were reported in 36% of patients and included pain (7.1%), urinary retention (6.9%), bleeding (5.0%), septic events (4.4%), and staple line complications (3.5%). Postoperative defaecatory urgency was noted in 20% of patients, although a similar number of patients, but not necessarily the same patients, also report urgency as a preoperative symptom. Postoperative faecal incontinence was noted in 1.8% of patients. There was no case of rectovaginal fistula although one serious adverse event of rectal necrosis necessitating colostomy was reported. The final report of the European STARR Registry with 12-month follow-up data was published in 2009 and concluded that PPH-01 STARR for ODS was safe and effective, at least in the short-term, with significant improvements in obstructed defaecation symptoms and quality of life (12).

There have been few studies comparing PPH-01 STARR with other treatment modalities (13), which is somewhat disappointing, and only one randomised controlled trial by Lehur et al. comparing STARR with biofeedback therapy (14). This randomised 119 patients to either PPH-01 STARR (59 patients) or biofeedback therapy (60 patients). Notably, 50% of patients in the biofeedback arm failed to complete the course of treatment and a proportion were subsequently treated with STARR. As expected, the morbidity was higher in the STARR group (15%), although all morbidity was relatively minor and self-limiting in nature. A significant improvement in ODS score was observed in the STARR group as well as those that completed biofeedback. However, the patient reported satisfaction was considerably higher following STARR (81.5%) than biofeedback (33%). Thus, it would appear from this study that a greater proportion of patients benefit from STARR than biofeedback therapy, albeit at the risk of minor morbidity.

Transtar

It should be emphasised that the indications for Transtar are the same as for PPH-01 STARR ie both techniques are suitable for patients with ODS associated with internal rectal prolapse with or without rectocele. Both techniques produce a full-thickness distal rectal resection with excision of the internal rectal prolapse and removal of the anatomical cause of obstruction.

Preoperative preparation

The preoperative preparation for Transtar is exactly the same as for PPH-01 STARR (see above).

Operative technique

An initial EUA confirms the presence of internal rectal prolapse with or without rectocele, and excludes a fixed enterocele/sigmoidocele and any coexistent pathology.

Once the operator is satisfied to proceed, the Contour30 Transtar™ kit is opened. This contains a circular anal dilator (CAD), an obturator, an anal retractor, and the Coutour30 stapling device. Re-loadable stapler cartridges are supplied separately. On average, a total of 5–6 stapler cartridges are required.

Four retaining sutures (1/0 silk) are placed at the anal verge in the 12, 9, 6, and 3 o'clock positions. The anal canal is gently dilated and the CAD with obturator fully inserted into the anorectum. The obturator is removed and the CAD secured to the anal verge with the four retaining sutures. The apex of the prolapse is identified by inserting a dry swab on a sponge holder into the distal rectum and slowly removing it. Four or five traction sutures are placed around the entire circumference of the apex of the prolapse, taking full thickness bits of the distal rectal wall, and running between the 2 and 12 o'clock, the 11 and 9 o'clock, the 8 and 6 o'clock, and the 5 and 4 o'clock positions. The traction sutures are loosely tied so as not to restrict the rectal lumen (Fig. 19.2A). A gap is left between the 4 and 2 o'clock positions for insertion of a 'deep' suture, which marks the depth of the prolapse to be resected. This suture is tied tightly.

The prolapse resection begins at the 'deep' suture at the 3 o'clock position. The Contour30 device is inserted into the distal rectum and the 'deep' suture used to pull the lateral prolapse into the jaws of the stapler which is closed, the vagina check for

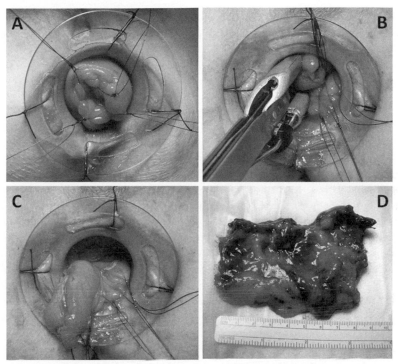

Fig. 19.2 A–D Transtar (A) Four or five gathering sutures are placed around the circumference of the apex of the prolapse and tied loosely, leaving a gap between the 2 and 4 o'clock sutures for a deep 'marking' suture. (B) Resection of the prolapse proceeds in a circumferential manner with successive firings of the Contour30 stapler. (C) The prolapse emerges from the CAD as a 'sausage-shaped' resection specimen. (D) The specimen is opened to reveal a full-thickness resection containing rectal mucosa, muscle wall, and extra-rectal adipose tissue.

inadvertent inclusion, and after a 30 second wait for tissue compression the device is fired. This effectively 'opens up' the prolapse. The Contour30 is withdrawn and the apex of the staple line is marked with a suture, which serves to indicate the beginning and end point of the resection and helps to avoid 'spiralling' of the resection.

A circumferential, full thickness resection of the prolapse is performed, working in an anti-clockwise direction, with successive firings of the Contour30 device (Fig. 19.2B). The stapler is re-loaded with a new stapler cartridge between each firing. Care is taken to keep the height of the resection the same distance from the anal verge with each firing and to end the resection at the 3 o'clock marking suture. An adequate resection results in a complete 'sausage-shaped' resection specimen, which is opened to check for incorporation of peritoneum of the Douglas Pouch (Fig. 19.2C and D).

The anastomotic line is checked for haemostasis and any bleeding points under-run with a dissolvable suture (3/0 vicryl). It is prudent to add reinforcing sutures at the points of overlapping staple lines i.e. the transition points between successive stapler firings. The CAD is removed and an appropriate local anaesthetic is infiltrated into the anoderm and around the sphincter complex.

Postoperative care

The postoperative care following Transtar is the same as that after PPH-01 STARR (see above).

Outcomes following Transtar

Due to its recent introduction into clinical practice, there is little literature regarding the outcomes following Transtar. What exists is comprised of small personal series (15,16) and one multicentre study (17). The first reported series was that by Renzi et al. in 2008, who reviewed the results of 33 patients who had undergone Transtar (15). The operation was deemed to be successful in 86% of patients, with a reduction in ODS score at 6-months follow-up and no major complications. A multicentre European study reported on 75 patients who had undergone Transtar in 2007 and found a significant reduction in ODS symptoms at both 3 and 12-months follow-up, with 77% of patients reporting an improvement (17). However, there was an intra-operative complication rate of 9%, which included staple line dehiscence and 'spiralling' of the anastomosis. Postoperative complications occurred in 3% of cases, and included 3 reports of bleeding. New onset defaecatory urgency was reported in 13% of patients, however, in those patients with preoperative urgency a resolution in symptoms occurred in 22%. Overall, the cohort experienced an improvement in continence score, with 44% reporting an improvement and 5% reporting deterioration.

One of the advantages claimed for Transtar over PPH-01 STARR is the ability to resect a larger prolapse, as the Transtar is not restricted by the limited stapler housing of the PPH-01 device. Theoretically, therefore, it might be expected that Transtar will produce a better anatomical correction, particularly in those patients with a large prolapse. To date, this has not been tested by randomized controlled trial but has been analysed in two retrospective reviews. Wadhawan et al. compared 25 patients who had undergone PPH-01 STARR with 27 patients who had undergone Transtar (16). On short-term follow-up, both techniques produced a significant reduction in ODS scores. Although Transtar resulted in a larger resection specimen, symptom resolution was similar, being 64% following PPH-01 STARR and 67% following Transtar. In a larger study of 150 patients (68 PPH-01 STARR and 82 Transtar), Isbert et al. showed an almost doubling in the volume of the resection specimen following Transtar but with no difference in the ODS scores at 12-months follow-up when compared to PPH-01 STARR (18). Complications were similar with both techniques, although a trend to increased postoperative pain was noted following Transtar.

PPH-01 STARR or Transtar?

There is currently much debate about which technique, the PPH-01 STARR or Transtar, is best suited for STARR. Whilst Transtar offers the advantages of better visualisation of resection, the avoidance of lateral 'dog-ears', and the ability to tailor the amount of resection to suit the degree of prolapse, to date the limited evidence available has not shown that this translates into a clinical benefit. It may be that any benefit is not apparent in the short-term analyses reported, but will become obvious on longer follow-up with fewer patients subsequently relapsing. Certainly, the Transtar technique is technically more challenging and there is a need to prove a clinical advantage before it is accepted as a replacement for PPH-01 STARR. In practice, it is likely that both techniques will remain in use. The safety profile of PPH-01 STARR is reasonably well established and it will continue to be used at least in patients with lesser degrees of prolapse and probably also in the few male patients with ODS. In contrast, it is likely that Transtar will be preferred in the patient with a large prolapse.

Key Points

◆ STARR is a relatively new technique for the treatment of obstructed defaecation associated with internal rectal prolapse with or without rectocele

◆ It may be performed by one of two transanal stapling techniques, PPH-01 STARR or Transtar, the aim of both techniques being to remove the anatomical obstruction to defaecation by performing a full thickness, circumferential resection of the distal rectum

◆ There is reasonable short-term evidence to support the use of PPH-01 STARR

◆ As yet, the evidence for Transtar is very limited, but initial results suggest at least a similar short-term efficacy with no increase in morbidity.

Editor's summary

Undoubtedly STARR and Transtar have a role to play in the treatment of pelvic floor disorders. STARR is easier to perform, has better reproducibility and is probably safer. However, they both suffer from the same limitations as all perineal procedures for prolapse, and they do not allow for co-treatment of concomitant pelvic floor abnormalities such as middle compartment prolapse and enterocele. Lack of experience, training, technical error and poor patient selection are responsible for bad outcomes. Faecal urgency occurs in 70%, is unpredictable and decays with time. However they possess the advantage of simplicity and the ability to be performed under regional anaesthesia. In properly informed patients, patient satisfaction is consistently high. STARR is effective in faecal incontinence associated with prolapse, early SRU and males. We take great care to assess support in the anterior and middle pelvic compartments, and for the presence of an enterocele, perineal descent, and complicated rectocele. In such cases we favour a laparoscopic ventral rectopexy. Patients who relapse after STARR should be considered for a rectopexy and vice-versa. However, the role of ventral rectopexy and STARR are probably complimentary rather than adversarial, and STARR may have a primary role in specific situations (eg males, isolated posterior compartment disorders, those unfit for general anaesthesia). Judgement is perhaps easier when all surgical approaches are available within the same MDT. The results of planned randomized controlled trials of STARR versus ventral rectopexy are awaited.

References

1. Gagliardi G, Pescatori M, Altomare DF et al. Results, outcome predictors, and complications after stapled transanal rectal resection for obstructed defecation. *Dis Colon Rectum* 2008;**51**(2):186–95.

2. Pescatori M, Gagliardi G Postoperative complications after procedure for prolapsed hemorrhoids (PPH) and stapled transanal rectal resection (STARR) procedures. *Tech Coloproctol* 2008;**12**(1):7–19.

3. Schwandner O, Stuto A, Jayne D et al. Decision-making algorithm for the STARR procedure in obstructed defecation syndrome: position statement of the group of STARR Pioneers. *Surg Innov* 2008;**15**(2):105–9.

4. Knowles CH, Eccersley AJ, Scott SM, Walker SM, Reeves B, Lunniss PJ Linear discriminant analysis of symptoms in patients with chronic constipation: validation of a new scoring system (KESS). *Dis Colon Rectum* 2000;**43**:1419–26.

5. Altomore DF, Spazzafuma L, Rinaldi M, Dodi G, Ghiselli R, Piloni V Set-up and statistical validation of a new scoring system for obstructed defaecation syndrome. *Colorect Dis* 2008;**10**:84–88.

6. *Transanal Stapling Techniques for Anorectal Prolapse*. DG Jayne & A Stuto(eds). Springer-Verlag: London, 2009.

7. Boccasanta P, Venturi M, Stuto A et al. Stapled transanal rectal resection for outlet obstruction: a prospective, multicenter trial. *Dis Colon Rectum* 2004;**47**(8):1285–96.

8. Schwandner O, Farke S, Bruch HP Stapled transanal rectal resection (STARR) for obstructed defecation caused by rectocele and rectoanal intussusception. *Viszeralchirurgie* 2005;**40**: 331–41.

9. Ommer A, Albrecht K, Wenger F, Walz MK Stapled transanal rectal resection (STARR): a new option in the treatment of obstructive defecation syndrome. *Langenbeck's Arch Surg* 2006;**391**: 32–37.

10. Renzi A, Izzo D, Di SG, Izzo G, Di MN.Stapled transanal rectal resection to treat obstructed defecation caused by rectal intussusception and rectocele. *Int J Colorect Dis* 2006;**21**(7):661–7.

11 National Institute for Health and Clinical Excellence (NICE) 2006 Interventional Procedure Guidance 169: Stapled Transanal rectal resection for Obstructed Defaecation Syndrome.

12. Jayne DG, Schwandner O, Stuto A. Stapled transanal rectal resection for obstructed defecation syndrome: one-year results of the European STARR Registry. *Dis Colon Rectum* 2009;**52**(7):1205–12.

13. Harris MA, Ferrara A, Gallagher J, DeJesus S, Williamson P, Larach S. Stapled transanal rectal resection vs. transvaginal rectocele repair for treatment of obstructive defecation syndrome. *Dis Colon Rectum* 2009;**52**(4):592–7.

14. Lehur PA, Stuto A, Fantoli M et al.. Outcomes of stapled transanal rectal resection vs. biofeedback for the treatment of outlet obstruction associated with rectal intussusception and rectocele: a multicenter, randomized, controlled trial. *Dis Colon Rectum* 2008;**51**(11):1611–8.

15. Renzi A, Talento P, Giardiello C, Angelone G, Izzo D, Di SG Stapled trans-anal rectal resection (STARR) by a new dedicated device for the surgical treatment of obstructed defaecation syndrome caused by rectal intussusception and rectocele: early results of a multicenter prospective study. *Int J Colorect Dis* 2008;**23**(10):999–1005.

16. Wadhawan H, Shorthouse AJ, Brown SR. Surgery for obstructed defaecation: does the use of the Contour device (Trans-STARR) improve results? *Colorect Dis*: 2010;**12**:885–90.

17. Lenisa L, Schwandner O, Stuto A et al. STARR with Contour Transtar: Prospective Multicentre European Study. *Colorect Dis* 2009;**11**(8):821–7.

18. Isbert C, Reibetanz J, Jayne D, Kim M, Germer CT, Boenicle L. Comparative study of Contour Transtar and STARR Procedure for the treatment of obstructed defaecation syndrome (ODS) - feasibility, morbidity and early functional results *Colorect Dis* 2009: 2010;**12**:901–8.

Chapter 20

Complete pelvic floor ultrasound

Marianne Starck and Sophie Pilkington

Introduction

Complete pelvic floor ultrasound is a novel and useful extension of the physical examination which allows the colorectal surgeon to assess the structure and function of the female pelvic floor in addition to the surface anatomy (1). The complete sequence of scans can be carried out in the clinic setting by the colorectal surgeon and provides additional information to confirm and document the physical findings (2). The 3D datasets and dynamic video clips can be reviewed after the physical examination and can be visualised at the pelvic floor multidisciplinary team meeting.

In general, pelvic floor patients are selected for surgery when they have significant symptoms and when anatomical correction can be expected to relieve their symptoms. Accurate and reliable imaging of pelvic floor dynamics is therefore important for determining treatment options for patients (3). Estimates suggest that one in every nine women will undergo surgery for pelvic floor disorders during their lifetime and that 30% of these will require additional surgery for the same condition (4,5). This implies that pelvic floor conditions are difficult to treat and have a high recurrence rate.

Currently the main imaging modalities used for evaluating pelvic floor disorders are barium proctography (6,7), magnetic resonance proctography (8,9), and 2-dimensional ultrasound with endoanal (10), endovaginal (11) and transperineal (2,12,13) probes. Over the last 10 years, 3-dimensional (3D) ultrasound has been gaining importance for evaluating the anal sphincter and urethra (14,15). Previous ultrasound investigation of the pelvic floor has been described by Dietz et al. using transperineal ultrasound focussing on the anterior compartment, especially the levator ani and gynaecological prolapse (2,12). However this technique uses a 4–8MHz transducer with three-dimension/four-dimension capability and 2.5mm slice intervals. Datasets were acquired during squeeze or Valsalva manoeuvres (16). It is not possible to see the superficial pelvic structures and anal sphincter morphology with this method. The definition can be improved by using 0.2mm intervals and a high frequency (13–16MHz) (1).

Complete pelvic floor ultrasound technique: a standardized approach

A complete pelvic floor ultrasound examination includes transperineal, endovaginal and endoanal ultrasound. It can be carried out using a 3D ultrasound machine such as B-K Medical Pro Focus UltraView™ with 8802, 2052 and 8848 transducers (Fig. 20.1a, 2a, 3a and 4a) and a 3D mover.

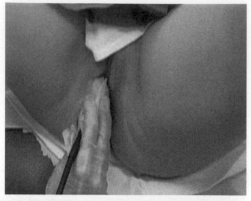

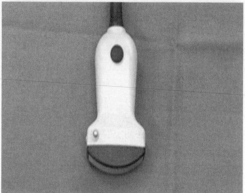

Fig. 20.1.a Transperineal examination with 8802 probe.

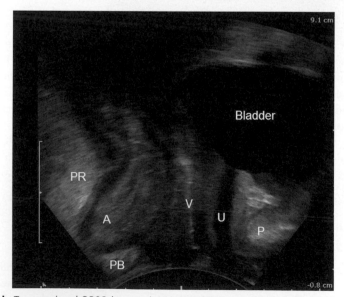

Fig. 20.1.b Transperineal 8802 image showing pubic bone (P), bladder, urethra (U), vagina (V), anal canal (A), perineal body (PB), puborectalis (PR).

The 8802 probe is a 6MHz curvilinear transducer and is used for transperineal scanning. The 2052 probe is a 6–16MHz 360° rotational transducer. It has a built-in motorized system that will automatically acquire a dataset of 300 transaxial images over a maximum distance of 60mm in 60 seconds. This is viewed as a 3D reconstruction that can be sliced in multiple directions. The 8848 probe contains sagittal and axial array transducers. The linear array has a long contact surface of 65 x 5.5mm, a frequency range of 5–12MHz, and a focal range of 3–60mm. By connecting the probe to a mover a 3D dataset can be acquired in an axial or sagittal plane.

A complete pelvic floor ultrasound examination takes about 10 minutes and has four main steps. No patient preparation is necessary. It is important to scan the patient in the gynaecological position with the legs elevated for ease of access and to maintain the normal symmetry of the structures around the midsagittal plane. The endoprobes must be inserted in a neutral position to avoid excessive pressure on surrounding structures that might lead to distortion of the anatomy. Dynamic images are taken at rest and during cough, squeeze and straining manoeuvres. Short video clips can be saved for later review.

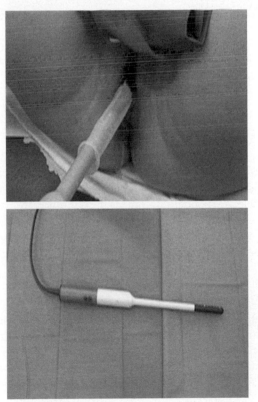

Fig. 20.2.a Endovaginal examination with 2052 probe.

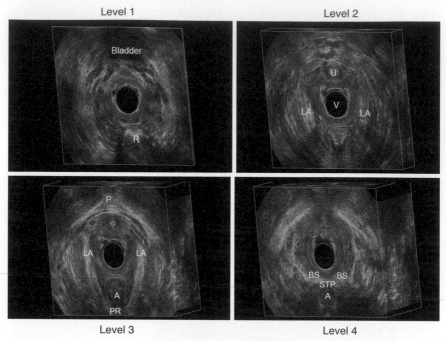

Fig. 20.2.b Endovaginal 360° examination with 2052 probe: Levels 1, 2, 3 and 4 showing base of bladder, rectum (R), urethra (U), vagina (V), levator ani (LA), pubic bone (P), puborectalis (PR), anal canal (A), bulbospongiosus (BS) and superficial transverse perineal (STP) muscles.

Step 1: Transperineal ultrasound with 8802 transducer (Fig. 20.1a and b)

Dynamic images are acquired in the midsagittal plane with the 8802 transducer placed in the transperineal or translabial position to give an overview of the structure and function of the pelvic floor (Fig. 20.1a and b). By moving the transducer from anterior to posterior a complete dataset of the pubic bone, bladder, urethra, vagina and anal canal including the puborectalis muscle can be acquired (Fig. 20.1b). During cough, squeeze and straining manoeuvres, movements of the pelvic organs can be assessed.

Step 2: Endovaginal 360° examination with 2052 transducer (Fig. 20.2a and b)

3D images are acquired with the 2052 transducer placed in the vagina. The probe should be orientated so that the pubic bone is located at 12 o'clock. The tip of the probe is positioned at the inferior aspect of the bladder just above the bladder neck. By pressing the start button, data acquisition will be collected automatically over a length of 60mm inferior to the starting point (Fig. 20.2b). Four standard levels of assessment have been described in the axial plane (1).

Level 1: Bladder base seen anteriorly and the rectum posteriorly.

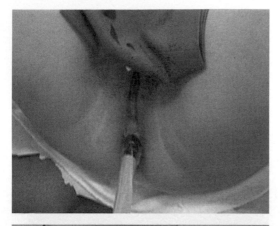

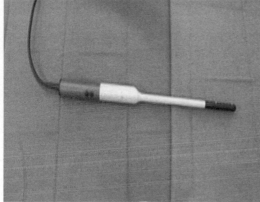

Fig. 20.3.a Endoanal 360°
examination with 2052
probe.

Level 2: Upper part of the urethra and the levator ani are seen.

Level 3: Pubic bone seen at 12 o'clock and levator ani attachment to it. Posteriorly the puborectalis is seen at the superior aspect of the anal canal.

Level 4: The superficial perineal muscles (bulbospongiosus and superficial transverse perineal muscles) are seen.

Step 3: Endoanal 360° examination with 2052 transducer (Fig. 20.3a, b, c and d)

3D images are acquired with the 2052 transducer (13–16MHz) placed in the anal canal. The tip of the probe should be located just above the puborectalis in the distal rectum. Proximally the puborectalis muscle can be assessed in the upper anal canal (Fig. 20.3b). In the mid anal canal, the internal and external anal sphincter and the transverse perineal muscles are seen (Fig. 20.3c). Distally the subcutaneous part of the external anal sphincter is visualised in the lower anal canal (Fig. 20.3d).

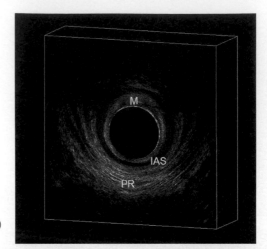

Fig. 20.3.b Upper anal canal with 2052 probe showing mucosa (M), internal anal sphincter (IAS) and puborectalis (PR).

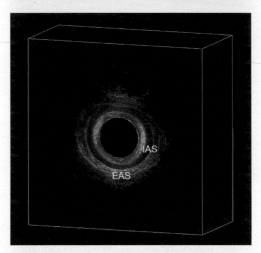

Fig. 20.3.c Mid anal canal with 2052 probe showing external anal sphincter (EAS) and internal anal sphincter (IAS).

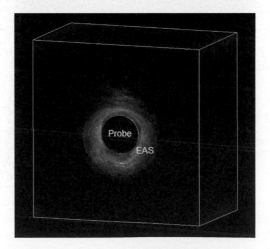

Fig. 20.3.d Lower anal canal with 2052 probe showing external anal sphincter (EAS).

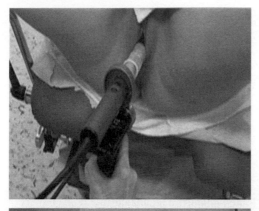

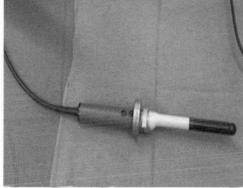

Fig. 20.4.a Endovaginal examination with 8848 probe and mover.

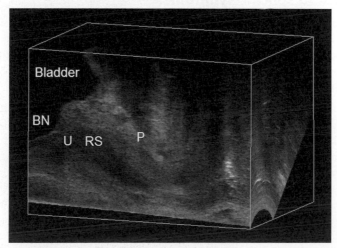

Fig. 20.4.b Anterior compartment showing bladder, bladder neck (BN), urethra (U), rhabdosphincter (RS), and pubic bone (P).

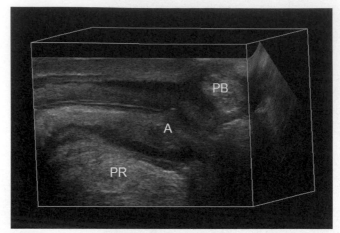

Fig. 20.4.c Posterior compartment showing puborectalis muscle (PR), anal canal (A) and perineal body (PB).

Step 4: Endovaginal examination with 8848 transducer (Fig. 20.4a, b and c)

3D datasets are acquired by attaching the 3D mover to the 8848 (12MHz) endovaginal probe (Fig. 20.4a). Both sagittal and axial planes can be scanned. Dynamic assessment in the midsagittal plane is performed after the 3D datasets. This is to avoid the passage of gas into the lower rectum, which causes artefacts and a poorer quality 3D dataset. Assessment of the anterior compartment shows the bladder neck, urethra, rhabdosphincter, and the pubic bone (Fig. 20.4b). Assessment of the posterior compartment shows the puborectalis muscle, anal canal, and perineal body (Fig. 20.4c).

Approach to specific syndromes

We recommend using the complete pelvic floor ultrasound technique for assessing all patients with pelvic floor dysfunction. In this section we will look at some common syndromes and provide some pointers about the important abnormalities to identify.

Faecal incontinence

In the investigation of faecal incontinence, it is necessary to define any underlying structural abnormalities and to assess the function of the entire pelvic floor rather than focussing exclusively on the anal sphincter. The transperineal images during squeeze and strain, give an overall impression of the movement of the pelvic floor which may be weakened in patients with faecal incontinence. The 3-D dataset from the endovaginal 360° examination with 2052 transducer allows assessment of the levator ani for defects and other signs of trauma such as asymmetry (Fig. 20.5). The transverse perineal muscles can also be assessed for defects (Fig. 20.6).

The finding of avulsion of puborectalis seen on the endovaginal 360° examination with 2052 transducer can be confirmed with the 3D endoanal ultrasound 2052 (Fig. 20.7). The 3D endoanal ultrasound is used to assess the anal sphincter complex for

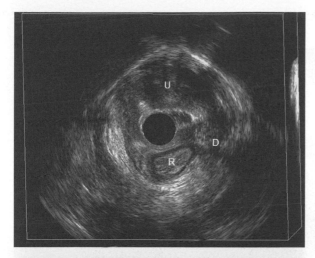

Fig. 20.5 Endovaginal 360°
examination with 2052
probe at Level 2 showing
rectum (R), urethra (U) and
a levator defect (D) on the
left with asymmetry.

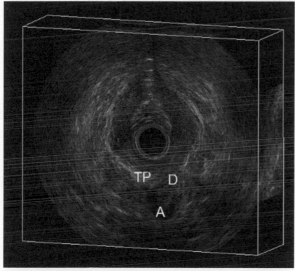

Fig. 20.6 Defect (D) in
transverse perineal muscle
(TP) on 3D dataset using
2052 probe.

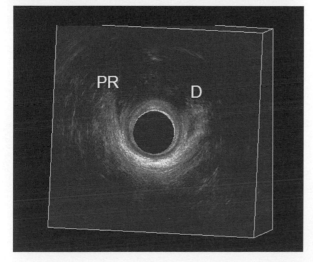

Fig. 20.7 Puborectalis
avulsion showing
puborectalis (PR) on the
right and a defect (D) on
the left.

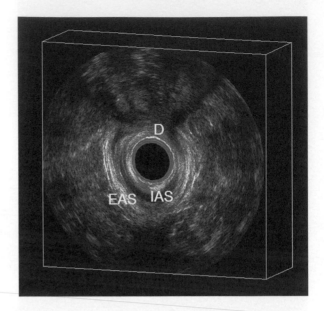

Fig. 20.8 Endoanal 3D dataset showing anal sphincter defect.

defects (Fig. 20.8) and length. The dynamic endovaginal 8848 datasets, particularly during squeeze, provide an assessment of puborectalis and sphincter contraction. Finally the 3D endovaginal 8848 datasets give more detailed structural information about the perineal body and transverse perineal muscles (Fig. 20.4c).

Obstructed defaecation

This is a complex disorder which is likely to have multifactorial causes. It is difficult to determine which abnormalities may be caused by excessive straining rather than being the underlying reason. Using complete pelvic floor ultrasound, it is possible to identify

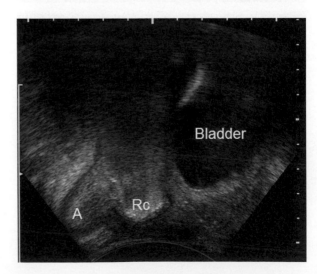

Fig. 20.9 Transperineal image showing rectocele (Rc), anal canal (A) and bladder.

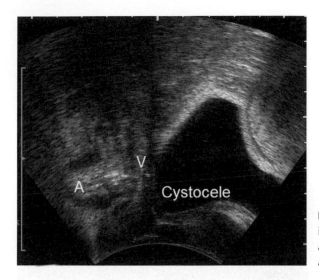

Fig. 20.10 Transperineal image on straining showing a cystocele, vagina (V) and anal canal (A).

anatomical abnormalities that may account for obstructive defaecation symptoms. The ultrasound datasets acquired during the dynamic manoeuvres are more informative than the static images.

Rectocele and cystocele can be seen during straining on the transperineal 8802 datasets (Fig. 20.9 and 10). Ultrasound assessment has been found to have a high positive predictive value in detecting rectocele and rectal intussusception but it has a low negative predictive value (17). During straining, the dynamic endovaginal 8848 datasets in the midsagittal plane may show a cystocele (Fig. 20.11), enterocele and rectal intussusception. Anismus, where there is no relaxation of puborectalis during straining, can be seen also.

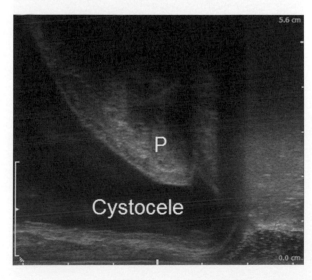

Fig. 20.11 Transvaginal 8848 image on straining showing a cystocele and pubic bone (P).

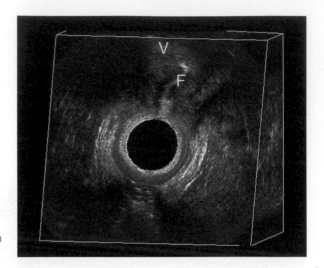

Fig. 20.12 Endoanal 2052 dataset showing a fistula (F) tracking between anal canal and vagina (V).

Anovaginal fistula

By combining endovaginal 8848 and endoanal 2052 ultrasound data, it is possible to delineate the anatomical course of complex fistulae-in-ano and those also involving the vagina (Fig. 20.12).

Urethral sling

Datasets from the transperineal 8802, 3D endovaginal 2052 and 8848 transducers can be used to show the position of urethral slings (Fig. 20.13). In patients who have failure

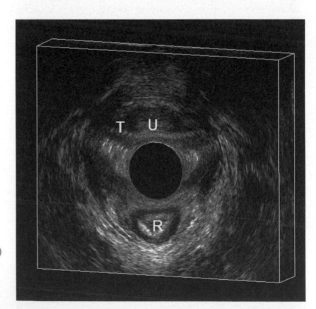

Fig. 20.13 Urethral tape (T) seen as a fine curved hyperechoic line posterior to urethra (U).

of symptom control after urethral sling placement, it is possible to assess sling migration and infection of the tape with complete pelvic floor ultrasound. The dynamic 8848 datasets can be used to assess the movement of the urethra in relation to the tape.

Summary

Complete pelvic floor ultrasound is a new imaging modality for investigation of pelvic floor disorders. By combining 3D and dynamic perineal, endovaginal and endoanal ultrasound, deep and superficial anatomical defects as well as functional disorders can be assessed.

Key points

- Complete pelvic floor ultrasound is a useful addition to physical examination in patients with pelvic floor disorders
- The patient should be positioned supine in a gynaecology bed with the legs raised
- No patient preparation is necessary
- A combination of transperineal, endovaginal and endoanal transducers are used
- Both 3D and dynamic datasets are acquired
- The dynamic datasets are acquired during rest, cough, squeeze and straining
- The technique is amenable to a 'one stop clinic' set-up with scanning performed by the colorectal surgeon.

Editor's summary

This new technology promises new insights into the pathoanatomy of pelvic floor disorders. Expertise is still developing and currently some structures (eg. rectocele) are more easily characterized than others (internal rectal prolapse). As the technique matures, dynamic ultrasound might possibly replace proctography and allow avoidance of any radiation dose at all. More research is required into the benefits and limitations of this technique.

References

1. Santoro GA, Wieczorek AP, Stankiewicz A, Wozniak MM, Bogusiewicz M, Rechberger T. High-resolution three-dimensional endovaginal ultrasonography in the assessment of pelvic floor anatomy: a preliminary study. *Int Urogynecol J Pelvic Floor Dysfunct* 2009; **20**(10):1213–22.
2. Dietz HP. Why pelvic floor surgeons should utilize ultrasound imaging. *Ultrasound Obstet Gynecol* 2006; **28**(5):629–34.
3. Maglinte DD, Bartram C. Dynamic imaging of posterior compartment pelvic floor dysfunction by evacuation proctography: techniques, indications, results and limitations. *Eur J Radiol* 2007; **61**(3):454–61.

4. Kenton K, Mueller ER. The global burden of female pelvic floor disorders. *BJU Int* 2006; **98** Suppl 1:1–5.

5. Delancey JO. The hidden epidemic of pelvic floor dysfunction: achievable goals for improved prevention and treatment. *Am J Obstet Gynecol* 2005; **192**(5):1488–95.

6. Mellgren A, Bremmer S, Johansson C, Dolk A, Uden R, Ahlback SO et al. Defecography. Results of investigations in 2,816 patients. *Dis colon rectum* 1994; **37**(11):1133–41.

7. Karasick S, Karasick D, Karasick SR. Functional disorders of the anus and rectum: findings on defecography. *AJR Am J Roentgenol* 1993; **160**(4):777–82.

8. Rentsch M, Paetzel C, Lenhart M, Feuerbach S, Jauch KW, Furst A. Dynamic magnetic resonance imaging defecography: a diagnostic alternative in the assessment of pelvic floor disorders in proctology. *Dis colon rectum* 2001; **44**(7):999–1007.

9. Mortele KJ, Fairhurst J. Dynamic MR defecography of the posterior compartment: Indications, techniques and MRI features. *Eur J Radiol* 2007; **61**(3):462–72.

10. Starck M, Bohe M, Fortling B, Valentin L. Endosonography of the anal sphincter in women of different ages and parity. *Ultrasound Obstet Gynecol* 2005; **25**:169–76.

11. Tunn R, Petri E. Introital and transvaginal ultrasound as the main tool in the assessment of urogenital and pelivc floor dysfunction: an imaging panel and practical approach. *Ultrasound Obstet Gynecol* 2003; **22**:205–13.

12. Dietz HP, Lekskulchai O. Ultrasound assessment of pelvic organ prolapse: the relationship between prolapse severity and symptoms. *Ultrasound Obstet Gynecol* 2007; **29**(6):688–91.

13. Beer-Gabel M, Teshler M, Barzilai N, Lurie Y, Malnick S, Bass D et al. Dynamic transperineal ultrasound in the diagnosis of pelvic floor disorders: pilot study. *Dis colon rectum* 2002; **45**(2):239–45.

14. Gold DM, Bartram CI, Halligren S, Humphries KN, Kamm MA, Kmiot WA. Three-dimensional endoanl sonography in assessing anal canal injury. *Br J Surg* 1999; **86**:365–70.

15. Athanasiou S, Khullar V, Boos K, Salvatore S, Cardozo L. Imaging the urethral sphincter with three-dimensional ultrasound. *Obstet Gynecol* 1999; **94**:295–301.

16. Dietz HP, Shek KL. Tomographic ultrasound imaging of the pelvic floor: which levels matter most? *Ultrasound Obstet Gynecol* 2009; **33**(6):698–703.

17. Perniola G, Shek C, Chong CC, Chew S, Cartmill J, Dietz HP. Defecation proctography and translabial ultrasound in the investigation of defecatory disorders. *Ultrasound Obstet Gynecol* 2008; **31**(5):567–71.

Chapter 21

Sacral neuromodulation

Mike Jarrett

Introduction

The first connection was made between electricity and muscular contraction by Luigi Galvani in 1791. Alessandro Volta, the inventor of the modern day battery, induced muscular contraction with his new discovery in 1800. From that time forward electrical stimulation has been trialled in various spheres of medicine to attempt to see if it could be used as a therapy for various pathologies and conditions. The evolution of such trials and experimentation have led to the use of electrical stimulation over a broad range of medicinal situations such as for pain relief (eg TENS machines: transcutaneous electrical nerve stimulation); in cardiac pacemaker and defibrillator devices; deep brain stimulation for advanced Parkinson's disease and dystonia; as well as in the areas of both urinary and bowel dysfunction.

The majority of the early work was done in the field of urology. Saxtorph treated urinary retention patients with an electrode placed on a transurethral catheter as far back as 1878. More recently Brindley undertook work in patients with spinal cord transection to attempt to stimulate micturition with high amplitude stimulation to the anterior sacral roots with sacral deafferentation (division of the posterior nerve roots). This stimulator worked on the physiological basis that smooth muscles contract and relax more slowly than striated muscles. Hence there is a brief time when bladder and rectal smooth muscle contraction 'overpower' a brief striated sphincter contraction allowing micturition or defaecation to be instigated. Sacral nerve stimulation (SNS) works at much lower amplitudes and indeed the amplitude used in the Brindley-Finetech stimulator would not be tolerated by a patient with an intact or partially intact spinal cord.

Low amplitude SNS was first explored by Tanagho and Schmidt (1) in 1982 and became commercially available in Europe in 1992. FDA approval in the US has been gained for its use in the urological sphere, but not currently for use in bowel dysfunction.

It was during the original MDT-103 trial of SNS in urinary voiding disorders that beneficial effects in patients with concomitant bowel dysfunction were noted. The MDT-301 trial was then undertaken to look at the use of SNS in faecal incontinence (2) and the Incontrol trial to look at its use in functional constipation (30).

Indications

The indications have evolved with time. Patients with faecal incontinence caused by idiopathic sphincter degeneration (3,4); iatrogenic internal sphincter damage (5); partial spinal cord injury (4,6); scleroderma (7); post rectal prolapse repair (8); or low anterior resection (9–12) of the rectum have all been reported to benefit from SNS.

The first evidence that SNS might be beneficial for patients with idiopathic constipation was from a series of 250 patients with a permanent sacral nerve stimulation implant for bladder dysfunction. Data were collected retrospectively on 36 patients who had concomitant constipation. It was noted that 78% of these experienced an increase in bowel frequency and subjective improvement in defaecation (Medtronic Inc., unpublished data). Other reports concerning the use of SNS for urge urinary incontinence have also included reports of having helped patients with constipation (13).

Most of the published studies about the use of sacral nerve stimulation for faecal incontinence have come from specialist centres with a particular interest in the field and based on a standard procedure. In most centres using SNS for faecal incontinence a regimen of initial conservative treatment, standard investigations (endoanal ultrasound and anorectal physiology studies), specific treatment criteria, and standardized follow-up have been applied.

The use of SNS for constipation is still being evaluated and published studies (14–17) (30) are from research and trial settings.

Technique and adverse events

The techniques for temporary and permanent electrode insertion for sacral nerve stimulation have been modified over time. They seek to locate and place an electrode through a sacral foramen to stimulate the corresponding sacral nerve root. Most commonly electrode insertion is through the third sacral foramen although the second and fourth have also been used successfully.

The patient is placed in the prone jack-knife position with the toes exposed and free to move and the anus exposed. Surface anatomy allows one to predict where the S2 (level of posterior superior iliac spines), S3 (halfway between tip of coccyx and the top of the sacrum/level of the greater sciatic notches), and S4 (level of the sacral hiatus) foramina are located. The foramina lie approximately one finger breadth from the midline and 'cone in' slightly from above down.

A foramen needle is placed at 60° to the skin aiming in a caudal direction to allow the best chance of successful foramen cannulation. The foramen needle may then be stimulated to achieve either a motor (when the patient is under general anaesthetic without muscle relaxant) or sensory (when the patient is under local anaesthetic) response (Table 21.1).

When the optimum 'bellows' contraction (anal contraction and lifting up of the perineum) or perianal sensation has been achieved either a temporary test wire is placed through the hollow foramen needle or a guidewire is placed to allow a permanent electrode to be placed.

Peripheral nerve evaluation (PNE) test stimulation originally used a percutaneous wire electrode (Medtronic model 041830; Medtronic Inc., Minneapolis, Minnesota, USA)

Table 21.1 Common motor and sensory responses to sacral stimulation

Foramen	Motor Response	Sensory Response
S2	Internal rotation of ipsilateral leg/calf contraction/toe flexion	High buttock tingling or tapping
S3	'Bellows' contraction of perineum and flexion of hallux	Perianal/anal tingling or tapping
S4	Anal contraction alone	Anterior perineal/vaginal tingling or tapping

that attached to a portable stimulator (Medtronic model 3625) (Fig. 21.1). This wire was easily dislodged and led to some patients having a permanent electrode (Medtronic model 3080) implanted at open operation for temporary test stimulation, with connection to an external stimulator using an extension cable. The extension cable was removed prior to permanent implantable pulse generator (IPG) (Medtronic model 3023) placement and connection to the fixed electrode if the test period had proved successful. Subsequently a helical PNE electrode (Medtronic model 3057) was developed which, due to its increased flexibility and friction led to a reduction in the number of premature dislodgements. The helical test wire is now the most commonly employed test method in the UK (5) and is a relatively inexpensive way of selecting appropriate patients for definitive implantation (Fig. 21.1). This wire may be placed under local or general anaesthetic and as a day case procedure.

An element of inflammation or infection around a wire traversing the skin for a 2–3 week period is almost inevitable but this settles very quickly on wire removal at the end of the test phase. The helical wire can be removed without the need for an anaesthetic. If the lead is removed prematurely, before a decision can be made about efficacy, a fresh lead can be placed and the patient re-tested.

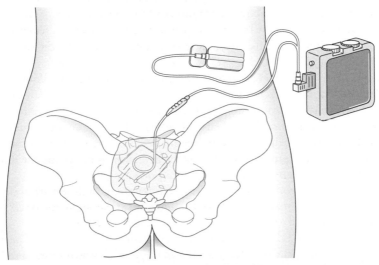

Fig. 21.1 Temporary peripheral nerve evaluation (PNE) in situ.

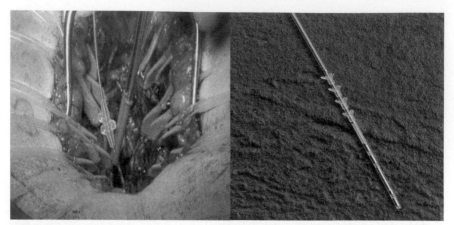

Fig 21.2 The old open technique and new 'tined' lead for permanent electrode placement.

In the past permanent electrodes were placed at open operation but they are now inserted using a percutaneous technique (18), necessitating only a small skin incision to place a 'tined' lead (Medtronic model 3093). This lead incorporates tines/barbs to prevent electrode displacement (Fig. 21.2). An incision is still required to make a subcutaneous pocket for the IPG. The use of the more recently developed percutaneous 'tined' lead appears to have reduced lead dislodgement although further audit is required.

With the new percutaneous tined lead technique there has been a resurgence of the staged procedure (an extension lead to connect the permanent electrode to an external pulse generator) (18). However, connection of the permanent electrode to an external stimulator has the potential to increase the chance of lead infection. Furthermore, the greater cost of the tined lead over the temporary test wire means that if the test period is unsuccessful a more expensive wire needs to be removed and its removal is more difficult due to the projecting barbs that prevent displacement, and the subcutaneous tunnelling.

Lead pain occurred in three patients when the IPGs were placed abdominally. This occurred at the point where the leads were tunnelled subcutaneously over the iliac crest. Local anaesthetic and steroid injections resolved the problem in all cases. Modifying the procedure by implanting the IPG below the superficial fascia in the buttock rather than in the anterior abdominal wall has eliminated the occurrence of this particular complication. Also, placing the IPG away from the midline minimises the patient feeling the IPG when lying or sitting down.

IPG pain was also common when it was set as the anode in the electrical circuit. By setting the system so that the anode and cathode are at the end of the tined lead this problem is minimised.

Operative time has been reduced both by the percutaneous technique of permanent electrode placement, and by placing the IPG in the buttock, which eliminates the need to turn the patient during the operation.

With the permanent lead and IPG placement the main potential complication is infection. Three patients from one centre were reported to have acquired an infection, requiring device removal (4). Once the device has been removed and the infection has settled a further implant can be placed. Judicious use of pre- and post-operative antibiotics and a strict aseptic technique should serve to minimise the risk of infection. A solution of gentamicin 80mg in 500ml normal saline can be used to soak all implanted equipment.

The use of bilateral foramen electrodes has been reported in one patient, both for temporary and permanent implants (9). A dual-channel impulse generator was used for the permanent system. A mild improvement was noted in this patient with bilateral compared to unilateral stimulation, although further work is required to fully evaluate this innovation.

Settings

Settings may be altered on the external stimulator device directly but the IPG settings are altered using the physician and patient telemetry devices (Fig. 21.3). The patient programmer has limited functions (on/off and voltage up/down). In studies to date the external stimulator or IPG has been set at a frequency of between 10 and 25 Hz, with a pulse width of 210μsec and amplitude set just below or above the threshold of patient sensation. The sensations felt by the patient include a tingling or tapping in the buttock, anus, down the leg, or in the vagina in women. There are four electrodes on each permanent wire, each of which can be set as the anode or cathode, although only one of each is set at any time. Electrode polarity is determined by the setting at which the lowest amplitude is required for the patient to feel the stimulation. The IPG is no longer used as an anode as this led to pain at the implantation site. The IPG used to be switched on and off using a magnet. If this facility is switched off using the patient programmer, potential interference from environmental electromagnetic forces is reduced.

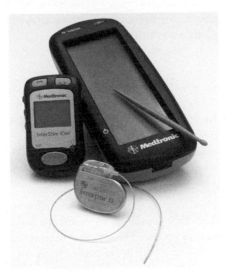

Fig 21.3 Physician and patient telemetry programmers. Used with permission from Medtronic.

Stimulation may be set to be continuous or cyclical (20 seconds on; 8 seconds off to prolong battery life). It is not altered at the time of defaecation. In some cases the IPG has been switched off at night to attempt to prolong battery life with no adverse effects on continence.

In the studies, no adverse event led to any longstanding problems for patients. All of the complications that arose were able to be rectified. Even in cases of implant infection it was possible to remove and then re-implant a new device once the infection had resolved. As the fully implanted system is made up of three constituent parts (electrode, short extension lead, IPG) a single section can be replaced if it becomes dislodged, malfunctions or the battery life expires in the IPG. The battery life is thought to be about six to eight years depending on the settings.

Results

Faecal incontinence

The review of studies tabulated below included 266 patients, all of whom had failed maximal conservative therapy, and who had been enrolled and received PNE. 149 patients (56%) went on to receive permanent implants following successful test stimulation (Table 21.2). The study by Matzel et al. (12) only included patients who went on to permanent implantation and hence an apparent rate of progression from PNE to permanent implantation of 100 percent. Uludag et al. (19), Jarrett et al. (5) and Rosen et al.(4) had similar permanent implantation rates of 77%, 78% and 80% of patients tested by PNE. Leroi et al. (20) and Ganio et al.(3) had lower permanent implantation rates of 55% and 27% respectively, although Ganio et al. reported five patients with a successful PNE who refused a permanent implant.

Complete continence to solid and liquid motion was reported in between 41 and 75% of patients, while there was an equal to or greater than 50% improvement in the number of incontinent episodes in between 75 and 100% of patients after permanent implantation. Improvement in the ability to defer defaecation and Cleveland Clinic incontinence scores (21) are also shown in Table 21.2.

Quality of life

The faecal incontinence specific American Society of Colon and Rectal Surgery (ASCRS) quality of life evaluation was documented in three out of the six studies. Rosen et al. and Jarrett et al. (4,5) reported significant improvement in all categories at latest follow-up. Two of the six studies reported Short-Form (SF) 36 Health Survey quality of life questionnaire results. Results are shown in Table 21.3.

Anal manometry

The role of anorectal physiological measurements in patient selection or outcome evaluation remains unclear. From the larger series one can conclude that there appears to be a significant increase in squeeze pressure and heightened rectal sensation. This does not appear to hold true on a patient-by-patient basis. Most trials, however, have performed such measurements.

Table 21.2 Patient numbers, follow-up, and incontinence outcome measures

STUDY	Months of follow-up (Range)	Received PNEs	Received permanent implants (%)	Faecal incontinent episodes/week		Cleveland Incontinence Score		Ability to defer defaecation (mins)		% fully continent	% >50% improved
				Baseline	Follow-up	Baseline	Follow-up	Baseline	Follow-up		
Ganio (2002)	25.6# (1–56)	116	31 (27%)	7.5# (1–11)	0.15# (0–2)	14.6# (6–20)	4.2# (3–9) p < 0.01	-	-	-	-
Jarrett (2004)	12* (1–72)	59	46 (78%)	7.5* (1–78.3)	1* (0–39) p < 0.001	14* (5–20) [n = 27]	6* (1–12) p < 0.001	<1* (0–5) [n = 39]	5–15* (1–>15) [n = 39] p < 0.001	41% (19/46)	95% (44/46)
Leroi (2001)	6	11	6 (55%)	3# (+/- 2.7)	0.5# (+/- 0.6)	-	-	0.25# (+/- 0.5)	19.0# (+/- 13.9)	50% (2/4)	75% (3/4)
Matzel (2003)	32.5* (3–99)	16	16 (100%)	40% of movements	0% of movements p = 0.001	17 (11–20)	5* (0–15) p = 0.003	-	-	75% (12/16)	94% (15/16)
Rosen (2001)	15* (3–26)	20	16 (80%)	2* (1–5)	0.67* (0–1.67)	-	-	2* (0–5)	7.5* (2–15)	-	100% (16/16)
Uludag (2002)	11#	44	34 (77%)	8.66*	0.67*	-	-	Mean 10–15 minutes at latest follow-up. No baseline data given.		-	-
TOTAL	-	266	149 (56%)	-	-	-	-	-	-	50% (33/66)	95% (78/82)

* Median. # Mean.

Table 21.3 Quality of life results

STUDY		ASCRS quality of life score				Short–Form 36							
		Lifestyle	Coping/ behaviour	Depression/ self-perception	Embarrassment	PF	RP	BP	GH	Vit	SF	RE	MH
Ganio [n = 31]	Baseline	-	-	-	-	58	49	49	46	43	49	40	50
	Follow-up	-	-	-	-	64	70	57	57	51	58	51	50
Jarrett [n = 46]	Baseline	2	1.5	2.29	1.84	62	50	53	49	37	53	49	54
	Follow-up	3.10 $p < 0.0001$	2.67 $p < 0.0001$	3.14 $p < 0.0001$	2.84 $p < 0.0001$	65	60	55	55 $p < 0.05$	46 $p < 0.05$	67 $p < 0.05$	64 $p < 0.05$	64 $p < 0.05$
Matzel [n = 16]	Baseline	1.10	1.07	1.84	1.17	-	-	-	-	-	-	-	-
	Follow-up	3.74 $p = 0.7$	3.18 $p = 0.7$	4.02 $p = 0.7$	3.50 $p = 0.7$	-	-	-	-	-	-	-	-
Rosen [n = 16]	Baseline	2.1	2.0	2.6	1.7	-	-	-	-	-	-	-	-
	Follow-up	3.9 $p < 0.01$	3.7 $p < 0.01$	3.7 $p < 0.01$	3.8 $p < 0.01$	-	-	-	-	-	-	-	-
Uludag [n = 34]		States 'improvement in all categories' at 11 months				States 'improvement in all categories' at 11 months							

Further trial evidence

A small double blind crossover study was carried out by Vaizey et al. (22). Stimulator settings were set at a sub-threshold level ie the patient could not tell whether their IPG was switched on or off and the main investigator and patients were unaware of the settings (blind). In both patients in the study a marked worsening of faecal incontinence to baseline levels was noted when the implantable pulse generator (IPG) was switched off and the study demonstrated a maintained reversible benefit from SNS at nine months.

A more recent randomized controlled study was carried out by Tjandra et al. (23) in which 120 patients with severe faecal incontinence were randomized between being treated with SNS or best supportive conservative therapy over a 12 month period. Patient demographics were well matched between the two groups. 54 of the 60 patients (90%) receiving trial PNE stimulation were successful and 53 went on to permanent implantation. With SNS, mean incontinent episodes per week decreased from 9.5 to 3.1 ($p < 0.001$) and full continence was gained in almost 50% of patients. A corresponding significant improvement in faecal incontinence specific quality of life indices was found in all 4 domains studied. By contrast, there was no significant improvement in any of these parameters in the control group.

This paper included patients with external anal sphincter (EAS) defects and indeed several other papers have also shown that patients with EAS defects either *de novo* or following failed overlap repair can gain benefit from SNS (24–26).

Constipation

An identical SNS implantation technique to the one described in this chapter can also be used in a selected group of patients that have significant symptoms from idiopathic constipation and that have failed conservative treatment (dietary alterations, the use of laxatives, suppositories, or enemas, and biofeedback). In early studies on 250 patients with urinary voiding disorders 28 out of 36 subjects (78%) with coexisting symptoms of constipation reported as increased frequency of defaecation at 6 month follow-up (27–29). Other small but more directed studies (15–17) demonstrated some potential benefit prior to a prospective multicentre European trial being recently published (REF EPUB AHEAD OF PRINT). 62 patients underwent PNE testing and 45 (73%) proceeded to permanent SNS implantation. After a median follow-up period of 28 months (range1–55 months) defaecatory frequency increased from 2.3 to 6.6 evacuations per week ($p < 0.001$) as well as a significant reduction in time spent toileting, in needing to strain, in feelings of incomplete evacuation, and in a subjective rating of abdominal pain and bloating ($p < 0.001$).

SNS appears to be successful in the treatment of idiopathic slow and normal transit constipation and colonic transit was found to have normalised in half of those with baseline slow transit ($p = 0.014$).

Conclusion

Sacral nerve stimulation has proven itself to be a first line surgical treatment for patients with either faecal incontinence or more recently with idiopathic slow or normal transit constipation who have been resistant to conservative treatment measures.

Key Points

- The mechanism of action is unclear, but sacral neuromodulation has no demonstrable effect on anal sphincter pressures
- Sacral neuromodulation has displaced anterior sphincter repair and neosphincter from the first and second line of surgical interventions for faecal incontinence
- Its role in the treatment of chronic constipation is less clear and the outcome for this indication is somewhat inferior to those for faecal incontinence.

Editor's summary

Sacral neuromodulation is a very promising technological advance in the management of pelvic floor disorders. It has been used predominantly in faecal incontinence, where it has relegated anterior sphincter repair to an increasingly uncommon surgical intervention, and threatens to make neosphincter procedures redundant. It also promises benefit in chronic constipation and some chronic pelvic pain disorders. It is simple and safe but very expensive and this is its chief drawback. More research is needed into its mechanisms of action.

References

1. Tanagho E, Schmidt R. Bladder Pacemaker; scientific basis and clinical future. *J Urol* 1982; **20**(6):614–9.
2. Matzel KE, Kamm MA, Stosser M, Baeten CG, Christiansen J, Madoff R et al. Sacral spinal nerve stimulation for faecal incontinence: multicentre study. *Lancet* 2004; **363**(9417):1270–6.
3. Ganio E, Realis Luc A, Ratto C, Doglietto GB, Masin A, Dodi G et al. Sacral nerve modulation for fecal incontinence: functional results and assessment of quality of life. URL: http://www.colorep.it (2003)
4. Rosen HR, Urbarz C, Holzer B, Novi G, Schiessel R. Sacral nerve stimulation as a treatment for fecal incontinence. *Gastroenterology* 2001;**121**(3):536–41.
5. Jarrett ME, Varma JS, Duthie GS, Nicholls RJ, Kamm MA. Sacral nerve stimulation for faecal incontinence in the UK. *Br J Surg* 2004;**91**(6):755–61.
6. Jarrett ME, Matzel KE, Christiansen J, Baeten CG, Rosen H, Bittorf B et al. Sacral nerve stimulation for faecal incontinence in patients with previous partial spinal injury including disc prolapse. *Br J Surg* 2005;**92**(6):734–9.
7. Kenefick NJ, Vaizey CJ, Nicholls RJ, Cohen R, Kamm MA. Sacral nerve stimulation for faecal incontinence due to systemic sclerosis. *Gut* 2002;**51**(6):881–3.
8. Jarrett ME, Matzel KE, Stosser M, Baeten CG, Kamm MA. Sacral nerve stimulation for fecal incontinence following surgery for rectal prolapse repair: a multicenter study. *Dis Colon Rectum* 2005;**48**(6):1243–8.

9. Matzel KE, Stadelmaier U, Bittorf B, Hohenfellner M, Hohenberger W. Bilateral sacral spinal nerve stimulation for fecal incontinence after low anterior rectum resection. *Int J Colorectal Dis* 2002; **17**(6):430–4.

10. Jarrett ME, Matzel KE, Stosser M, Christiansen J, Rosen H, Kamm MA. Sacral nerve stimulation for faecal incontinence following a rectosigmoid resection for colorectal cancer. *Int J Colorectal Dis* 2005; **20**(5):446–51.

11. Uludag O, Dejong HC. Sacral neuromodulation for faecal incontinence. *Diseases of the Colon & Rectum* 2002; **45**(12):A34–6.

12. Matzel KE, Bittorf B, Stadelmaier U, Hohenberger W. Sacral nerve stimulation in the treatment of faccal incontinence. *Chirurg* 2003; **74**(1):26–32.

13. Caraballo R, Bologna RA, Lukban J, Whitmore KE. Sacral nerve stimulation as a treatment for urge incontinence and associated pelvic floor disorders at a pelvic floor center: a follow-up study. *Urology* 2001; **57**(6:Suppl 1):121.

14. Kenefick NJ, Vaizey CJ, Cohen CR, Nicholls RJ, Kamm MA. Double-blind placebo-controlled crossover study of sacral nerve stimulation for idiopathic constipation. *British Journal of Surgery* 2002; **89**(12):1570–71.

15. Kenefick NJ, Nicholls JR, Cohen R.G., Kamm MA. Permanent sacral nerve stimulation for the treatment of idiopathic constipation. *Br J Surg* 2002; **89**:882–8.

16. Malouf AJ, Wiesel PH, Nicholls T, Nicholls RJ, Kamm MA. Short-term effects of sacral nerve stimulation for idiopathic slow transit constipation. *World Journal of Surgery* 2002; **26**(2):166–70.

17. Ganio E, Masin A, Ratto C, Basile M, Realis Luc A, Lise G et al. Sacral Nerve Modulation for Chronic Outlet Constipation. URL:http://www.colorep.it (2003)

18. Spinelli M, Giardiello G, Arduini A, van den Hombergh U. New percutaneous technique of sacral nerve stimulation has high initial success rate: preliminary results. *Eur Urol* 2003; **43**(1):70–74.

19. Uludag O, Darby M, Dejong CH, Schouten WR, Baeten CG. Sacral neuromodulation is effective in the treatment of fecal incontinence with intact sphincter muscles; a prospective study. *Ned Tijdschr Geneeskd* 2002; **146**(21):989–93.

20. Leroi AM, Michot F, Grise P, Denis P. Effect of sacral nerve stimulation in patients with fecal and urinary incontinence. *Diseases of the Colon & Rectum* 2001; **44**(6):779–89.

21. Jorge JM, Wexner SD. Etiology and management of fecal incontinence. *Dis Colon Rectum* 1993; **36**(1):77–97.

22. Vaizey CJ, Kamm MA, Roy AJ, Nicholls RJ. Double-blind crossover study of sacral nerve stimulation for fecal incontinence. *Dis Colon Rectum* 2000; **43**(3):298–302.

23. Tjandra JJ, Chan MK, Yeh CH, Murray-Green C. Sacral nerve stimulation is more effective than optimal medical therapy for severe fecal incontinence: a randomized, controlled study. *Dis Colon Rectum* 2008; **51**(5):494–502.

24. Chan MK, Tjandra JJ. Sacral nerve stimulation for fecal incontinence: external anal sphincter defect vs. intact anal sphincter. *Dis Colon Rectum* 2008; **51**(7):1015–24.

25. Jarrett ME, Dudding TC, Nicholls RJ, Vaizey CJ, Cohen CR, Kamm MA. Sacral nerve stimulation for fecal incontinence related to obstetric anal sphincter damage. *Dis Colon Rectum* 2008; **51**(5):531–7.

26. Conaghan P, Farouk R. Sacral nerve stimulation can be successful in patients with ultrasound evidence of external anal sphincter disruption. *Dis Colon Rectum* 2005; **48**(8):1610–4.

27. Hassouna MM, Siegel SW, Nyeholt AA, Elhilali MM, van Kerrebroeck PE, Das AK et al. Sacral neuromodulation in the treatment of urgency-frequency symptoms: a multicenter study on efficacy and safety. *J Urol* 2000; **163**(6):1849–54.

28. Jonas U, Fowler CJ, Chancellor MB, Elhilali MM, Fall M, Gajewski JB et al. Efficacy of sacral nerve stimulation for urinary retention: results 18 months after implantation. *J Urol* 2001; **165**(1):15–19.

29. Schmidt RA, Jonas U, Oleson KA, Janknegt RA, Hassouna MM, Siegel SW et al. Sacral nerve stimulation for treatment of refractory urinary urge incontinence. *Sacral Nerve Stimulation Study Group. J Urol* 1999; **162**(2):352–7.

30. Kamm MA, Dudding TC, Melenhorst J, Jarrett M, Wang Z, Buntzen S et al. Sacral nerve stimulation for intractable constipation. *Gut* 2010; **59**(3):333–40.

Chapter 22

Anal bulking

Mark Mercer-Jones

Background

Faecal incontinence (FI) characterized by involuntary loss of control of gas, liquid and
solid stool takes two forms: active/urge, and passive incontinence. A subgroup of
patients complains of staining of their underclothes, or faecal leakage (FL) without
frank incontinence.

Medical treatment of passive FI and FL includes dietary advice, stool bulking, anti-
diarrhoeal drugs, and biofeedback. In general, the internal anal sphincter (IAS), a thin
smooth muscle under tension, is not amenable to repair (1).

Alternative strategies involve compensating for loss of IAS function eg sacral nerve
stimulation (SNS), dynamic graciloplasty, or artificial sphincter. All are expensive and
in the case of the latter two approaches, have significant morbidity. For patients with
infrequent, mild to moderate FI and FL there are few alternatives.

Following their success in treating female urinary stress incontinence, there has
been interest in exploring the use of injectable bulking agents in the treatment of
patients with passive FI and FL. A variety of compounds have been injected, both
submucosally and intersphincterically into the anal canal to correct asymmetry,
and bulk-up the anal cushions. Results have been variable, largely because of false
expectations and poor patient selection. Key to their success is an understanding of the
pathophysiology of passive FI/FL and patient selection.

Pathophysiology of passive FI and FL

Assuming normal cortical sensory awareness, rectal compliance, stool consistency and
an absence of a local disease process, or, occult prolapse, then abnormalities of the
sphincter/anal canal cause FI and FL. It is useful to classify patients accordingly: traumatic or degenerative, neurogenic, combined, or idiopathic. (Idiopathic FI is diagnosed when there is a normal sphincter and normal anal canal sensation.)

Traumatic/degenerative

Traumatic IAS defects are commonly found post-partum and following perianal
surgery. They may be single (commonly associated with guttering) or multiple, and
cause asymmetry of the anal canal. It is possible to record the anal canal asymmetry
index (AI) during the recording of resting pressure at stationary pull-through.
Although values of 20% are regarded as normal, patients with IAS defects alone, or
in combination with defects in their EAS have AIs > 40% (2). Degeneration may

be primary, or secondary, and is usually associated with circumferential thinning or fragmentation (3) and less asymmetry.

Neurogenic

Both motor and sensory autonomic neuropathies affect continence. Pudendal neuropathy may result in external anal sphincter (EAS) weakness and a reduction in maximum resting pressure (MRP). Neuropathies can also reduce anal canal sensation; this may impair the sampling reflex and the ability to distinguish content. IAS tone is mostly regulated by the autonomic nervous system; sacral parasympathetic fibres are inhibitory whilst sympathetic thoraco-lumbar outflow fibres are excitatory (4).

Idiopathic

Passive FI is usually associated with a reduced MRP, particularly in traumatic and degenerative pathologies. However, 1/3 of patients with idiopathic FI have normal MRPs (5). Passive FL in contrast, is frequently idiopathic and associated with normal or even high MRPs especially in males (6) and patients with reduced rectal sensation (7).

Components of MRP include: striated EAS activity (30%), nerve induced IAS activity (45%), myogenic IAS activity (10%) and the anal cushions (15%) (8). When one considers that the IAS cannot completely seal the anal canal, (even at maximum contraction there is a gap of 7–8 mm), then the importance of the anal cushions is to be realized (9). Two processes may contribute to a widening of this gap and hence idiopathic FI/FL: atrophy, or iatrogenic loss of the anal cushions removes the ability to form a tight seal; and aging causes an increase in IAS thickness, inner and outer diameters (10). Thus, irrespective of the size of the anal cushions, increasing age may widen the gap with resultant incontinence.

The proposed mechanism of action of anal bulking

Anal bulking has the potential to improve symptoms of passive FI and FL by altering the morphology of the anal canal. In patients with discrete IAS defects, there is asymmetry of the canal whilst in those with neuropathy, degeneration, anal cushion atrophy and aging there is widening of the canal at rest. By correcting asymmetry, increasing the length of the high-pressure zone (2), restoring/enlarging the anal cushions, or by pushing the existing cushions into the anal canal, the deficiency is plugged. It is probable that bulking has little to do with increasing MRP.

Patient selection and exclusions

A valid criticism of most series on anal bulking is that variation in outcome is related to patient selection eg heterogeneity of aetiology, extent of disruption, severity of incontinence, inclusion of FI and FL. Whilst these make interpretation of results difficult, trends regarding suitable patient selection have emerged.

Treatment should be confined to patients with passive FI or FL who have failed all conservative measures. Whilst there is some evidence for efficacy in patients with severe FI (11,12), the only randomized placebo-controlled trial showed no benefit in patients with severe FI and IAS defects or degeneration (13). There is evidence that patients with severe FL may benefit (11). For patients with mild or infrequent passive FI and those who have discrete IAS defects or circumferential degeneration, evidence for efficacy is mostly level III. Neuropathy does not preclude a good outcome (11) nor does the additional presence of a small defect in the EAS (2). The group who benefit the most are those with idiopathic FI and FS, or those with generalised thinning of the IAS, lending support to the theory of anal cushion atrophy and age related widening of the gap (11,14). Exclusions to anal bulking include: urge FI or those with significant EAS defects, pregnancy, immunosuppression, perianal sepsis, haemorrhoids, high-grade recto-anal intussusception, cancer, and Crohn's disease.

Types of agent

Bulking agents are either biologic or non-biologic, and should be at least 80μm in diameter to prevent migration. The most commonly used agents in the UK are Permacol™, PTQ™, and Durasphere®.

◆ Permacol™ (Covidien, UK) is a non-allergenic, acellular implant manufactured from porcine dermal collagen. Cross-linkage of the collagen prevents degradation by human collagenases for up to 18 months. The collagen acts as a scaffold to allow fibroblast infiltration and host collagen deposition. Pre-loaded syringes (2.5 ml) are used with a disposable 18 G needle. Therapeutic doses range between 2.5–9 ml.

◆ PTQ™ (Uroplasty Ltd, Geleen, Holland) is a polydimethylsiloxane elastomer suspended in a bio-excretable hydrogel carrier of polyvinylpyrrolidone; particles are 100–450 μm. Particles again form a template for host collagen deposition. Vials (2.5 ml) are used with a ratchet gun and a 2.5inch, 18G needle. Therapeutic doses range between 2.5–10 ml.

◆ Durasphere® (Carbon Medical Technologies, St Paul, Minnesota, USA) contain carbon-coated zirconium oxide beads suspended in a carrier gel. Particles range from 90–212 μm in diameter and in theory they should not migrate. There have been reports of migration into lymph nodes following transurethral injection (company data) and hypersensitivity reactions (15). Therapeutic doses range between 2–10 ml.

◆ Others include: Bovine, cross-linked collagen (14,16) which requires skin-testing as it is antigenic in 5% of individuals; calcium hydroxyl apatite ceramic micro-spheres (17); polyacrylamide hydrogel (18); and stabilized non-animal hyaluronic acid with dextranomer (19).

Site of injection

There are two sites described (submucosal, or intersphincterically) and two injection techniques (via the anal margin or the trans-sphincter route). Bulking agent is always injected at and above the dentate line.

Submucosal injection

This has been described for all agents (3,12,14–20). This is performed with the needle entering the anal canal at the anal margin and advancing it to the submucosa using an anoscope. With correct placement the operator will see the mucosa bulge inwards.

Because there is a risk of infection, leakage and ulceration, this technique should only be used for collagen bulking (3) and with Durasphere® (21). The preferable method for non-biologics is to place the needle 2.5 cm from the anal verge and pass it through the EAS into the submucosa ie trans-sphincteric.

Intersphincteric injection

This has been described for PTQ™ (2,11,13,15,22) and is a more difficult technique as it is harder to judge correct placement. A finger placed within the anal canal acts as a guide to the course of the needle. The needle should be introduced 2.5cm from the anal verge and passed across the EAS. If placed correctly, the mucosa will not bulge but a slight indentation will be felt within. Using endoanal ultrasound prior to injection, it is possible to place 25G marker needles directly into the inter-sphincteric plane at the appropriate sites and use these as guides for subsequent injection; it is difficult to inject whilst the ultrasound probe is within the anus. There is evidence from one randomized trial that ultrasound guided intersphincteric injection gives superior results compared to blind injection (11). There is evidence that for FL, intersphincteric (PTQ™) gives superior results to submucosal (Durasphere®) (15).

Technique and peri-operative care

In some patients with an identified IAS defect, the bulking agent is injected at this site and geometrically opposite. The rational behind this appears sound in that correction of anal canal asymmetry will improve continence. The amount injected is often large (7.5 ml) at the site of the defect, and smaller opposite (2.5 ml) (Fig. 22.1 and 2) (11,15,20); peri-operative ultrasound is advisable. Where the IAS is circumferentially thinned, or the FI/FL is idiopathic it is recommended that injections (1–3 ml) be placed in sites corresponding to the anal cushions (3,12–20).

75% of published interventions were performed under local anaesthesia. Pre-operative enemas were used in 50% (2,13,15,18,23), and postoperative lactulose in 20% (2,11,23); the rationale being to prevent hard stool from disrupting the implants in the early post-operative period. Although there is no evidence in support of this, at the very least, a single pre-operative enema is advised. Eighty per cent received antibiotics and in 50% they were continued for 3–7 days. One study using PTQ™ (20), two using Durasphere® (21,24) and one using Contigen® (14) used no antibiotics; all had submucosal implants and no infective complications followed. A single per-operative dose of antibiotic is justifiable when using PTQ™. Warfarin and all anti-platelet drugs should be stopped pre-operatively.

Complications

Anal bulking is safe with only one reported type III hypersensitivity reaction to Durasphere® (15). Local complications range from abscess formation and anal ulceration, to pain and pruritis-ani. Abscesses are reported following 2.8–5% of PTQ™ implants. Abscesses occur with submucosal and intersphincterically injected PTQ™, but in all cases the deployment method was trans-sphincteric injection (2,12,20).

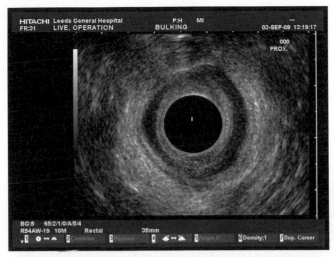

Fig. 22.1 Endoanal ultrasound of a woman with an internal anal defect (11–1 o'clock) and passive faecal incontinence (mild).

Submucosal PTQ™ injected via the anal margin is not recommended as anal ulceration is reported in 40% (3). Anal erosion and leakage of implants has only been reported following submucosal Durasphere® in 3–10% of patients (15,21,24). The lowest complication rate is seen with submucosal collagen; 0.5% abscess formation and no reported leakage. Anal pain is experienced in 5–30% of patients irrespective of the material or position of injection.

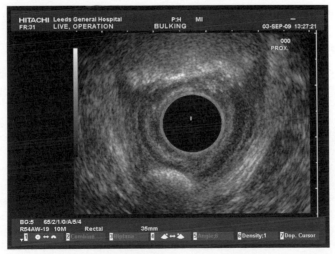

Fig. 22.2 Appearances after intersphincteric injection of PTQ™ of 7.5 ml at the site of the defect, and 2.5 ml opposite.

Clinical effectiveness, longevity, and reinjection rates

In total 18 case-series (including 3 trials) are discussed (Table 22.1 and 2); four discuss FL and the remainder FI. Objective improvement was seen in 60–83% of FL patients at 1 yr (15,16,20). In one study (20) non-responders (33%) were re-injected (at 1 month). Two studies report sustained improvement in objective scores after 6 months (Durasphere® (submucosal) and PTQ™ (intersphincteric) (15,21)). There is no long-term data published on FL. For FI, objective improvement was reported in 12 of the 16 series with follow-up ranging from 2–24 months. In four series, objective improvement was considered non-significant (3,13,18,22), and in the remainder improvement ranged from 50–91% (2,11,14,17,19,23,24).

In some series, patients who failed to respond to the initial injection were re-injected at three months. For example, in one study (24), 45% were re-injected with submucosal Durasphere® after complaining of leakage of the beads. In another (17), 33% were re-injected with submucosal Coaptite®, and in another (13) 33% of patients were re-injected with inter-sphincteric PTQ™ (with no improvement). There is evidence for FL that improvement may develop after 6 months (11). For non-responders it would thus seem reasonable to wait at least 6 months (unless the bulking agent has been lost) before considering re-injection.

Whilst data on long-term outcome is lacking, submucosal Permacol™ is still effective in 61% of patients with FI at 14 months (25). Re-injection rates for patients who initially responded, are 27% for submucosal Contigen® (median 15 months) (14) and 42% for submucosal Permacol™ (median 12 months) (26), Deterioration in objective scores at two years has been reported in two studies using submucosal PTQ™ (12,25). In a follow-up report on 189 patients injected with inter-sphincteric PTQ™, efficacy was sustained at two years but there was a notable deterioration at three years (26). Deterioration over time does not appear to be related to loss of the implant but rather tissue accommodation to the bulk of the injectable (26). The results on efficacy and deterioration over time are similar to intramural urethral bulking for stress urinary incontinence.

Summary

The problem in advising on the use of bulking agents for FI and FL is the lack of objective data and more importantly level I evidence. The National Institute for Clinical Effectiveness (NICE) reported in 2007 that the evidence for their use was inadequate for safety and effectiveness. This was based on a review of 158 patients in seven case-series. Surprisingly two were case-series using autologous fat! Since then, 13 case-series, one randomized-controlled trial and one randomized placebo-controlled trial have been reported (additional 531 patients). Further recommendations are therefore warranted.

The only level I evidence comes from a 2007 blinded, randomized, placebo-controlled trial comparing inter-sphincteric PTQ™ versus saline for moderate and severe passive FI (13). At three months, the percentage of subjects experiencing a successful treatment (defined as a Cleveland Clinic-Faecal Incontinence score < 8) was no different between PTQ™ (n = 22) and saline (n = 22) groups. Importantly, the placebo-related effect was 27%. This was a well-conducted trial that included patients with passive FI and IAS defects/degeneration but not FL, and excluded patients with urge FI and

Table 22.1 Studies treating passive faecal leakage.

Reference	Year	No./Age	Bulking Agent	Site of Injection	Aetiology	Exclusions- Urge/EAS defects	Objective outcome	Subjective outcome	Median follow-up (months)	Comments
Kumar D et al.[25]	1998	n=17 53 (42–76)	Bovine collagen (Glutaraldehyde cross-linked)	Submucosal 2 ml at 1–3 sites	IAS defect n=8 Idiopathic n=9	All passive FL EAS defect excluded	65% cure 6% partial cure 30% failure	ND	8 (4–12)	All failed conservative treatment. All had low MRP. Non-standardized FI/FL scoring system
Davis K et al.[24]	2003	n=18 60 (31–87)	Durasphere®	Submucosal 1.8 ml (0.5–3 ml) at IAS defect	IAS defect n=17 Neuropathic n=1	All passive FL EAS defect in 7	Wexner score at 12 months fell 11.9 ± 5.10 to 8.07± 3.68[b]	FIQL at 12 months	28.5 mean (11–40)	All failed conservative treatment. MRP normal 3 patients withdrew
Van der Hagen SJ et al[28]	2006	n=24 55 (median) (33–79)	PTQ	Submucosal 6.7 ml (2.5–18 ml) at IAS defect	IAS defect n=24	All passive FL EAS defect not excluded	Daily soiling frequency fell from 2.0 (1–5) to 1.5 (0–3) at 12 months[a], Vaizey score fell from 4.2 (0–8) to 2.1 (0–6) at 12 months[a]	NS	12	Conservative treatment not recorded. All had normal anrectal function. Al had keyhole defects Repeat injections in 8
Tjandra JJ et al[23]	2009	n=40 59.2 (36–74)	PTQ™ (n=20) vs Durasphere® (n=20)	Interspinctheric PTQ™, 2.5 ml at 4 sites (or 7.5 ml at site of IAS defect and 2.5 ml opposite) Submucosal Durasphere®, 2.5 ml at 4 sites (or 7.5 ml at site of IAS defect and 2.5 ml opposite	IAS defect n=5 Neuropathic n=27 Idiopathic n=8	All passive FL excluded only if EAS defect >120°	In PTQ group, Wexner score at 12 months fell 11.45±2.63 to 3.80±2.76[a] in Durasphere group, Wexner score at 12 months fell 11.45±2.35 to 7.00±2.77[a]	FIQL at 12 months in PTQ group[b]	12	All failed conservative Treatment. MRP low or borderline. Randomised, blinded. More PTQ patients achieved>50% improvement in continence than Durasphere

Age is mean (range), unless otherwise indicated. Amount injected is mean (range). Objective outcomes are mean ± SD unless indicated.
[a] The P-values for each outcome are <0.001.
[b] The P-values for each outcome are <0.05. ND is not done. And NS is not significant. EAS is external anal sphincter. FIQL is Fecal Incontinence Quality of Life. FL is faecal leakage. IAS is internal anal sphincter. MRP is Mean Resting Pressure.

Table 22.2 Studies of bulking for passive FI

Reference	Year	No./Age	Bulking Agent	Site of Injection	Aetiology	Exclusions-Urge/EAS defects	Objective Outcome	Subjective Outcome	Median Follow-up (months)	Comments
Malouf AJ et al[4]	2001	n=10 median 64 (41–80)	PTQ	Submucosal 5 ml at site of IAS defect or 5–11.5 ml circumferentially	IAS defect n=4 Idiopathic n=6	All passive FI EAS defect not excluded	20% marked improvement 10% minor improvement	ND	6	Failed conservative treatment. Poor study with a change in injection technique part way through. Non-standardised objective scoring system. Anal ulceration in 40%
Tjandra JJ et al[13]	2004	n=82 median 66 (34–89)	PTQ	Intersphincteric Randomised to ultrasound guided (n=42) vs palpation (n=40) 2.5 ml at 4 sites cicumferentially or 7.5 ml at site of IAS defect and 2.5 ml opposite	IAS defect n=11 Idiopathic n=23 Neuropathic n=48	All severe passive FI 21 patients had previous sphincteroplasty	At 6 months, Wexner score in ultrasound guided group fell from median 14.5 (10–20) to 5 (2–13)[b] Wexner score in palpation group fell from 14.5 (11–20) to 8 (2–12)[b]	Ultrasound guided group showed improvement in SF-12 and FIQL Palpation group showed improvement in FIQL	6 (1–12)	Failed conservative treatment. Low MRP in all, that improved after treatment. At 3 months, more ultrasound guided patients had >50% improvement in Wexner score than palpation patients. Good short term results in patients with an intact IAS and severe FI. Interesting why the results of the described randomised trial comparing PTQ to saline were never published
Stojkovic SG et al[20]	2006	n=73 median 63 (52–70)	Contigen	Submucosal 1.7 ml at 3 sites circumferentially, total volume 5 ml	IAS defect n=9 Idiopathic n=49 Neuropathic n=13	Urge FI not excluded 3 patients with EAS defects	At 12 months, Wexner score (median) fell from 10 (i.q.r. 6–16) to 6 (i.q.r. 3–10)[a]	ND	12 (i.q.r. 9–16)	No evidence that patients failed conservative management. Low MRP reported only in the first 37 patients. Only idiopathic group showed significant improvement. 20 patients reinjected at a median of 15 months (i.q.r. 9–24)

Table 22.2 (continued) Studies of bulking for passive FI

Study	Year	n	Agent	Technique/dose	Sphincter defect	FI type	Outcome	QoL	Follow-up (months)	Comments
De la Portilla F et al[18]	2006	n=20 median 57 (55–65)	PTQ	Submucosal 2.5 ml at 3 sites circumferentially	IAS defect or degeneration n=19	All severe passive FI. EAS defect excluded	At 6 months, Wexner score fell from 13.5±5.31 to 5.06±4.6[a]	FIQL NS	6 (6–24)	All patients failed conservative management. No neurological investigation reported. All low MRP. Longer follow-up data showed significant benefit at 1 yr, but not at 2 yrs
Maeda Y et al[26]	2007	n=10	Permacol (n=5) vs Bulkamid (n=5)	Submucosal Both at 3 sites circumferentially Permacol 15 ml (15–17.5) Bulkamid 9 ml (8–9)	IAS defect or degeneration n=7	All passive FI Urge FI not excluded EAS defect n=2	At 6 months, St Mark's score in Permacol group fell from 16 (11–24) to 15 (8–22). In Bulkamid group it fell from 15 (12–17) to 12 (5–18)	FIQL in both groups[b]	6	All patients had failed conservative management. Unusually large amounts of agent injected, especially permacol. Small numbers make comparison meaningless
Siproudhis L et al[1]	2007	n=44 64±9	PTQ vs Saline	Intersphincteric Randomised to PTQ n=22 vs Saline n=22 2.5 ml at 3 sites circumferentially	IAS defects or degeneration in all patients	All severe FI Urge FI and EAS defects excluded	At 3 months, Wexner score for PTQ group fell from 13.8±2 to 11.7±5, and for saline group from 14.6±3 to 11.4±5 Both NS	FIQL showed no improvement in either group	3	All patients had failed conservative management. A blind, randomised trial. Randomisation process not described. No record of neurological investigation. MRP reduced in all. Could ultrasound guidance have improved results? A placebo-related effect was seen in 27% of the saline injected patients. Short follow-up

(continued)

Table 22.2 (continued) Studies of bulking for passive FI

Reference	Year	No./Age	Bulking Agent	Site of Injection	Aetiology	Exclusions-Urge/EAS defects	Objective Outcome	Subjective Outcome	Median Follow-up (months)	Comments
Soerensen MM et al[15]	2007	n=33 median 53 (21–75)	PTQ	Intersphincteric 2.5 ml at 3 sites circumferentially	IAS defect n=5 Idiopathic n=17	Both urge and passive FI EAS defects n=3 Combined IAS/EAS n=8	At 12.9 months, Wexner score fell from 12.7 (6–18) to 10.4 (2–17)[b]	SF-36 NS	12.9 mean (3–22)	All patients failed conservative management. No record of neurological investigation. Heterogenous group. Improvement could have been placebo-related
Altomare DF et al[16]	2008	n=33 61.5 (22–83)	Durasphere	Submucosal 8.8 ml (total) (2–19 ml) At 4 sites circumferentially	Unclear as EAUS not done in all patients	Urge FI not excluded EAS defects not excluded	At median of 20.8 months, Wexner score (median) fell from 12 to 8[a]	FIQL NS	20.8 (10–22)	All patients failed conservative management. No record of neurological investigation Unclear aetiology. A poor study
Ganio E et al[14]	2008	n=10 62.9 (48–75)	Coaptite	Submucosal 1 ml at 4 sites circumferentially	IAS defect or thinning in all patients	All passive FI Urge FI not excluded EAS defects not excluded 2 patients previous sphincteroplasty 1 patient previous gracioplasty	At 12 months, FISS score fell from 85.9±9.4 to 28.0±29.0[b]	FIQL[b]	12	All patients failed medical management. No record of neurological investigation. 80% showed a marked improvement. All low MRP which improved with treatment

Table 22.2 (*continued*) Studies of bulking for passive FI

Study	Year	n	Age	Agent	Amount / Technique	Patient type	FI type	Outcome	QoL outcome	Follow-up (months)	Comments
Aigner F et al[17]	2009	n=11	66 (56–74)	Durasphere	Submucosal 2.82 ml (8–12 ml)	Idiopathic n=11	Urge and passive FI. EAS defects excluded	At 2 yrs, Wexner score fell from 12.27±0.97 to 4.91±0.87[b]	At 6 months 3 out of domains of FIQL improved[b]	24	All failed conservative management except medical management not reported. All low MRP. No neurological investigations and no rectal sensitivity recorded. 73% complained of urgency pre-injection
Oliveira LCC et al[3]	2009	n=35	60.3 (19–80)	PTQ	Intersphincteric 2.5 ml at 3 sites circumferentially	IAS defect n=20; IAS and EAS defect n=15	Urge and passive FI. EAS defects not excluded	At 1 month, Wexner score fell from 11.3 to 4.3[a], the scores at 1 yr are similar. Asymmetry index at 2 cms[a]	FIQL[b] at 3 months	12	No record of failed medical management. All low MRP. No neurological investigations. Improvement in the high pressure zone and asymmetry index noted
Danielson J et al[27]	2009	n=34	median 61 (34–80)	NASHA Dx gel	Submucosal 1 ml at 4 sites circumferentially	IAS defect n=3; Idiopathic n=7; Neurogenic n=23	Urge and passive FI	At 12 months, Miller score fell from 14 (6–18) to 11 (1–16)[a]	Patient reported outcome excellent/good 44% at 1 yr	12	All patients failed conservative management. 18 patients reinjected. Only passive FI patients showed a significant decrease in FI scores at 1 yr. Treatment response (50% reduction in incontinence episodes) seen in 56% at 1 yr

Age is mean (range), unless otherwise indicated. Amount injected is mean (range) unless indicated. Objective outcomes are mean ± SD unless indicated.

[a] The P-values for each outcome are <0.001.

[b] The P-values for each outcome are <0.05. ND is not done. And NS is not significant. FIQL is Fecal Incontinence Quality of Life.

SF-36 is short form −36. MRP is mean resting pressure. I.q.r. is interquartile range.

EAS is external anal sphincter. FI is faecal incontinence. IAS is internal anal sphincter.

EAS defects. However, injections were not placed using ultrasound guidance and the follow-up may not have been long enough to judge true effectiveness; ultrasound guidance improves efficacy for intersphincteric PTQ^{TM}, and improvement continues for one year (11). The interesting difference between this trial and that of Tjandra and co-investigators (11), (where moderate and severe FI responded to intersphincteric PTQ^{TM}), was patient selection. Only 10% of Tjandra's patients had IAS defects, while over 60% had a pudendal neuropathy. In addition in those patients with an IAS defect, inter-sphincteric injection was of 7.5 ml of PTQ^{TM} at the site of the defect and 2.5 ml on the opposite side. In the randomized placebo-controlled trial (13) it was 2.5 ml in the three areas corresponding to the anal cushions. In conclusion, current evidence does not support anal bulking in patients with a combination of moderate/severe FI and IAS defects.

It is clear that anal bulking is safe with minimal local and systemic side effects and that injection should not preclude repeated injections or alternative surgical strategies. It would appear that its effectiveness and longevity is comparable with results reported following its use in stress urinary incontinence. Patient selection should focus on those with FL (irrespective of aetiology and severity) and those with mild FI. Patients with moderate and severe idiopathic FI should also be considered. The patient's age should also be taken into account. The elderly are often unfit or unwilling to undergo major surgical intervention, and a treatment that can be given under local anaesthesia is attractive. Younger patients should be advised that the long-term outcome is not known and that repeat injections will be required.

The choice of agent depends upon the aetiology of the FI or FL and the expertise of the surgeon. PTQ^{TM} should be injected trans-sphincterically into the intersphincteric plane at the sites of the anal cushions, and this is best guided by ultrasound. For patients with IAS defects and FL, or patients with mild FI, inter-sphincteric injections can be either injected at the site of the defect (5–7.5 ml) and opposite (2.5 ml), or circumferentially at the site of the anal cushions. There is no evidence that either technique is superior. For Permacol^{TM}, Durasphere®, Coaptite®, and NASHA^{TM} Dx, submucosal placement is easier to perform.

Key points

- Bulking is a useful adjunct in the treatment of passive FI and FL
- Injectable agents are safe
- The mechanism of action is probably by providing a tighter anal canal seal and correcting asymmetry
- Evidence suggests that bulking is of no benefit to patients with severe and moderate FI and IAS defects
- Evidence suggests that those that benefit most are those with an idiopathic or neuropathic aetiology
- The effects of bulking diminish with time.

Editor's summary

Patients with mild or moderate passive faecal incontinence who have no prolapse and have failed conservative therapies are considered for anal bulking. Patients with any degree of severity of faecal leakage are also considered. Patients with severe passive faecal incontinence should only be treated if elderly, or if unsuitable for a sacral nerve test-wire (particularly if the IAS is not severely disrupted). A normal MRP (or occasionally high MRP in males) does not preclude treatment.

Patients with faecal incontinence should undergo physiology and anal ultrasound. Patients with post-defaecatory soiling or idiopathic faecal incontinence require a defaecating proctogram. Haemorrhoids and internal rectal prolapse require recognition and exclusion as causes of faecal incontinence before anal bulking agents are used.

References

1. Morgan R, Patel B, Benyon J, Carr N. Surgical management of anorectal incontinence due to internal anal sphincter deficiency. *Br.J.Surg.* 1997;**84**(2):226–30.
2. Oliveira LCC, Jorge JMN, Yussuf S, Habra-Gama A, Kiss D, Cecconello. Anal incontinence improvement after silicone injection may be related to restoration of sphincter asymmetry. *Surg Innov* 2009;**16**(2):155–61.
3. Malouf AJ, Vaizey CJ, Norton CS, Kamm MA. Internal anal sphincter augmentation for faecal incontinence using injectable silicone biomaterial. *Dis Colon Rectum* 2001;**44**: 595–600.
4. Mills K, Chess-Williams. Pharmacology of the internal anal sphincter and its relevance to faecal incontinence. *Autonomic Autocoid Pharmacol* 2009;**29**:85–95.
5. Stojkovic SG, Balfour L, Burke D, Finan PJ, Sagar PM. Role of resting pressure gradient in the investigation of idiopathic faecal incontinence. *Dis Colon Rectum* 2002;**45**(5):668–73.
6. Titi M, Jenkins JT, Urie A, Molloy RG. Prospective study of the diagnostic evaluation of faecal incontinence and leakage in male patients. *Colorectal Dis* 2007;**9**:647–52.
7. Hoffmann BA, Timmcke AE, Gathright JB jr, Hicks TC, Opelka FG, Beck DE. Fecal seepage and soiling: a problem of rectal sensation. *Dis Colon Rectum* 1995;**38**(7):746–8.
8. Lestar B, Penninckx F, Kerremans R. The composition of anal basal pressure. An *in vivo* and *in vitro* study in man. *Int J Colorectal Dis* 1989;**4**(2):118–22.
9. Lestar B, Penninckx F, Rigauts H, Kerremans R. The internal anal sphincter can not close the anal canal completely. *Int J Colorectal Dis* 1992;**7**(3):159–62.
10. Huebner M, Margulies RU, Fenner DE, Ashton-Miller JA, Bitar KN, DeLancey JO. Age effects on internal anal sphincter thickness and diameter in nulliparous females. *Dis Colon Rectum* 2007;**50**:1405–11.
11. Tjandra JJ, Lim JF, Hiscock R, Rajendra P. Injectable silicone biomaterial for fecal incontinence caused by internal anal sphincter dysfunction is effective. *Dis Colon Rectum* 2004;**47**:2138–46.
12. De la Portilia F, Fernandez A, Leone E, Rada R, Cisneros N, Maldonado VH, Vega J, Espinosa E. Evaluation of the use of PTQ implants for the treatment of incontinent patients due to internal anal sphincter dysfunction. *Colorectal Dis* 2007;**10**:89–94.

13. Siproudhis L, Morcet J, Lane F. Elastomer implants in faecal incontinence: a blind randomized placebo-controlled study. *Aliment Pharmacol Ther* 2007;**25**(1):1125–32.

14. Stojkovic SG, Lim M, Burke D, Finan PJ, Sagar PM. Intra-anal-collagen injection for the treatment of faecal incontinence. *Br J Surg* 2006;**93**:1514–8.

15. Tjandra JJ, Chan MKY, Yeh HCH. Injectable silicone biomaterial (PTQ) is more effective than carbon-coated beads (Durasphere) in the management of faecal incontinence. *Aliment Phrmacol Ther* 2008;**18**:237–43.

16. Kumar D, Benson MI, Bland IE. Glutaraldehyde cross-linked collagen in the treatment of faecal incontinence. *Colorectal Dis* 1998;**10**:268–72.

17. Ganio E, Marino F, Giani I, Realis Luc A, Clerico G, Novelli E, Trompetto M. Injectable synthetic calcium hydroxylapatite ceramic microspheres (Coaptite) for passive faecal incontinence. *Tech Coloproctol* 2008;**12**:99–102.

18. Maeda Y, Vaizey CJ, Kamm MA. Pilot study of two new injectable bulking agents for the treatment of faecal incontinence. *Colorect Dis* 2007;**10**:268–72.

19. Danielson J, Karlbom U, Sonesson AC, Wester T, Graf W. Submucosal injection of stabilizing non-animal hyaluronic acid with dextranomer: a new treatment option for fecal incontinence. *Dis Colon Rectum* 2009;**52**:1101–6.

20. Van der Hagen SJ, van Gemert WG, Basten CG. PTQ implants in the treatment of faecal soiling. *Br J Surg* 2007;**94**:222–3.

21. Davis K, Kumar D, Poloniecki J. Preliminary evaluation of an injectable anal sphincter bulking agent (Durasphere) in the management of faecal incontinence. *Aliment Phamacol Ther* 2003;**18**:237–43.

22. Sorensen MM, Lunby L, Buntzen S, Laurberg S. Intersphincteric injected silicone biomaterial implants: a treatment for faecal incontinence. *Colorectal Dis* 2008;**11**:73–6.

23. Altomare DF, La Torre F, Rinaldi M, Binda GA, Pescatori M. Carbon-coated microbeads anal injection in outpatient treatment of minor fecal incontinence. *Dis Colon Rectum* 2008;**51**:432–5.

24. Aiger F, Conrad F, Margreiter R, Oberwalder M. Anal submucosal carbon bead injection for treatment of idiopathic fecal incontinence: a preliminary report. *Dis Colon Rectum* 2009;**52**:293–8.

25. De la Portilla F, Vega J, Rada R, Segovia-Gonzales MM, Cisneros N, Maldonado VH, Espinosa E. Evaluation by three-dimensional anal endosonography of injectable silicone biomaterial (PTQ) implants to treat fecal incontinence: long-term localization and relation with deteroration of continence. *Tech. Coloproctol* 2009;**13**:195–9.

26. Tjandra JJ, Tan J, Lim JF, Murray-Green C. Long-term results of injectable silicone biomaterial for passive fecal incontinence–a randomized trial. *DisColon Rectum* 2006;**49**:730–1.

Chapter 23

Anterior sphincter repair

Sophie Pilkington

Introduction

The commonest cause of an anal sphincter defect in women is obstetric trauma. There is a wide variation in the reported incidence of sphincter injury after childbirth, but approximately 11% of postpartum women are likely to be affected (1). Most injuries are identified at the time of delivery and repaired. Women who present later with faecal incontinence and fail conservative management may undergo 'secondary' anterior sphincter repair. Although this improves initial incontinence rates by 60 to 97% (2), in the long term the functional outcome deteriorates (1,3).

Early reports of anal sphincter repair focused on narrowing the anal orifice. The first description of an overlapping sphincter repair to restore a functioning anal sphincter was by Parks in 1971(4). In this technique, the scar tissue was excised and the freed ends of undamaged muscle were sutured in an overlapping configuration. A preoperative diverting colostomy was used. The technique was modified by Slade who found that not excising the scar and avoiding a stoma improved the functional outcome (5).

Enthusiasm for anterior sphincter repair, which was initiated in the 1970s, has been tempered by reports of deteriorating long-term function and the risk of worsening symptoms after surgery (3). In addition the therapeutic options for patients with faecal incontinence have increased over the last decade with the development of neuro-modulation and artificial sphincters. It is not clear from the current literature whether sphincter repair should be performed before or after neuromodulation to produce successful control of symptoms for the maximum length of time. The role of anterior sphincter repair in the era of sacral nerve stimulation needs further evaluation (6).

Patient selection

Fewer patients are being selected for anterior sphincter repair. The recognition of a less than perfect outcome and long-term deterioration in function in combination with the recent development of alternative less invasive treatment (neuromodulation) has driven this decline.

When selecting patients for anterior sphincter repair, a detailed history is essential with particular attention to severity of symptoms of anal incontinence and the impact on quality of life. A physical examination including the perineum, anal canal and rectum is carried out. Anorectal physiology to document sphincter function and endoanal ultrasound to assess the anatomy of the sphincters, including the presence of a defect (Fig. 23.1.a and b), is performed. The sensitivity of 2- and 3-dimensional

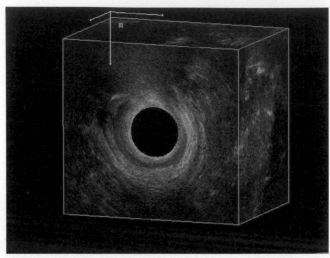

Fig. 23.1.a Three-dimensional endoanal ultrasound dataset showing sphincter defect.

ultrasound for diagnosing sphincter injuries is similar (7). However 3-dimensional ultrasound is able to accurately assess the length as well as radial extent of the defect (8) (Fig. 23.1.a). The role of pudendal nerve terminal motor latency is controversial and it is not reliable for predicting outcome (9,10).

Other causes of faecal incontinence, including colorectal cancer and inflammatory bowel disease, must be excluded with flexible sigmoidoscopy.

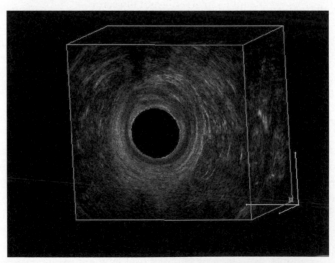

Fig. 23.1.b Endoanal ultrasound dataset showing immediate postoperative appearances in the same patient after anterior Sphincter repair.

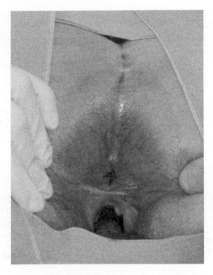

Fig. 23.2.a Prone jack-knife position.

Description of operation

Full mechanical bowel preparation is not used universally with some institutions avoiding its use (11) and others recommending it (12,13). The procedure is carried out under general anaesthesia in the prone jack-knife position (Fig. 23.2.a). A single dose of prophylactic antibiotics is usually given at induction. A curvilinear incision is made in the perineum (Fig. 23.2.b) and the external anal sphincter is mobilised anteriorly with sharp dissection (Fig. 23.2.c). Mobilization is continued laterally between external anal sphincter and surrounding fat. However the muscle is not dissected posterolaterally so as to avoid damage to the pudendal nerves in this position. The levator ani muscles are identified bilaterally and dissection is continued superiorly to

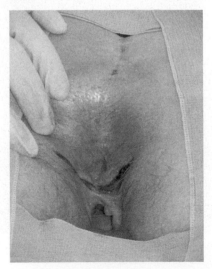

Fig. 23.2.b Curvilinear perineal incision.

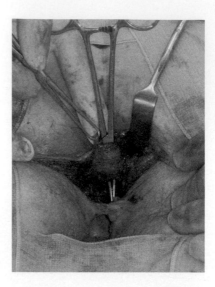

Fig. 23.2.c External anal sphincter (EAS) mobilized.

the level of the pelvic floor. The external anal sphincter is divided at the site of the scar but the scar tissue is not excised (Fig. 23.2.d). A tension-free overlapping repair of the external anal sphincter is carried out using delayed-absorbable mattress sutures (Fig. 23.2.e). The anal canal should admit the little finger after the repair. Interrupted absorbable sutures are used for skin closure (Fig. 23.2.f). A little gap may be left in the closure to allow drainage, or alternatively a small drain may be used.

Although some centres recommend separate dissection of the internal anal sphincter and direct suturing of defects (11,12), this is often not possible as the normal tissue planes are obliterated in the scarred sphincter (13). Repair of an isolated internal anal sphincter injury does not improve symptoms (14,15). Levatorplasty or plication of puborectalis is frequently added to the overlapping repair to lengthen the anal canal

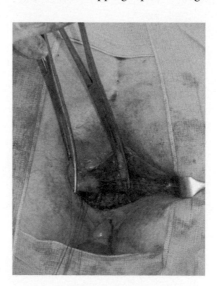

Fig. 23.2.d EAS divided at site of scarring but no scar excision.

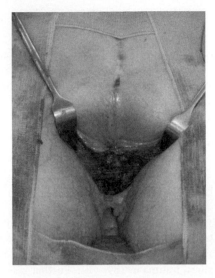

Fig. 23.2.e Completed overlapping repair of external anal sphincter.

and recreate the perineal body (12,13). A high incidence of dyspareunia has been reported after rectocele repair when levatorplasty is included (16,17). Sexual function has not been rigorously assessed after secondary sphincter repair but the majority of patients may have improved sexual function due to reduced anal incontinence (11).

Outcome of anterior sphincter repair

Up to 80% of patients have an initial improvement in their symptoms after sphincter repair (2,9,18) but only 20% remain continent to solid and liquid stool at 10 years (1). The reason for this deterioration in function is not clear. The anal sphincter has been the focus for operative intervention in patients with faecal incontinence especially since the introduction of endoanal ultrasound to identify sphincter defects.

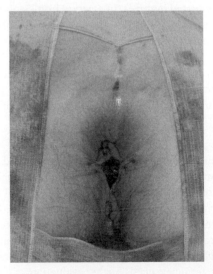

Fig. 23.2.f Skin Closure.

Table 23.1 Long-term results after anterior sphincter repair (follow-up greater than 5 years)

Reference	Patients contributing to results/total study group (percentage)	Length of follow-up months (range)	Percentage with solid or liquid incontinence
Malouf (3) 2000	38/55 (69%)	77 (60–96)	89
Halverson (23) 2002	49/71 (69%)	69 (48–141)	54
Gutierrez (22) 2004	135/191 (71%)	120 (84–192)	78
Barisic (30) 2006	56/65 (86%)	80 (26–154)	52
Zutshi (24) 2009	31/44 (71%)	129 (113–208)	100

However, these defects rarely exist in isolation and damage to other pelvic floor structures representing a global pelvic floor problem are increasingly recognized. Three-dimensional endoanal ultrasound detects external anal sphincter injury in 11% of deliveries and additional perineal trauma in 18% (19). Further research is needed to assess whether dynamic and 3-dimensional 'complete pelvic floor' scanning can improve patient selection and outcome assessment for secondary sphincter repair.

Many published series assessing outcome after anterior sphincter repair have relied on patient recall and subjective measures of improvement and satisfaction. A more reliable assessment of outcome is provided by the completion of pre- and post-operative symptom severity scores and quality of life questionnaires such as the Cleveland Clinic Incontinence Score (20) and Fecal Incontinence Quality of Life Questionnaire (21). The largest series of published secondary sphincter repairs (n = 191) showed that at a median follow-up of 10 years only 6% were fully continent and 58% were incontinent to solid stool (22). Table 23.1 summarizes the long-term functional outcome in studies with a follow-up period of greater than 5 years. In this table, the results of Halverson (23) and Zutshi (24) represent the same cohort of patients followed up at 5 and 10 years. The faecal incontinence rate deteriorated over this time period from 54 to 100% of patients.

Secondary repair significantly increases the mean resting pressure, mean squeeze increment and anal canal length as estimated by length of high pressure zone during anorectal physiology (25,26).

A poor clinical outcome is associated with a persistent sphincter defect on endoanal ultrasound (27). A repeat secondary repair may improve function (28,29) although there is a risk of worsening the scarring and nerve damage to the sphincter.

Summary

Treatment of faecal incontinence due to obstetric injury has focussed primarily on the anal sphincter. More recently it has been recognized that external anal sphincter defects rarely exist in isolation. Damage to the rest of the pelvic floor frequently coexists with the sphincter defect and is likely to contribute to symptoms. This may explain in part why repairing the sphincter defect has an unpredictable effect on continence.

There is still a place for secondary repair of sphincter defects in patients with faecal incontinence that affects their quality of life. However, in the era of neuromodulation the timing of anterior sphincter repair needs further evaluation.

Key points

◆ Prone jack-knife position facilitates secondary repair
◆ A defunctioning stoma is not necessary
◆ Good short-term functional outcome although perfect continence is rarely achieved
◆ Long-term function deteriorates
◆ There is a need for further evaluation of patient selection for sphincter repair in era of neuromodulation.

Editor's summary

Anterior sphincter repair remains an excellent procedure for selected patients with faecal incontinence, particularly the younger patient presenting relatively soon after obstetric trauma. The older patient with a delayed presentation is probably better suited to sacral neuromodulation (SNS). Patients with incontinence and a cloacal deformity represent the prime indication for sphincter repair over other techniques. Technically speaking, the internal anal sphincter should be identified separately and imbricated if possible, and ideally a nerve-stimulator is very useful to distinguish skeletal muscle. Any method to reduce the high incidence of wound breakdown (oblique or introital incisions) is commended. Sphincter repair should not be undertaken without a thorough interrogation of the pelvic floor.

References

1. Dudding TC, Vaizey CJ, Kamm MA. Obstetric anal sphincter injury: incidence, risk factors, and management. *Ann Surg* 2008; **247**(2):224–37.
2. Zorcolo L, Covotta L, Bartolo DC. Outcome of anterior sphincter repair for obstetric injury: comparison of early and late results. *Dis Colon Rectum* 2005; **48**(3):524–31.
3. Malouf AJ, Norton CS, Engel AF, Nicholls RJ, Kamm MA. Long-term results of overlapping anterior anal-sphincter repair for obstetric trauma. *Lancet* 2000; **355**(9200):260–5.
4. Parks AG, McPartlin JF. Late repair of injuries of the anal sphincter. *Proc R Soc Med* 1971; **64**(12):1187–9.
5. Slade MS, Goldberg SM, Schottler JL, Balcos EG, Christenson CE. Sphincteroplasty for acquired anal incontinence. *Dis Colon Rectum* 1977; **20**(1):33–5.
6. Nicholls J. Sphincter repair for incontinence. *Colorectal Dis* 2009; **11**(6):545–6.
7. Christensen AF, Nyhuus B, Nielsen MB, Christensen H. Three-dimensional anal endosonography may improve diagnostic confidence of detecting damage to the anal sphincter complex. *Br J Radiol* 2005; **78**(928):308–11.
8. Gold DM, Bartram CI, Halligan S, Humphries KN, Kamm MA, Kmiot WA. Three-dimensional endoanal sonography in assessing anal canal injury. *Br J Surg* 1999; **86**(3):365–70.
9. Engel AF, Kamm MA, Sultan AH, Bartram CI, Nicholls RJ. Anterior anal sphincter repair in patients with obstetric trauma. *Br J Surg* 1994; **81**(8):1231–4.

10. Gearhart S, Hull T, Floruta C, Schroeder T, Hammel J. Anal manometric parameters: predictors of outcome following anal sphincter repair? *J Gastrointest Surg* 2005; **9**(1):115–20.

11. Maslekar S, Gardiner AB, Duthie GS. Anterior anal sphincter repair for fecal incontinence: Good longterm results are possible. *J Am Coll Surg* 2007; **204**(1):40–46.

12. Grey BR, Sheldon RR, Telford KJ, Kiff ES. Anterior anal sphincter repair can be of long term benefit: a 12-year case cohort from a single surgeon. *BMC Surg* 2007; **7**:1.

13. Tjandra JJ, Han WR, Goh J, Carey M, Dwyer P. Direct repair vs. overlapping sphincter repair: a randomized, controlled trial. *Dis Colon Rectum* 2003; **46**(7):937–42.

14. Leroi AM, Kamm MA, Weber J, Denis P, Hawley PR. Internal anal sphincter repair. *Int J Colorectal Dis* 1997; **12**(4):243–5.

15. Morgan R, Patel B, Beynon J, Carr ND. Surgical management of anorectal incontinence due to internal anal sphincter deficiency. *Br J Surg* 1997; **84**(2):226–30.

16. Kahn MA, Stanton SL. Posterior colporrhaphy: its effects on bowel and sexual function. *Br J Obstet Gynaecol* 1997; **104**(1):82–86.

17. Mellgren A, Anzen B, Nilsson BY, Johansson C, Dolk A, Gillgren P et al. Results of rectocele repair. A prospective study. *Dis Colon Rectum* 1995; **38**(1):7–13.

18. Young CJ, Mathur MN, Eyers AA, Solomon MJ. Successful overlapping anal sphincter repair: relationship to patient age, neuropathy, and colostomy formation. *Dis Colon Rectum* 1998; **41**(3):344–9.

19. Williams AB, Bartram CI, Halligan S, Spencer JA, Nicholls RJ, Kmiot WA. Anal sphincter damage after vaginal delivery using three-dimensional endosonography. *Obstet Gynecol* 2001; **97**(5 Pt 1):770–5.

20. Jorge JM, Wexner SD. Etiology and management of fecal incontinence. *Dis Colon Rectum* 1993; **36**(1):77–97.

21. Rockwood TH, Church JM, Fleshman JW, Kane RL, Mavrantonis C, Thorson AG et al. Fecal Incontinence Quality of Life Scale: quality of life instrument for patients with fecal incontinence. *Dis Colon Rectum* 2000; **43**(1):9–16.

22. Bravo GA, Madoff RD, Lowry AC, Parker SC, Buie WD, Baxter NN. Long-term results of anterior sphincteroplasty. *Dis Colon Rectum* 2004; **47**(5):727–31.

23. Halverson AL, Hull TL. Long-term outcome of overlapping anal sphincter repair. *Dis Colon Rectum* 2002; **45**(3):345–8.

24. Zutshi M, Tracey TH, Bast J, Halverson A, Na J. Ten-year outcome after anal sphincter repair for fecal incontinence. *Dis Colon Rectum* 2009; **52**(6):1089–94.

25. Fleshman JW, Peters WR, Shemesh EI, Fry RD, Kodner IJ. Anal sphincter reconstruction: anterior overlapping muscle repair. *Dis Colon Rectum* 1991; **34**(9):739–43.

26. Oliveira L, Pfeifer J, Wexner SD. Physiological and clinical outcome of anterior sphincteroplasty. *Br J Surg* 1996; **83**(4):502–5.

27. Pinedo G, Vaizey CJ, Nicholls RJ, Roach R, Halligan S, Kamm MA. Results of repeat anal sphincter repair. *Br J Surg* 1999; **86**(1):66–69.

28. Giordano P, Renzi A, Efron J, Gervaz P, Weiss EG, Nogueras JJ et al. Previous sphincter repair does not affect the outcome of repeat repair. *Dis Colon Rectum* 2002; **45**(5):635–40.

29. Vaizey CJ, Norton C, Thornton MJ, Nicholls RJ, Kamm MA. Long-term results of repeat anterior anal sphincter repair. *Dis Colon Rectum* 2004; **47**(6):858–63.

30. Barisic GI, Krivokapic ZV, Markovic VA, Popovic MA. Outcome of overlapping anal sphincter repair after 3 months and after a mean of 80 months. *Int J Colorectal Dis* 2006; **21**(1):52–56.

Chapter 24

Neosphincters and artificial sphincters for treating faecal incontinence

Steven Brown

Introduction

The preservation of continence is one of the core underlying principles of a colorectal surgeon. It is not only important for the patient as the inability to control the release of stool is an extremely debilitating problem, but there are huge economic implications. The direct costs of pads, appliances and other prescription items and long-term care issues are a huge drain on limited resources. And yet preservation of continence after injury can be challenging. Maintenance of faecal continence is a complex process which is dependant on such wide ranging factors as stool consistency and transit, rectal sensation and compliance, and higher centre control. Compromised sphincter function is one of the commonest causes of faecal incontinence. Compromise can occur after simple structural defects (eg damage after childbirth), because of a weak but intact sphincter (neuropathic sphincter due to diabetes, neurological disorders, spinal trauma), or after complex disruptions (eg congenital anorectal malformations, trauma).

Reflecting these varied causes are the various treatment options, ranging from conservative measures aimed at symptomatic control through to surgical options aimed at fixing a mechanical cause. These options include repairing any defect; stimulating the nerve supply; bowel irrigation methods allowing more convenient and complete evacuation; or sphincter bypass with a stoma. At the ultra-invasive end of the surgical spectrum are the procedures that augment the pelvic floor using a neo-sphincter (1).

Therapeutic strategy

When should neo-sphincter formation be considered? Certainly careful investigation is required first. Advances in imaging over the last two decades now allow a detailed assessment of the best treatment option. For example, patients with a damaged sphincter may be selected for repair; whilst alternative options can be considered where no defect is seen. The development of conservative therapies, especially biofeedback means surgery is usually a last resort. Even after failure of non-surgical therapies, the conservative trend is often continued with less invasive procedures, such as sacral nerve stimulation, considered first.

Nevertheless, there is still a role for more invasive procedures. Neosphincter formation should probably be considered in three groups of patients. The main group is those in whom the less invasive treatment options have been exhausted or excluded. In a small group of patients with loss of a large proportion of the native sphincter (after trauma or congenital absence of sphincter) neosphincter formation may even be the primary procedure. The third group where neosphincter formation is the only option for restoration of continence is the group undergoing total anorectal reconstruction after, for instance, abdominoperineal resection for rectal cancer.

In all cases patients should be prepared psychologically, emotionally, and financially to undergo multiple operations with the possibility of ultimate failure and acceptance of a permanent stoma.

Methods of augmenting the pelvic floor using a neosphincter

The principle of anal sphincter augmentation involves the fashioning of a biological or artificial material or device around or above the non-operational sphincter. This wrap or band not only acts to improve retention in the rectum but may also have the functional ability to act as a neosphincter. Biological materials that can be used for such a wrap or band include muscle transposed to the site and wrapped around the sphincter. Artificial devices include various encircling appliances, the earliest and simplest version being a silver wire, described by Thiersch over 100 years ago. More recently pressure activated devices have been used that allow a more functional operation.

Muscle wraps

Gracilis muscle

The Gracilis is very well suited to transposition around the anal canal. Not only is it a long thin muscle suited to wrapping, but it has a very constant innervation from the obturator nerve and a blood supply from the profunda femoris vessels. These enter through one neurovascular bundle in the proximal end of the muscle, allowing easy mobilization without damage. The gracilis is also the most superficial muscle in the medial aspect of the thigh making it convenient for harvesting by detaching its insertion into the medial distal tibia. Its loss does not result in a functional deficit in the lower limb after transposition (2).

The technique involves mobilization through one long or more commonly 2 or 3 smaller incisions in the medial aspect of the thigh. The muscle is detached from its insertion into the tibial tuberosity and the neurovascular bundle isolated. The muscle is then transposed around the anal canal through two small perianal incisions and the tendon fixed either to the ischial tuberosity or the skin after a 360° or 540° configuration (Fig. 24.1).

Gluteus maximus wrap

The second most commonly used muscle used to treat faecal incontinence is the gluteus maximus muscle. Single, and latterly bilateral, wrap techniques have been described (2). Advocates of the use of this muscle argue that the glutei are natural synergists of the anal sphincter and are often used to maintain continence by patients with compromised sphincters. However, the nerve and vascular supply is much more

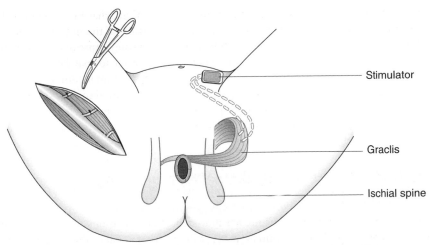

Fig. 24.1 Formation of a gracilis neosphincter. Mobilization of the right gracilis. The left gracilis has been wrapped around the sphincter in the most common gamma configuration with the distal end sutured to the ischial tuberosity (N=stimulator, G=gracilis, T=ischial spine). Reproduced from Koch SMG, Baeten C. (2003) Sphincter replacement grafts. *Chirurg*;74:15–19, with kind permission from Springer Science and Business Media.

variable than the gracilis making the transposition procedure more difficult and subsequent function more unreliable. In addition, the functional deficit after transposition is greater than that caused by transposition of the gracilis.

Other muscles

The use of 2 gracilis muscles may be advantageous in terms of function but increases potential morbidity to the legs (3). Other muscles including the semitendinosus and the long head of the biceps femoris have been considered and have some advantages even over the gracilis muscle. However, both are major flexors of the knee joint, and loss is likely to impair knee movement and stability. Other described muscle transpositions include the obturator internus and the Palmaris longus from the forearm used as a free graft, neither of which have proved superior to the gracilis with time.

Effect of stimulation; the dynamic neosphincter

The technique of muscle transposition has been around for over 50 years. However, initial descriptions were of an adynamic procedure with effectiveness due to a degree of mechanical obstruction caused by the tightness of the wrap. Published studies have shown inconsistent results (4). One problem relates to the function of the muscle. Although it is possible to voluntarily contract the muscle, maintenance of the contraction for long periods is difficult as the muscle fatigues easily.

In the early 1990s, Baeten (5) and Williams (6) pioneered the use of electrical stimulation to the muscle or nerve to convert the neosphincter into a dynamic functioning neosphincter. The underlying physiological principle behind the stimulation is the conversion of the predominantly type II fibres of the gracilis muscle into type I fibres similar to those found in the anal sphincter. These fibres can undergo prolonged repetitive contractions and are resistant to fatigue thus allowing improved function of the neosphincter as the prolonged muscle contraction should improve the anal tone.

It is important at this stage to note there are some variations in technique when it comes to implanting the stimulating apparatus (7). The stimulating electrodes are usually placed in the muscle close to the entry of the nerve. Some advocate placing an electrode directly onto nerve claiming better functional results. The stimulator is usually implanted in the subcutaneous tissues of the abdominal wall but recent experience suggests there is less erosion of the device if it is placed below the rectus sheath. The procedure may be performed in two stages with transposition of the muscle followed by implantation of the stimulating device 6–8 weeks later. However, more recently others have advocated a single stage procedure suggesting less morbidity and that immediate stimulation of the muscle may improve function.

Outcomes after dynamic graciloplasty

During the subsequent 17 years since the introduction of the dynamic neosphincter there have been numerous studies with nearly 1000 participants that have examined the success of the graciloplasty (8). As with many studies concerning faecal incontinence it is very difficult to combine and compare results because of the variation between them (there are differences in participants; inclusion and exclusion criteria; the technique itself; assessment criteria; and outcome measures). With these caveats in mind there are a few trends that can be extrapolated from the literature.

Follow-up has ranged from 6 months to over 6 years and what has been deemed to be an improvement in continence ranging from 0% to 100% (8). The most recent studies suggest an overall success rate of below 50%. This is even lower in patients with congenital abnormalities (anorectal agenesis) with failure rates exceeding 66% even in the most experienced hands (8). In almost all studies there is a recognized and significant surgical revision rate, explantation rate and a high complication rate. Combining the data from the 20 most recent studies this amounts to about half of all patients undergoing at least one surgical revision with about one third eventually failing (8).

Almost 90% will suffer complications. These complications fall into 3 main groups; technical, infectious, and physiological (8). Technical complications usually relate to the stimulator device and leads and are usually easily remedied, although there will be significant cost implications. Other technical complications such as loose or too tight an anal wrap leading to erosion are improved with experience of the operator. Avoidance of infectious complications requires strict attention to sterile technique, including skin preparation and careful handling of the device. There is no evidence to suggest that a two-stage technique or defunctioning the patient reduces the infection rate. Physiological complications, particularly obstructed defaecation are more difficult to rectify but colonic irrigation may offer an effective therapy (9).

Given the limited long-term benefit, the considerable potential for complications, and the considerable cost; one might consider that continuation of the procedure is not justified by the improved continence that some enjoy. An alternative view is to consider that the procedure does have a place in the armamentarium of continence surgery, but only at the extreme end of the spectrum of refractory incontinence. However, with the complexity of the operation, the variation in success and the limited numbers of patients that are appropriate for the procedure, it is common sense to suggest that, the procedures should be confined to a small number of centres where adequate patient volume, appropriate patient selection, and counselling and surgical expertise optimize morbidity and satisfactory outcome rates.

Artificial devices

The artificial bowel sphincter most commonly used is the Acticon® device (American Medical Systems, Minneapolis, MN) and is similar in construction to the artificial sphincter used for urinary incontinence. It consists of an inflatable cuff placed around the upper anal canal usually through a transverse perineal incision, a pressure regulating balloon implanted extraperitoneally, and a subcutaneously positioned pump placed in either the scrotum or labia (Fig. 24.2). When the cuff is inflated to a pressure of about 80–120 mmHg the anal canal is closed and the pressure maintained by the reservoir. Squeezing the pump 4–5 times empties the cuff and opens the anal canal, allowing evacuation.

The procedure was first reported in 1987 (10). The indications are similar to those of the dynamic muscle wraps, namely end stage faecal incontinence refractory to less invasive therapies. There are some contra-indications: for example Crohn's disease or conditions that result in scarring of the perineum and rectovaginal area. Excluding these

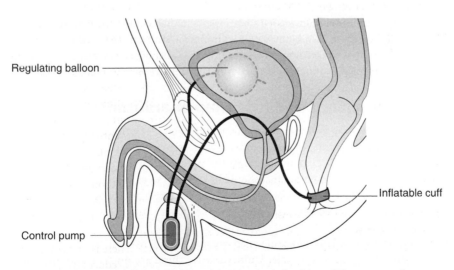

Fig. 24.2 Design of the Acticon ® neosphincter. The inflatable cuff is connected to a pump placed in the scrotum or labia with the balloon reservoir placed in the pre-vesical space. Reproduced from Muller C, Belyaer O, Deska T, et al. (2005) Fecal incontinence: an up-to-date critical review of surgical treatment options Langenbecks *Arch Surg.* 2005;**390**:544–52, with kind permission from Springer Science and Business Media.

patients, the procedure is certainly technically easier, more cosmetic, and less surgeon-dependant than the dynamic muscle wrap.

Outcomes of an artificial bowel sphincter

The technical ease of insertion of an artificial sphincter compared with a muscle wrap does not necessarily translate into better results. Again the literature is difficult to compare particularly due to different outcome definitions. In addition, the data tends to be reports of case series, although there is one very small study that is randomized controlled trial (11). With these caveats in mind data from all the relevant trials over the last 14 years is combined in table 24.1.

There are some consistent themes from all of these studies. Firstly the complication rate is high. Infection is the commonest complication, with rates over 50% in many series, often resulting in erosion of the device and eventual explantation. Other complications include device related malfunction resulting in surgical revision in about half of all patients. A third group of complications relate to function. As with the stimulated muscle wraps there appears to be a significant incidence of obstructed defaecation. The cause is unknown but may relate to pre-existing evacuation dysfunction or to the cuff size and tension (8). Whatever the cause, fortunately most seem to respond to conservative therapy in the form of enemas and/or laxatives (12). Overall complication rates exceed 100% with one study reporting 454 complications in 115 patients suggesting many patients undergo multiple procedures (12). Even with increasing experience there is a constant explantation rate of over 30% although the revision rate does improve (8).

The high complication rate has led some experts in the field to believe that the procedure only continues to exist because of its commercial support. Nevertheless, there is a group of patients who undergo successful implants and who continue to have good long-term control of continence with a significant improvement in their quality of life.

Which neosphincter? Muscle wrap or artificial?

Both the muscle wrap and the artificial bowel sphincter techniques are indicated for end stage faecal incontinence, where other less invasive techniques have been tried or are inappropriate and the patient accepts the potential for complications and even failure. Of course a third option that should be considered in these patients is a stoma. This option is simple to perform but not without complications of its own. It has a significant impact on body image and quality of life and with some patients, may be resisted at all costs.

If a stoma is refused the choice of which neosphincter to use will depend to a certain extent on the expertise available. Unfortunately there are no direct comparisons between the two techniques in terms of outcome and quality of life. Technically it is generally accepted that a muscle wrap may be preferred in patients with a very thin or scarred perineum (8). In terms of expense, mathematical models suggest the artificial bowel sphincter is more cost effective than the dynamic graciloplasty. A stoma is the most financially effective procedure over a 5-year time horizon but becomes less effective with time as stoma costs remain ongoing (13).

Table 24.1 Data summary of all relevant studies since 1996 looking at outcome after an artificial bowel sphincter. Where possible, patients with total anorectal reconstruction have been excluded. (Data from reference 8.)

Paper	Year	No of patients	Mean age (years)	Follow-up (years)	Success	Surgical revisions	Explantations (total)	Complications (total)
Wexner	2009	47	48.8	3.3	34	na	13	na
Ruiz-Cormona	2009	17	46.0	5.7	9	19	11	43
Galles	2009	44	na	na	22	16	9	na
Melenhorst	2008	33	55.3	1.5	26	26	8	38
Michot	2007	9	43.0	1.8	8	0	1	1
La Torre	2004	7	na	na	5	5	2	2
Da Silva	2004	11	25.3	1.7	8	1	0	5
Altomare	2004	28	58.0	4.2	6	14	11	47
Casal	2004	10	56.0	2.4	2	4	3	7
O'Brien	2004	7	66.0	0.5	6	3	1	5
Ortiz	2003	8	34.4	3.7	2	5	3	10
Michot	2003	25	51.1	2.8	12	8	5	10
Parker	2003	47	39.5	5.4	12	25	22	47
Devesa	2002	53	46.0	2.2	13	16	14	77
Lehur	2002	16	43.0	2.1	11	2	5	7
Wong	2002	115	49.0	1.0	51	81	41	454
Ortiz	2002	22	47.0	2.3	4	6	9	17
Lehur	2000	24	44.0	1.7	18	9	8	14
Dodi	2000	8	na	0.9	6	0	2	4
O'Brien	2000	13	44.0	na	9	4	3	8
Christiansen	1999	17	46.0	7.0	8	6	7	5
Lehur	1998	13	40.0	2.5	4	8	4	9
Vaizey	1998	6	53.0	0.8	2	1	1	9
Gelet	1997	1	61.0	2.0	1	2	0	2
Wong	1996	12	55.0	4.8	9	7	7	4
Total		593	47.5	2.7	48%	49%	32%	164%

Total anorectal reconstruction

Neoanal reconstruction has been carried out successfully after construction of a neorectum following proctocolectomy or abdominoperineal resection. This has been termed total anorectal reconstruction (14). As well as reconstruction with a gracilis neosphincter, the use of an artificial bowel sphincter has also been described (15). Physiological complications tend to be greater in this group as patients have lost the ability to sense rectal filling and the sampling reflex associated with the dentate line.

For cancer patients it is important to stage the cancer accurately. Although most experts would advocate reconstruction in a patient with a T2 N0 lesion, the procedure for a T3 or N1 lesion is more controversial. Some advocate a mandatory disease free survival of at least two years before reconstruction. This provides the advantage of oncological certainty but secondary reconstruction is significantly more difficult technically.

Alternative neosphincters and the future

Just as a neosphincter can be applied to a perineal colostomy site in patients undergoing total anorectal reconstruction, some have advocated the use in an abdominal colostomy in the hope of creating a continent colostomy and improve quality of life. Some recent successful trials have been carried out using a stimulated rectus flap in pigs and dogs (16).

The prosthetic artificial sphincter

The prosthetic artificial sphincter (PAS) device consists of a sphincter device that is linear rather than circular. It is positioned intra-abdominally and when inflated, flattens and angulates the bowel against a soft gel filled pillow, thus reproducing the action of the puborectalis muscle and, because of the angulation of the rectum, allowing better control of continence at pressures lower than that likely to cause ischaemia. The device has a reservoir and a pump similar to the Acticon® sphincter (17) (Fig 24.3). The action of the device, which has similarities to normal physiology, makes it potentially less likely to cause ischaemia; and the intra-abdominal position means that theoretically there should be less infection and erosion potential. However, there are two obvious potential drawbacks. The intra-abdominal position of the device make it more invasive than the perineal procedure (although invasiveness could be reduced with the use of laparoscopy) and its position above the sphincters leave the potential for a dead space and problems with faecal seepage. Data so far is limited to a small case series of 12 patients;it was successful in nine patients after a median of 59 months follow-up, with three undergoing explantation (two for infection). Further data is awaited for this promising technique.

The puborectalis sling operation

This technique relies on the original theory of Parks that suggests an important component of continence is the anorectal angle formed by the puborectalis sling. Polyester or Teflon slings have been used to reconstruct the sling (18). Although simple to carry out, few patients have been assessed and the procedure remains experimental.

Pudendal nerve anastomosis

Combination of a pudendal nerve anastomosis to a peripheral nerve and subsequent wrap of the innervated muscle is a novel experimental procedure that has been described (19). There are a number of advantages of such a technique if it works; it is more physiological and integrates intact sensory mechanisms, it may also avoid the need for permanent stimulator implants. The technique has been shown to be feasible in animal models and human cadavers using the gracilis wrap (20).

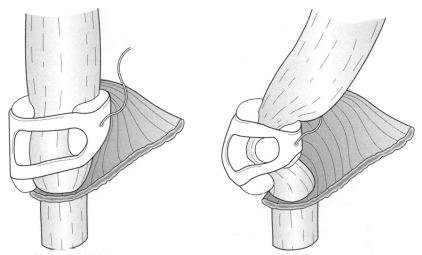

Fig. 24.3 The design and positioning of the PAS device for faecal incontinence. The device is positioned above the anal canal causing angulation on inflation and aiding maintenance of continence. Reproduced with permission from Finlay IG, Richardson W, Hajivassiliou CA (2004). Outcome after implantation after a novel prosthetic anal sphincter in humans. *Br J Surg,* 2004;**91**:1485–92.

German artificial sphincter system (GASS)

Using the latest advances in microtechnology this device aims to incorporate some of the separate components of the standard artificial bowel sphincter into one unit that is easier to insert. The GASS unit consists of a support ring that includes two cuff elements; the fluid reservoir on the outside and a multichamber occluding cuff on the inner aspect (21) (Fig. 24.4). Defaecation is controlled through a subcutaneous generator that activates a micropump within the unit. The integration of the components of the unit may reduce the potential for complications and *in vivo* studies are awaited. The idea of a technologically advanced integrated device is also being developed in centres in China with studies so far remaining *in vitro* and experimental (22).

The future

Recent studies, again from China, have alluded to the use of Nickel Titanium metal alloys (shape metal alloys) and utilised their ability to bend in an arc when heated and return to their original shape when cooled. This property has been incorporated in a device that has been successfully trialled in animals (23).

Conclusions

One constant theme throughout the literature on the treatment of faecal incontinence is the lack of good quality, randomly designed, controlled trials (1). The small number of these trials together with their small sample sizes and poor methodology makes any evidence based summary of the literature and guide to practice very difficult. Opinion is therefore based almost completely on uncontrolled data and individuals' experience.

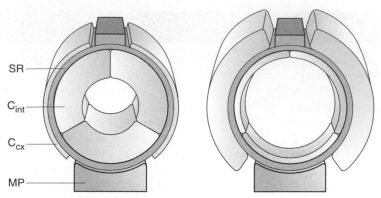

Fig. 24.4 The GASS unit. An example of a novel artificial sphincter.

The inherent bias should therefore be taken into account when considering any of the included information not only in this chapter but most of the rest of this book.

What can be said with certainty is that the main types of neosphincter included in this chapter certainly have very limited applications. The high level of complications associated with both techniques, even in expert hands need to be taken into account whenever either technique is contemplated. It is really when all other options have been exhausted that such procedures should be considered and even then only carried out after careful counselling particularly concerning the option of a stoma.

This is an area where developments may change everything very quickly. Already options such as sacral nerve stimulation have reduced the indications for invasive continence surgery. The use of microtechnology combined with a better understanding of dynamics of the anorectal unit may lead to further more reliable options for neosphincter formation in the future.

Key points

- Consider a neosphincter if other options have been excluded/exhausted, there is loss of a large proportion of native sphincter or for total anorectal reconstruction
- The stimulated gracilis neosphincter is the most common muscle wrap neosphincter, with an overall success of less than 50% (50% requiring at least 1 surgical revision and one third eventually failing)
- The commonest artificial sphincter is the Acticon® neosphincter
- Complications of both the Acticon® neosphincter and the gracilis neosphincter approach 100% and include technical, infectious and physiological issues
- The choice of neosphincter depends on local expertise with the muscle wrap being indicated if there is a scarred or thinned perineum
- A stoma should not be overlooked as an alternative procedure.

Editor's summary

With advancing technological developments such as sacral neuromodulation, (considerably less morbid and very effective) the indications for a neosphincter are diminishing. The longer-term efficacies are reasonable and although the true frequency of postoperative complications is difficult to know, morbidity (infection, erosion, obstructed defaecation), surgical reoperations and explants are high following both gracilis and artificial neosphincter. Despite this, some highly selected and motivated patients can benefit, experiencing some improvement in anal incontinence and quality of life. Each country probably should have access to no more than one or two super-specialized centres offering these procedures.

References

1. Brown SR, Nelson RL. Surgery for faecal incontinence in adults. *Cochrane Database Syst. Rev.* 2007 Apr **18**(2):CD001757.

2. Christiansen J, Hansen CR, Rasmussen O. Bilateral gluteus maximus transposition for anal incontinence. *Br J Surg* 1995;**82**:903–5.

3. Devasa JM, Madrid JM, Gallego BR, et al. Bilateral gluteoplasty for faecal incontinence. *Dis Colon Rectum* 1997;**40**:883–7.

4. Yoshoika K, Keighley MRB. Clinical and manometric assessment of gracilis muscle transplant for fecal incontinence. *Dis Colon rectum* 1988;**31**:767–9.

5. Baeten CG, Konsten J, Spaans F, et al. Dynamic graciloplasty for treatment of faecal incontinence. *Lancet* 1991;**338**:1163 5.

6. Williams NS, Patel J, George BD, et al. Development of an electrically stimulated neoanal sphincter. *Lancet* 1991;**338**:1166–9.

7. Chapman AE, Geerdes B, Hewett P, et al. Systematic review of dynamic graciloplasty in the treatment of faecal incontinence. *Br J Surg* 2002;**89**:138–53.

8. Belyaev O, Muller C, Uhl W. Neosphincter surgery for faecal incontinence: A critical and unbiased review of the relevant literature. *Surgery Today* 2006;**36**:295–303.

9. Koch SM, Uludag O, El Naggar K, et al. Colonic irrigation for defaecation disorders after dynamic graciloplasty. *Int J Colorectal Dis* 2008;**23**:195–200.

10. Christiansen J, Lorentzen. Implantation of artificial sphincter for anal incontinence. *Lancet* 1987;**2**(8553):244–4.

11. O'Brien PE, Dixon JB, Skinner S, et al. A prospective, randomized, controlled clinical trial of placement of the artificial bowel sphincter (Acticon neosphincter) for the control of fecal incontinence. *Dis Colon Rectum* 2004;**47**:1852–60.

12. Wong WD, Congliosi SM, Spencer MP, et al. The safety and efficacy of the artificial bowel sphincter for fecal incontinence: results from a multicenter cohort study. *Dis Colon Rectum* 2002;**45**:1139–53.

13. Tan EK, Vaisey C, Cornish J, et al. Surgical strategies for faecal incontinence- a decision analysis between dynamic graciloplasty, artificial bowel sphincter and end stoma. *Colorectal dis* 2007;**10**:577–86.

14. Geerdes BP, Zoetmulder FA, Heineman E, et al. Total anorectal reconstruction with a double dynamic graciloplasty after abdominoperineal reconstruction for low rectal cancer. *Dis Colon Rectum* 1997;**40**:698–705.

15. Marchal F, Doucet C, Lechaux D, et al. Secondary implantation of an artificial sphincter after abdominoperineal resection and pseudocontinent perineal colostomy for rectal cancer. *Gastroenterol Clin Biol.* 2005;**29**:425–8.

16. Stadelmann, WK, Majzoub RK, Bardoel JW, et al. Electrically stimulated rectus abdominis muscle flap to achieve enterostomal continence: development of a functional canine model. *Plast Reconstruct Surg.* 2007;**119**:517–25.

17. Finlay IG, Richardson W, Hajivassiliou CA. Outcome after implantation of a novel prosthetic anal sphincter in humans. *Br J Surg* 2004;**91**:1485–92.

18. Yamana T, Takahashi T, Iwadae J. Perineal puborectalis sling operation for faecal incontinence: preliminary report. *Dis Colon Rectum* 2004;**47**:1982–9.

19. Congliosi SM, Johnson DR, Medot M, et al. Experimental model of pudendal nerve innervation of skeletal muscle neosphincter for faecal incontinence. *Br J Surg* 1997;**84**:1269–73.

20. Pirro N, Sielezneff I, Malouf A, et al. Anal sphincter reconstruction using a transposed gracilis muscle with a pudendal nerve anastomosis: a preliminary anatomic study. *Dis Colon rectum* 2005;**48**:2085–9.

21. Schrag H-J, Padilla FF, Goldschmidtboing F, et al. German artificial sphincter system; first report of a novel and highly integrated sphincter prosthesis for therapy of major faecal incontinence. *Dis Colon Rectum* 2004;**47**:2215–8.

22. Zan P, Yan G-z, Liu H. Modelling of human colonic blood flow for a novel artificial sphincter system. *J Zhejiang Univ Sci B.* 2008;**9**:734–8.

23. Liu H, Yun L, Masaru H, et al. Biochemical evaluation of an artificial anal sphincter made from shape memory alloys. *J Artif Organs* 2007;**10**:223–7.

24. Koch SMG, Baeten C. Sphincter replacement grafts. *Chirurg* 2003;**74**:15–19.

25. Muller C, Belyaev O, Deska T, et al. Fecal incontinence: an up-to-date critical review of surgical treatment options. *Langenbecks Arch Surg* 2005;**390**:544–52.

Index

Page numbers in *italics* indicate figures and tables.